# EMOTIONAL SCHEMA THERAPY

# Also from Robert L. Leahy

Cognitive Therapy Techniques:
A Practitioner's Guide
*Robert L. Leahy*

Contemporary Cognitive Therapy:
Theory, Research, and Practice
*Edited by Robert L. Leahy*

Emotion Regulation in Psychotherapy:
A Practitioner's Guide
*Robert L. Leahy, Dennis Tirch,
and Lisa A. Napolitano*

Overcoming Resistance in Cognitive Therapy
*Robert L. Leahy*

Psychological Treatment of Bipolar Disorder
*Edited by Sheri L. Johnson and Robert L. Leahy*

Roadblocks in Cognitive-Behavioral Therapy:
Transforming Challenges into Opportunities for Change
*Edited by Robert L. Leahy*

Treatment Plans and Interventions
for Bulimia and Binge-Eating Disorder
*Rene D. Zweig and Robert L. Leahy*

Treatment Plans and Interventions
for Depression and Anxiety Disorders: Second Edition
*Robert L. Leahy, Stephen J. F. Holland,
and Lata K. McGinn*

# Emotional Schema Therapy

Robert L. Leahy

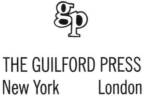

THE GUILFORD PRESS
New York     London

© 2015 The Guilford Press
A Division of Guilford Publications, Inc.
370 Seventh Avenue, Suite 1200, New York, NY 10001
www.guilford.com

Printed in the United States of America

This book is printed on acid-free paper.

Last digit is print number:   9   8   7   6   5   4   3   2   1

The author has checked with sources believed to be reliable in his effort to
provide information that is complete and generally in accord with the standards
of practice that are accepted at the time of publication. However, in view of the
possibility of human error or changes in behavioral, mental health, or medical
sciences, neither the author, nor the publisher, nor any other party who has
been involved in the preparation or publication of this work warrants that the
information contained herein is in every respect accurate or complete, and they
are not responsible for any errors or omissions or the results obtained from the
use of such information. Readers are encouraged to confirm the information
contained in this book with other sources.

**Library of Congress Cataloging-in-Publication Data**
Leahy, Robert L.
  Emotional schema therapy / Robert L. Leahy.
    pages cm
  Includes bibliographical references and index.
  ISBN 978-1-4625-2054-1 (hardback : acid-free paper)
  1. Schema-focused cognitive therapy.   2. Emotions—Psychological
aspects.   I. Title.
  RC455.4.S36L43 2015
  616.89′1425—dc23

                                                            2014042002

*For Helen*

# About the Author

Robert L. Leahy, PhD, is Director of the American Institute for Cognitive Therapy in New York and Clinical Professor of Psychology in the Department of Psychiatry at Weill Cornell Medical College. His research focuses on individual differences in emotion regulation. Dr. Leahy is Associate Editor of the *International Journal of Cognitive Therapy* and past president of the Association for Behavioral and Cognitive Therapies, the International Association for Cognitive Psychotherapy, and the Academy of Cognitive Therapy. He is the 2014 recipient of the Aaron T. Beck Award from the Academy of Cognitive Therapy. Dr. Leahy has published numerous books, including, most recently, the coauthored volumes *Treatment Plans and Interventions for Bulimia and Binge-Eating Disorder*; *Treatment Plans and Interventions for Depression and Anxiety Disorders, Second Edition*; and *Emotion Regulation in Psychotherapy*.

# Preface

Therapists from all approaches are concerned to some extent with the emotional experience that patients bring to therapy. Those who use cognitive restructuring hope that new ways of viewing things will change how people feel, dialectical behavior therapy encourages patients to learn how to regulate emotions that often seem chaotic and frightening, acceptance and commitment therapy encourages flexibility and tolerance of emotion while pursuing a valued life, metacognitive therapy focuses on the role of problematic reliance on worry and rumination to cope with difficulty, and behavior activation stresses the importance of proactive and rewarding behavior rather than passivity, isolation, and avoidance. And, in the psychoanalytic realm, mentalization therapy emphasizes the value of increased awareness of and reflection on the mental or internal states of self and others, while more traditional psychodynamic models attempt to access emotions and memories that are associated with long-lasting difficulties. Emotions are what lead people to seek out help, regardless of the theoretical orientation one takes, but little has been said about how the patient thinks about and strategizes regulating those emotions.

Before I met Aaron Beck and pursued work in cognitive therapy, I was actively involved in work on social cognition—that is, how people explain the causes of behavior, their use of trait concepts in describing others, recognition of variability in others and in the self, and judgments of intentionality and responsibility. Social cognition has relevance to cognitive-behavioral therapy in that one's emotions—and the strategies one uses to regulate them—may be related to the "theory" one has about emotions.

The emotional schema model proposes that once emotions are activated we often have interpretations of those emotions, and these interpretations are related to strategies we use to cope with the emotions.

This book develops a model of how people think about their own emotions and those of others. Throughout this book, I describe a number of feelings, desires, or experiences, and refer to them as "emotions"—sadness, anxiety, anger, confusion, envy, jealousy, resentment, and sexual feelings. I use the term "emotional schemas" to describe beliefs about the causes, legitimacy, normality, duration, and tolerance of complexity of emotion. Once an emotion arises—for example, anxiety—the individual then assesses the nature of this emotion: "Is this emotion going to last indefinitely?", "Do other people feel the same way that I feel?", "Should I feel ashamed of my feelings?", "Is it OK to have mixed feelings?", "Can I express my feelings?", "Will other people validate me?", "Do my feelings make sense?", and a range of other interpretations and evaluations of one's own emotional experience. Does the individual believe some emotions, such as anger, are "legitimate," whereas other emotions, such as anxiety, are not? And, once an emotion arises, what strategies does the individual activate to deal with these emotions? Does the individual seek out reassurance, withdraw from others, ruminate, blame others, avoid, retreat into passivity, abuse substances, interpret things differently, engage in problem solving, activate useful behavior, seek distraction, self-mutilate, dissociate, binge, accept the emotion, or engage in other responses?

Moreover, these emotional schemas are also related to how one thinks about and responds to the emotions of others. For example, when one's intimate partner is upset, does one think one's partner's emotions make no sense, does one pathologize these emotions and label them as "abnormal," does one believe these emotions will go on indefinitely, does one discourage expression, or does one believe that emotions interfere with rationality and solving the problem? And, based on these interpretations, does one criticize and ridicule that person, tell one's partner that he or she is complaining too much, withdraw and stonewall, or try to convince one's partner that he or she should not have these feelings?

In this book, I describe a model of how people might theorize about emotion and how these "theories" of emotion contribute to a wide range of psychopathology. While recognizing the importance of theories about how negative interpretations of reality can lead to sadness or anxiety or how avoidance and passivity can contribute further to depression, the emotional schema model attempts to extend our understanding further by proposing that once an emotion arises, the individual's implicit theory of emotion is activated, and this leads to either helpful or unhelpful strategies of coping. Quite simply, "Once you feel sad, what do you think about this sadness and what do you do next?" For example, if I think my sadness will go on indefinitely or escalate further, I might be desperate to find a "quick fix" by abusing substances or by simply withdrawing. Alternatively, if I think my sadness is a temporary experience and that my emotions depend on what I do and with whom I interact, then I might activate adaptive behavior. Interpretations lead to strategies, and strategies may make things worse—or better.

We are fortunate to have so many cognitive-behavioral therapy approaches that have value—that empower the patient with understanding and skills, and give a sense of hope in the face of what often seem insurmountable odds. The emotional schema approach attempts to add to the wide range of conceptualizations and tools at the disposal of the therapist. Thus, those from a wide range of theoretical orientations in cognitive-behavioral therapy and even in the psychodynamic tradition may find some value in the observations and suggestions offered here.

# Acknowledgments

One of the pleasures in writing a book is to thank the many people who have made this work possible. I have been fortunate to have worked on many books with my colleagues at The Guilford Press; I am especially grateful to Jim Nageotte, my editor for many years, and to Jane Keislar, Marie Sprayberry, and Laura Specht Patchkofsky, who have diligently worked on the final edits and been very helpful in getting this book into better shape.

Over the years, I have been quite fortunate to have excellent colleagues at the American Institute for Cognitive Therapy in New York City (*www. CognitiveTherapyNYC.com*), with whom I have shared and revised many of the ideas put forth in this volume. In particular, I wish to thank Laura Oliff, Dennis Tirch, Jenny Taitz, Mia Sage, Nikki Rubin, Victoria Taylor, Melissa Horowitz, Ame Aldao, Peggilee Wupperman, Maren Westphal, and many other clinical colleagues. Poonam Melwani and Sindhu Shivaji have been outstanding in working on the bibliography, assisting with the edits, and seeking out materials to make the final product a reality.

There are many other colleagues in the field to whom I am most grateful, beginning with Aaron T. Beck, the founder of cognitive therapy. Others include Lauren B. Alloy, David H. Barlow, Judith S. Beck, David A. Clark, David M. Clark, Keith S. Dobson, Christopher G. Fairburn, Arthur Freeman, Paul Gilbert, Leslie S. Greenberg, Steven C. Hayes, Stefan G. Hofmann, Stephen J. Holland, Steven D. Hollon, Marsha M. Linehan, Lata K. McGinn, the late Susan Nolen-Hoeksema, Cory F. Newman, Jacqueline B. Persons, Christine Purdon, John H. Riskind, Paul M. Salkovskis, Zindel

V. Segal, John D. Teasdale, Adrian Wells, and J. Mark G. Williams. We are immensely blessed to have so many outstanding therapists addressing these important issues. I would also like to thank my good friend and colleague Philip Tata, who has always been a great source of support and wisdom, and whose friendship I deeply cherish. And, finally, I thank my lovely wife, Helen, who continues to inspire me and help me reach for the best that I can hope to be. This book is dedicated to her.

# Contents

## PART IV

### SOCIAL EMOTIONS AND RELATIONSHIPS

# PART I

# EMOTIONAL SCHEMA THEORY

# CHAPTER 1

# The Social Construction of Emotion

You may often be seen to smile, but never heard to laugh while you live.

—Lord Chesterfield, *Letters to His Son, 1774*

Imagine the following. Ned has been dating Brenda for 3 months, and it has been a roller-coaster ride for him. Arguments have been followed by intense intimacy, which has been followed by indifference from Brenda and her claims of ambivalence. He has now received a text message from Brenda telling him that the relationship is over and that she wants no further communication from him. Ned is perplexed, since this seems like a callous way to end a relationship, and his first response is one of anger. As he thinks about this more during the day, he begins to feel anxious, and to worry that he will always be alone. He then becomes sad, feeling empty and confused. He also notices moments when he feels better—even relieved that the relationship is over—but then he wonders whether he is just fooling himself and his emotions will soon flood him with misery again. Ned thinks he should have only one feeling, not this entire range of feelings. He cannot understand why his feelings are so strong, since he has been with Brenda for "only" 3 months. He dwells on his negative feelings while sitting alone in his apartment, drinking, and bingeing on junk food. Ned begins to think that if he doesn't get rid of these feelings, he might go insane; he remembers how his aunt had to go to the hospital when he was a kid. Ashamed to tell his friend, Bill, about the depths of his feelings, he isolates himself and does not want to be a burden. "What is wrong with me?" he muses as he pours himself another Scotch. "Will I ever feel better?"

Just a few blocks away in the city, Michael has been going through a similar roller-coaster relationship with Karen, from whom he has just received a text message telling him that the relationship is over. Michael is angry with Karen's insensitivity, and his emotions during the next 2 days run the gamut from anger, sadness, anxiety, loneliness, emptiness, and confusion to moments of relief that the relationship is over. Now Michael is more reflective and more accepting of things in life than Ned is, and he reflects on his emotions: "Well, it makes sense that I would have a lot of different feelings, since the relationship was confusing. In fact, the relationship was all about intense feelings—it *was* a roller-coaster ride. I can only imagine that a lot of other people might feel the same way." He turns to his friend, Juan, who has always had a sympathetic ear, and tells him about the turmoil he is going through. It's a bit intense, this discussion, but Juan and Michael have been through a lot together. As he talks, Juan nods his head in understanding. Limiting himself to a couple of beers, Michael goes home to get some rest. He thinks, "I've been through tough times before. My feelings are intense right now, but I can handle things." He also realizes that the reason he has such strong feelings is that relationships matter to him. He really wants a committed relationship, and he won't give up on that just because this one ended. Emotions are the cost of caring.

What distinguishes our unfortunate "Ned the Neurotic" from "Michael the Mensch" is that Ned has a negative theory of his emotions, whereas Michael accepts and uses his emotions in more constructive ways. These two approaches to the same event reflect what I call "emotional schemas"—that is, individual theories about the nature of emotion and how to regulate them. One person may try to suppress emotions because he or she views them as incomprehensible, overwhelming, endless in duration, and even shameful; another person may accept emotions as temporary, rich in complexity, part of being human, and telling us about our values and needs. The therapeutic model I describe in this book, "emotional schema therapy," focuses on identifying an individual's idiosyncratic theory of the emotions of self and others, examining the consequences of these constructions of emotions, differentiating helpful from unhelpful strategies of emotion regulation, and helping the individual integrate emotional experience into a meaningful life.

Almost everyone has experienced emotions such as sadness, anxiety, or anger, but not everyone develops major depression, generalized anxiety disorder, or panic disorder. What gives rise to the persistence of emotions that then develop into psychological disorders? I emphasize throughout this book that it is not only the experience of emotion that matters, but also the interpretations of those emotions and the strategies one employs to cope with or regulate them. There are pathways from painful emotions to psychopathology, and different pathways from painful emotions to adaptive life strategies. The view advanced here is that one's interpretations and responses to painful emotions will determine whether psychopathology arises from the experience. For instance, one can experience intense sadness without developing major depressive disorder.

There are numerous theories of emotion, and these vary widely. Emotions have been viewed as innately programmed responses to the evolutionarily relevant environment (Darwin, 1872/1965; Nesse & Ellsworth, 2009; Tooby & Cosmides, 1992); as electrochemical processes that occur in various parts of the brain (Davidson & McEwen, 2012); as the consequences of "irrational" thinking (D. A. Clark & Beck, 2010; Ellis & Harper, 1975); as the results of appraisals of threat or stressors (Lazarus & Folkman, 1984); as determining the ability to process information (the affect infusion model; Forgas, 1995); as "containing" information about needs and thoughts that are related to those needs (the emotion-focused model; Greenberg, 2002); or as primary—that is, as preceding cognition (Zajonc, 1980). Each of these models—and many others—has contributed greatly to our understanding of the importance of emotion in daily life and the development of psychopathology. The model proposed here, which I refer to alternatively in this book as the "emotional schema model" or as "emotional schema theory," extends our understanding of emotion by proposing that essential aspects of the process of emotion experience include the individual's interpretation and evaluation of emotions, and his or her strategies of emotion control. From this perspective, emotion is not only an experience; it is also an *object* of experience. Although emotions have evolved through evolutionary adaptation and may be universal experiences, one's interpretations, evaluations, and responses are also socially constructed.

Fritz Heider (1958) proposed that individuals maintain beliefs about themselves and others regarding the nature of causes of behavior, intentionality, and the organization of the self. Heider observed that the ordinary person is a "psychologist" in his or her own right, utilizing models of attribution and evaluation, and inferring traits and personal qualities. This "naive psychology" (or common sense), as it was called, became the basis of the field of "social cognition" (which has morphed into "theory of mind"). I describe how "naive psychology" may be extended to a model of how individuals conceptualize emotions in themselves and others, and how these specific models of emotion may lead to problematic strategies of emotion regulation.

Emotional schema theory is a social-cognitive model of emotion and emotion regulation. It proposes that individuals differ in their evaluation of the legitimacy and shame about emotion, their interpretations of the causes of emotion, their need to control emotion, their expectations about the duration and danger of emotion, and their standards regarding the appropriateness of emotion display (Leahy, 2002, 2003b; Leahy, Tirch, & Napolitano, 2011). Even if emotion has a strong biological determination, and even if emotion is related to specific eliciting stimuli, the *experience* of emotion is often followed by an interpretation of that emotion: "Does my anxiety make sense?", "Would other people feel the same way?", "Will this last indefinitely?", "How can I control this?", or "Will I go insane?" These interpretations of emotion, which I refer to as "theories of emotion," are the central content of "emotional schemas"—that is, beliefs about the emotions of ourselves and others, and how these emotions can be regulated. I refer to emotional schema theory as a social-cognitive model because emotions are both personal and social phenomena that are interpreted by ourselves and others; as such, changes in interpretations (our own and others') will result in changes in emotional intensity and dysregulation.

In this chapter, I briefly review how emotion and rationality have been viewed in the Western philosophical tradition, and how Western ideas about emotions and emotional displays have changed in the last several hundred years, suggesting that the "construction of emotion" has been in continual flux. I also discuss how current models of affective forecasting suggest that "naive" theories of emotion may have an impact on decision making and the current experience of emotion. The argument throughout is that not only our experience of emotion, but also our interpretations of that experience and what we believe it predicts, matter.

## A BRIEF HISTORY OF EMOTION
## IN WESTERN PHILOSOPHY AND CULTURE

### Primacy of the Rational

In *The Republic*, Plato uses the metaphor of the charioteer who attempts to control two horses—one that is amenable to direction, and the other that charges off out of control. Plato viewed emotions as impediments to rational and productive thinking and action, and thus as detracting from the pursuit of virtue. Plato (1991) describes the initial impact of events that lead to emotion as "the fluttering of the soul." If we think of the progression of a rational response to events, the first movement may begin with a jolt or "fluttering of the soul." Subsequent movements involve stepping back and observing what is happening, next considering the virtue that is relevant (e.g., "courage"), and then considering the actions and thoughts that might lead one to a virtuous response. As we will see later, the emotional schema model acknowledges that a first response to an emotion may be characterized by a sense of "disruption" or "surprise." This process is also likely to reflect automatic or unconscious processes (Bargh & Morsella, 2008; LeDoux, 2007)—that is, Plato's "fluttering of the soul." However, individuals can also stand back and evaluate what is currently happening, what their options are, how this is related to valued goals, and how their emotions might rise or fall depending on their interpretations and what they do. Aristotle viewed virtue as the character trait and practice that represents the ideal "mean" between the two extremes of a desired personal quality. In the emotional schema model—as in the model underlying acceptance and commitment therapy (Hayes, Strosahl, & Wilson, 2012)—there is the recognition that values (or virtues) can determine how one views emotions and the ability to tolerate discomfort in the context of valued action. The goal is not simply a particular emotion, but rather the meaning, value, or virtue that one wishes to attain.

Aristotle (1984, 1995) emphasized flourishing (*eudaimonia*) to pursue "the good life"—a sense of happiness or well-being that one is acting in accord with virtues and the valued meaning of one's life. Aristotle defined "virtues" as those qualities of character that one admires in another person; that is, the goal is to become the person that you would admire. The emotional experience of "happiness" is the result of daily practice of virtues, such as temperance, courage, patience, modesty, and other qualities. Thus feeling "good" is a consequence of *pursuing* the good and *practicing* the behavior—that is, *virtue*. The emotional schema model draws on Aristotle's view that practicing valued habits or virtues can facilitate greater adaptation and fulfillment.

Stoics, such as Epictetus, Seneca, and Cicero, viewed rationality as superior to emotion and suggested that emotions lead one to overreact and lose sight of important values; they thus detract from virtue and ultimately enslave the individual (Inwood, 2003). The emphasis among the Stoics was on rational conduct, elimination of overattachment to the external world, discipline over one's desires, and freedom from material need and the need for approval. Stoic exercises included practicing hunger, physical discomfort, and poverty to learn that one could survive without material riches; contemplating the elimination of valued objects or persons in one's life to recognize their value; reflecting each day on what one did well and how one could improve; standing back from an emotion and considering the course of rational action; recognizing that thoughts are what make life bad, not reality itself; and beginning each day, as the Emperor Marcus Aurelius did, with the following recognition of the limits of reality and the importance of acceptance while pursuing virtue: "Begin each day by telling yourself: Today I shall be meeting with interference, ingratitude, insolence, disloyalty, ill-will, and selfishness—all of them due to the offenders' ignorance of what is good or evil" (Marcus Aurelius, 2002).

The primacy of cognition gained further support during the European Enlightenment, with a growing emphasis on rational discourse, reason, individual freedom, science, and exploration of the unknown. Locke, Hume, Voltaire, Bentham, Mill (Gay, 2013), and others attempted to free thinking from what they viewed as the limitations of superstition, authority, and emotional appeals. New discoveries in science questioned the authority of Christian doctrine. Kant's emphasis on a rational and virtuous life based on the categorical imperative freed moral reasoning from dictates of the

Church. Locke's contract theory located legitimacy in agreements rather than brute authority. And the exploration of new worlds led to a recognition that cultural norms were possibly arbitrary arrangements rather than eternal truths. However, in contrast to the privileged status of rationality and science, Hume argued that reason is the slave of emotion, since reason cannot tell us what we *want*; it can only tell us how to *get there*. Emotion, in Hume's view, plays a more central role. According to Hume, emotions tell us about what matters, whereas rationality may help us achieve the goals set by emotion.

In the 20th century, the emphasis on rationality, practicality, and the discovery of "facts" rather than faith became central to pragmatism, logical positivism, ordinary-language philosophy, and the general area of analytic philosophy. Gilbert Ryle (1949), in *The Concept of Mind*, rejected the idea that there is a "ghost in the machine"; he criticized the idea that souls, minds, personalities, and other "inferred entities" determined anything. Logical positivists, such as the young Wittgenstein (1922/2001), Ayer (1946), Carnap (1967), and others, proposed that the only criterion of truth is verifiability, that knowledge is derived from experience, and that emotional appeals are misleading and need to be submitted to the test of logical discourse and clear definition. Austin (1975) and Ryle (1949) advanced the idea that philosophy should concentrate on the ordinary use of language to clarify, through logical analysis, the meanings of statements. The emphasis was on clarification, logic, empiricism (in some cases), and— if possible—reduction to mathematical statements of logic. Emotion was viewed as noise.

## Primacy of Emotion

Although rationality and logic have always constituted a major influence in philosophy (and in Western culture in general), emotion has always been a counterpart, serving a dialectical function throughout history. Plato's emphasis on logic and rational thought was in contrast to the great tradition of Greek tragedy. Indeed, Euripides's *The Bacchae* (1920) represented the tragic view that if one ignores the god (Dionysius or Bacchus) who gathers followers in song, dance, and a sense of total abandon, then, ironically, one will face complete destruction in madness. One ignores emotion at one's own peril. The emotional schema model suggests that the goal is not "feeling good," but the capacity for feeling *everything*. There is no higher or lower "self" in this model; rather, all emotions are included in the "self." This model argues for the inclusion of emotions—even "disparaged" emotions such as anger, resentment, jealousy, and envy—and for the acceptance of those emotions as part of the complexity of human nature.

The tragic vision recognizes that suffering is inevitable; that the mighty can fall; that forces beyond one's control or even imagination can destroy;

that injustice is often inevitable; and that the suffering of others matters to oneself because it exemplifies what can happen to anyone. All of us are part of the same community of fragile, fallible, and mortal people. In contrast to the tragic vision, Plato privileged rationality as the way to power and control, and tragedy as the great leveler through its appeal to emotion.

In the 19th century, Nietzche (1956) suggested that the great contrast in culture and philosophy was between the Apollonian and the Dionysian—that is, between the emphasis on structure, logic, rationality, and control, and the emphasis on the emotional, the intense, the individual, and the wild expression of total freedom. The latter was reflected in the Romantic movement, which embraced emotion completely—emphasizing emotional intensity, individual experience, heroics, magical thinking, metaphor, myth, the personal and private, revolutionary thinking, nationalism, and intense individual love. Nature was given precedence over the constructed world of the Enlightenment, with an emphasis on natural instincts, the "noble savage," natural landscapes, and freedom from constraint. Logic was viewed as a distraction from the lived experience. Leading Romantic philosophers included Hegel, Schopenhauer, and Rousseau, leading poets included Shelley, Byron, Goethe, Wordsworth, Coleridge, and Keats. Romanticism also had a significant influence on music, as represented by Wagner, Beethoven, Schubert, and Berlioz (Pirie, 1994).

One element of the Romantic movement was the 18th-century movement of sentimentalism, which emphasized intensity of individual expression rather than rationality or accepted norms, with intense expression representing authenticity, sincerity, and the strength of one's feelings. Indeed, it was not uncommon for members of the House of Lords in Britain to argue their positions while weeping. Suicide was the ultimate expression of this romantic intensity.

In the late 19th and 20th centuries, existentialism became a major counterforce to British and American rationalist models in philosophy, with existentialists emphasizing the role of individual purpose, choice, recognition of mortality, the arbitrary nature of existence, and emotions. Kierkegaard (1941) described the existential dilemmas of dread, "the sickness unto death," and the crisis of individual choice. Heidegger (1962) proposed that philosophy needed to address the implications of individual "thrownness" into life and history and the individual's dilemma in constructing meaning. And Sartre (1956) argued that individuals must resolve the dilemmas that are a result of their given situation by exercising their freedom. The emotional schema model proposes that individuals struggle with their freedom of choice, often having difficulty with the "given" that is arbitrarily part of their everyday lives, while recognizing that the choices people face often involve dilemmas or tradeoffs that are emotionally difficult. Choice, freedom, regret, and even dread are viewed as essential components of life in this model, and these "realities" cannot be simply eliminated by cost–benefit analyses, rationalization, or pragmatism. Although rational evaluation is important, every tradeoff involves a cost. And costs are often unpleasant and difficult.

This brief review cannot do justice to the dichotomized view of emotion and rationality in Western culture (and, of course, does not address the importance of these factors in other cultures). As Nussbaum (2001) has suggested each "realm"—the rational and the emotional—has its value, and each informs the other. The emotional schema model recognizes that emotions and rationality are often in a struggle with one another—often in a dialectic tension as to what will influence choice. Yet both are essential.

## Cultural and Historical Factors in Emotion

The emerging field in history referred to as "emotionology" traces the changes in how emotions have been viewed in different societies at different historical periods and how emotions are socialized. Indeed, the study of the history of emotion provides considerable evidence about the social construction of emotion—especially which emotions were valued, which were suppressed, and how rules for display of emotions changed. In 1939, Austrian social historian Norbert Elias wrote a monumental study of the emergence of internalization and self-control in Western European society (republished many years later as *The Civilizing Process: Sociogenetic and Psychogenetic Investigations*; Elias, 1939/2000). Elias traced the changes in rules of conduct regarding speech, eating, dress, greetings, sexual conduct, aggressive conduct, and other social forms of behavior from the 13th century to the early 20th century. With the consolidation of power in the hands of the King and the rise of courtly society where knights would live for part of the year in the King's court, rules of self-control became more significant. Elias argued that greater internalization of emotion and behavior ensued. Indeed, the word "courtesy" is derived from the word "court." Loud displays of emotion, confrontation, and sexual behavior were no longer acceptable, as these emotional experiences became increasingly internalized. Moreover, there was an increased emphasis on personal and private affection; the rise of a sense of a private emotional self, through the spread of reading and the use of personal diaries; and a greater sense of shame and guilt. Max Weber (1930), in *The Protestant Ethic and the Spirit of Capitalism*, further expanded the idea that internalization of emotion both provided the emotional conditions for capitalism and was a by-product of capitalism. Thus delay of gratification, emphasis on work and productivity, the value of success as a reflection of individual merit, coordination with market forces, and the seller–buyer relationship all led to greater control of emotion. All of these developments reflected the social construction of emotion.

We can see the further development of emotional control in the North American Puritan culture of the 16th and 17th centuries, with an emphasis on control of anger and passion, denial of worldly pleasure, emphasis on modesty, and greater emphasis on both shame and guilt. The 18th and 19th centuries in America and Britain also saw the rise of "conduct books," which attempted to instruct the reader on proper behavior. During this time, especially in America, there was greater emphasis on the idea of the "self-made man," along with the rise of commerce; the decline of the aristocracy; and the emergence of a new class of tradespeople, entrepreneurs, businesspeople, and professionals. Presumably, a man was not limited by his class status and could rise in the social class system if he mastered the right conduct. Women, on the other hand, would need to rely on opportunistic marriages to advance their status. Benjamin Franklin's *Poor Richard's Almanac* (1759/1914) provided daily advice to readers on delay of gratification, the importance of savings, the benefits of hard work, and the importance of reputation. It was Franklin who coined an early version of the phrase "No pain, no gain," in proposing that everyone should exercise 45 minutes each day.

A future American president, John Adams, who aspired to rise in the social class hierarchy of the 18th-century colonies, would stand in front of a mirror observing his facial expression and posture, attempting to control his expression so as not to show any unnecessary emotion. Control over one's face, one's body, one's hand movements, and the intonation of one's voice was all part of the new emphasis on self-control. Perhaps the most influential book advocating self-control was the British aristocrat Lord Chesterfield's *Letters to My Son* (1774/2008), which urged readers to do the following: "Maintain a sense of reserve," "Don't show your true feelings," "Frequent and loud laughter is the characteristic of folly and ill manners," "Be wiser than other people, if you can, but do not tell them so." Other books advised women to hide their sexuality and true feelings behind a veneer of courteous indifference, with an emphasis on modesty. The standard was to be friendly but not flirtatious, and not to show too much interest in a man. Women had to control men's passions. Blushing was approved of for women because it showed embarrassment about any sexual or flirtatious content. Again, the emphasis was on the control of body, face, and verbal expression. Increasingly, in the 18th and 19th centuries the emphasis was that one should not show any intensity of emotion, and should certainly not rely on emotion.

Christopher Lasch, in *Haven in a Heartless World* (1977), describes the rise of a domestic, home-centered venue for emotional intimacy during the Victorian period and after. Emotions went behind closed doors, where domestic "harmony" was emphasized. The Victorian period also saw the rise of the "gendering of emotion"—that is, sex-typing of emotion.

Men occupied the "public" sphere of commerce, while women were now confined to the "private" sphere of the home. Thus, in the public sphere, men were allowed to be competitive, conflicted, and ambitious, whereas at home both men and women would focus on affection, trust, and intimacy. There was greater emphasis on love between spouses, "mother love," and family harmony (anger was not tolerated); jealousy was condemned, since it disrupted the harmony of family life. In this divided world, anger was not seen as appropriate for home life, but was viewed as appropriate for men to direct outward to motivate them. In the socialization of children in the 19th century, it was viewed as appropriate to be afraid—but boys were told to use courage to overcome fear. Courage was not expected for girls. There was also an increased emphasis on guilt rather than shame.

During the late 19th century and early 20th century, emotional norms changed further. With the decline of infant mortality, parents could hope that their infants would live until adulthood; this led to decreased birth rates. An individual infant could get more attention and thereby foster a stronger parental bond of love. Thee was also a greater emphasis on childhood as a distinct stage of life, with clothes especially designed for children, a new emphasis on protection of their welfare, and expectations that children were not simply little adults (Ariès, 1962; Kessen, 1965). In addition, the rise of the commercial economy—especially the increasing emphasis on services and trade—meant that emotional expression needed to adapt to shifting buyer–seller relations (Sennett, 1996). Finally, in the 20th century, with the emergence of gender equality, sexist views of women as hysterical, weaker, or more emotional and less rational were increasingly regarded as outmoded, even though they persisted in early psychoanalytic theory (Deutsch, 1944–1945).

Between the 1920s and the 1950s there emerged new theories of emotion socialization, influenced both by Watson's (1919) research showing that fears are learned, and by the psychoanalytic argument tracing neurosis to childhood difficulties. A popular interpretation of Watson's behaviorism was that avoidance is the best strategy for dealing with fear. There was no longer an emphasis on using courage to face hardship or fear; there was a reduced emphasis on tolerating difficult feelings; and there was more emphasis on what might be characterized as an expressive and reassurance culture. The influence of psychoanalytic theory led to the emphasis on a "safe," reassuring environment, as exemplified in the popular writings of pediatrician Benjamin Spock, with his exhortations on reassurance, expression, coddling, and overprotection as ways to handle a child's fears (e.g., Spock, 1957). As emotions became feared experiences and the goal was to protect a child from experiencing difficulty, there was also the rise of "coolness" in popular culture—that is, the emphasis on being self-contained, in control of emotion, unsentimental, or even aloof and unreachable (Stearns,

1994). Popular cartoon heroes showed no fear (they were "cool"); they did not have to overcome fear or face fear. Characters like Superman appeared so invulnerable that they did not have to show courage.

Of course there was a counterpart to all this internalization, self-control, and muted expression of emotion, as reflected in counterculture mores of self-expression, spontaneity, intensity of individual experience, and sexual freedom. More rebellious elements of popular culture emerged: the popularity of jazz from the 1920s onward; the age of Prohibition with a wide underground of lawbreakers; the 1950s beatniks; the rise of rock and roll; the 1960s hippies; the protest music of the Vietnam era; the "turn on and tune out" message of the drug culture advocated by Timothy Leary and others; and the eventual emergence of "gangsta' rap" and other intense individual expressions that appeared to celebrate complete emotionality and the rejection of self-control.

Thus emotion has been repeatedly constructed and deconstructed in Western culture over the past 3,000 years. The history of emotions reflects this growing awareness of how emotions are viewed, how socialization and norms influence emotional expression, and how some emotions fall out of favor (such as jealousy). All these shifts suggest that emotions are largely products of *social construction*. The history of emotion and the philosophical schools that privilege emotion or rationality all suggest that emotions are not simply innate, spontaneous, universal phenomena (although certainly there is a universal predisposition toward them), but that the evaluation of emotion and rules for emotion display vary considerably within our culture and across cultures.

This brief overview suggests that interpretations or cognitive appraisals of emotion—and the influence of emotions on thinking—are important psychological phenomena in their own right. I now turn to a brief description of current approaches in social psychology that describe common biases in the "naive psychology" of emotion. These approaches reflect the interface between social cognition and the interpretation and prediction of emotion.

## COGNITIVE APPRAISALS OF EMOTIONS

Consider the examples at the beginning of this chapter: two men, each going through a breakup in a relationship. The sadder of the two may feel sad and lonely at the present time, and, when asked how he anticipates he will feel in a few months, may predict that he will continue to be sad—perhaps even sadder than he is now. This is an example of "affective forecasting," which refers to predicting that an emotion will be more extremely negative or positive than it turns out to be (Wilson & Gilbert, 2003).

Research on affective forecasting suggests a number of biases or heuristics that lead to overpredicting emotional responses. One such factor is "focalism"—that is, the tendency to focus on a single feature of the event, rather than to consider other possible features that could reasonably mitigate one's emotional response to the event (Kahneman, Krueger, Schkade, Schwarz, & Stone, 2006; Wilson, Wheatley, Meyers, Gilbert, & Axsom, 2000). For example, some individuals may believe that if they move from a cold and overcast environment like Minnesota to sunny California, they will feel immensely happy for many years. However, they discover that after a brief period of feeling better, their happiness returns to the same level that they experienced in Minnesota. This is because they are focused on one factor (sunshine) while ignoring other important factors, such as their primary relationships and their work environments.

Another central feature of affective forecasting is "impact bias," which refers to the tendency to overestimate the emotional effects of events (Gilbert, Driver-Linn, & Wilson, 2002). That is, one may predict that a positive event will lead to lasting positive affect, while a negative event will lead to lasting negative affect. For example, an individual may predict that a breakup in a relationship will lead to everlasting negative feelings, but may believe that the beginning of a relationship will lead to feeling wonderful indefinitely. One dimension of predicting an emotion is how long it will last—the "durability effect." Wilson and Gilbert (2003) have since subsumed durability effect under impact bias. The durability effect reflects the belief that an emotion will continue for a long time.

Another factor affecting affective forecasting is "immune neglect"—that is, the tendency to ignore one's ability to cope with negative events. For example, Gilbert and colleagues (2002) found that participants would overpredict the duration of negative affect following six hypothetical situations: the breakup of a romantic relationship, the failure to achieve tenure, an electoral defeat, negative personality feedback, an account of a child's death, and rejection by a prospective employer. According to Wilson and Gilbert (2005), such individuals often ignore or underestimate their ability to cope; they do not recognize the powerful effects of coping strategies such as "dissonance reduction, motivated reasoning, self-serving attributions, self-affirmation, and positive illusions," which mitigate the effects of "negative life events" (Gilbert, Pinel, Wilson, Blumberg, & Wheatley, 1998, p. 619). For example, after a breakup with a girlfriend, a man may reduce the negative impact of the event by claiming he is better off without her (dissonance reduction), come up with negative attributions about the former partner (motivated reasoning), view himself as highly desirable now that he is single (self-serving attributions), bolster his hope by convincing himself and others that the best lies ahead (self-affirmation), and predict that his work and love life can only get better (positive illusions). Although one can argue that in each case these adjustments entail cognitive distortions or rationalizations, they may also mitigate the negative effects of the breakup. Moreover, unforeseen positive events may also occur, and these can also lead to a more positive outcome.

Moreover, individuals are prone to overvaluing a loss versus valuing a gain—a phenomenon known as "loss aversion" (Kahneman & Tversky, 1984). A common adage, "We suffer our losses more than we enjoy our gains," has support in the empirical literature. In a study of responses to gambling wins and losses, individuals overpredicted negative affect following a loss, not realizing that they would be able to rationalize their losses and that they were not as likely as they anticipated to dwell on these losses; that is, these people actually coped better with gambling losses than they anticipated they would (Kermer, Driver-Linn, Wilson, & Gilbert, 2006). As a result of loss aversion, individuals may often get stuck with an unpleasant situation, overestimating how bad they will feel if they ultimately regret giving it up.

Another factor in emotion prediction is the "affect heuristic"—a form of "emotional reasoning"—in which one uses a current emotion to predict a future emotion (i.e., uses the current emotion as an anchor) or predicts future emotional responses based on how one feels at the current moment (Finucane, Alhakami, Slovic, & Johnson, 2000). The affect heuristic helps account for greater risk taking for behaviors that "feel good." For example, if unprotected sex feels good, then it is viewed as less risky (Slovic, 2000; Slovic, Finucane, Peters, & MacGregor, 2004). It can also account for assessing the value or safety of things based on how one feels (e.g., "I know it's dangerous because I feel anxious").

In addition, individuals often estimate their future emotional responses based on their current appraisals of uncertainty; that is, the more uncertainty they feel, the greater the negativity anticipated (Bar-Anan, Wilson, & Gilbert, 2009). Intolerance of uncertainty is a key factor underlying worry, rumination, and obsessive–compulsive disorder (OCD), suggesting that uncertainty about negative outcomes may be a heuristic underpinning emotional schemas. For example, not knowing "for sure" how one will feel, when one is feeling poorly at the present time, may augment predictions of negative affect later.

Finally, many individuals discount the value of an alternative over time, such that they prefer a smaller gain now to a larger gain later. "Time discounting" refers to an emphasis on present events or availability of rewards, while reducing the value of delayed gratification (Frederick, Loewenstein, & O'Donoghue, 2002; McClure, Ericson, Laibson, Loewenstein, & Cohen, 2007; Read & Read, 2004). This bias toward the present may contribute to demands for immediate gratification, intolerance of discomfort, difficulty in persisting on difficult tasks, and demoralization about reaching goals (O'Donoghue & Rabin, 1999; Thaler & Shefrin, 1981; Zauberman, 2003). In its extreme form, decisions about emotion regulation may be myopic; that is, one may be so entirely focused on immediately reducing an uncomfortable emotion that one chooses (ultimately) self-defeating alternatives, such as substance misuse or binge eating. Future rewards are discounted to such an extent that the only valued alternative may seem like the one that is most immediate. One manifestation of myopic time discounting is the "contingency trap," where an individual gets locked into immediate contingencies, thereby developing an ultimately self-defeating habit. The model of contingency traps has been applied to addictive behavior: Withdrawal leads to immediate pain, whereas the use of the substance leads to immediate gratification, resulting in a greater momentum toward more substance use and a willingness to pay higher prices as one adjusts to higher levels of the substance (Becker, 1976, 1991; Grossman, Chaloupka, & Sirtalan, 1998).

Cognitive appraisals and heuristics such as these are essential components of emotional schemas. They contribute to the beliefs that emotions are durable, are out of control, and need to be eliminated or suppressed immediately. Ironically, emotions appear to have an evanescence: They often quickly fade rather than endure, lasting a short period until another emotion appears (Wilson, Gilbert, & Centerbar, 2003). Predictions about how long one will be miserable after a breakup, loss of a job, physical injury, or conflict with a good friend tend to overestimate how extreme one's emotions will be. Similar data suggest that happiness or unhappiness is not durable after significant life events. Indeed, the research on resilience suggests that an overwhelming percentage of individuals have returned to their pre-event baseline 1 year after major negative life events, suggesting that emotional "injuries" are resolved through various processes of coping (Bonanno & Gupta, 2009). Furthermore, individuals differ in the capacity to recover from trauma or loss, partly as a result of "regulatory flexibility"—that is, the ability to recruit adaptive processes to cope with difficulties that arise (Bonanno & Burton, 2013). This suggests that coping processes may be more important than the momentary experience of painful emotion.

Emotional schema therapy attempts to expand the range of regulatory flexibility, so that the occurrence of emotion need not result in extreme affective forecasting or self-defeating emotion regulation strategies, but rather can become the opportunity to recruit a wide range of adaptive interpretations and strategies for coping. Emotional schema therapy highlights problematic theories about a current emotion and shows how these are related to unhelpful coping styles that perpetuate further dysfunction. The chapters to come examine a variety of techniques to address a number of these beliefs about emotion, and suggest more helpful strategies for coping with emotions that appear troubling.

## THE PLAN OF THE BOOK

This chapter has shown how evolutionary theory, social construction, and historical and cultural contexts can influence the beliefs, strategies, and acceptability of various emotions. The next two chapters describe the core considerations in conducting emotional schema therapy (Chapter 2) and the general model of emotional schemas (Chapter 3). Part II (Chapters 4 and 5) reviews initial assessment and socialization to the model. Part III reviews specific emotional schemas and how to address them. Chapter 6 describes problematic beliefs about validation, their origin, and ways to address these beliefs in therapy. Chapter 7 reviews strategies for modifying several types of specific emotional schemas: those involving the dimensions of comprehensibility, duration, control, guilt/shame, and acceptance. Chapter 8 discusses the inevitability of ambivalence, examining how emotional perfectionism and intolerance of uncertainty make it difficult for some individuals to live with mixed feelings. Chapter 9, the final chapter of Part III, examines how the emotional schema model links uncomfortable emotions to the values and virtues that can help individuals tolerate the necessary challenges of a meaningful life. In Part IV of the book, "Social Emotions and Relationships," I have focused a chapter on jealousy (Chapter 10) and one on envy (Chapter 11), since these emotions can become so problematic that people kill themselves or others over them. I could have discussed a wide range of other emotions (such as humiliation, guilt, resentment, or anger), but jealousy and envy often include these other emotions—and, due to their social nature and putative evolutionary and cultural relevance, they appear most appropriate for this model. The last two chapters (12 and 13) review how emotional schemas can be relevant to couple relationships and to the therapeutic relationship, respectively.

## SUMMARY

Emotion and emotion regulation have gained increasing importance in psychology in the past decade with advances in neuroscience of emotion, cognitive models, dialectical behavior therapy, acceptance and commitment therapy, emotion-focused therapy, mentalization therapy, and other approaches ranging from cognitive behavioral therapy to psychodynamic therapy. In this chapter, I have introduced the idea that a component of the unfolding process of experiencing an emotion is the interpretation and evaluation of that emotion, along with the use of helpful or unhelpful strategies of emotion regulation. I refer to these concepts and processes as "emotional schemas." In Western philosophical and cultural traditions, there has been a continued dichotomization of emotion and rationality—with some arguing that emotion interferes with deliberative, rational, and virtuous action, and others viewing emotion as a source of meaning and interpersonal connection. Over the past several hundred years, Western concepts and recommended strategies for coping with emotion have changed substantially, with some emotions, such as jealousy and courage, losing "status." Finally, I have introduced the idea that the social psychology of emotion and choice can help illuminate some of the sources of bias in interpretations of emotion and prediction of future emotion. The remainder of this book examines how individual differences in emotional schemas may account for psychopathology, avoidance, noncompliance, and other problematic behaviors, and how assisting individuals in understanding and modifying these emotional schemas can deepen their experience of therapy and move them to confronting the difficult experiences required for growth. In the next chapter, I outline some of the main tenets of emotional schema therapy.

# CHAPTER 2

# Emotional Schema Therapy
## *General Considerations*

> He had seen everything, had experienced all emotions,
> from exaltation to despair, had been granted a vision
> into the great mystery, the secret places, the primeval
> days before the Flood.
> —*GILGAMESH*, ca. 2500 B.C.E.

In traditional cognitive models, emotion precedes, accompanies, or is a consequence of cognitive content (Beck, Emery, & Greenberg, 1985; Beck, Rush, Shaw, & Emery, 1979; D. A. Clark & Beck, 2010). For example, the cognitive model of depression suggests that a cognitive schema with self-negating content (e.g., "I am a loser") results in sadness, helplessness, or hopelessness. The cognitive model of panic disorder proposes that interpretations of interoceptive sensations (e.g., heart pounding, muscle tension, dizziness) result in an escalation of anxiety (D. M. Clark, 1996; D. M. Clark, Salkovskis, & Chalkley, 1985; D. M. Clark et al., 1999; Salkovskis, Clark, & Gelder, 1996). The cognitive model of OCD suggests that overappraisals of the threat of specific beliefs (e.g., "I am contaminated"), along with beliefs about personal responsibility for a thought and the need to neutralize or eliminate any possibility of an event, result in a vicious cycle of thought appraisal, threat appraisal, intolerance of uncertainty, and failed attempts at control (Salkovskis & Kirk, 1997). And, finally, the cognitive model of personality disorders emphasizes beliefs about personal qualities of self (e.g., "I am helpless" or "I am defective") and qualities of others (e.g., "They are untrustworthy" or "They are rejecting"), followed

19

by problematic strategies for coping (avoidance, compensation) (Beck, Freeman, & Davis, 2004).

The emotional schema model extends these cognitive models to appraisals of, and strategies to cope with, emotions. It is argued in this new model that emotions themselves may constitute *objects* of cognition; that is, they may also be viewed as *content* to be evaluated, controlled, or utilized by an individual (Leahy, 2002, 2003b, 2009b). This approach is derived from the field of social cognition, with its emphasis on naive psychology models of intentionality, normality, social comparison, and attribution processes (Alloy, Abramson, Metalsky, & Hartledge, 1988; Eisenberg & Spinrad, 2004; Leahy, 2002, 2003b; Weiner, 1974, 1986). Heider (1958) and those who followed him in social cognition were particularly interested in how laypersons conceptualized personality, intentions, the causes of behavior, and concepts of responsibility. The emotional schema model follows in this tradition. If one can argue that the metacognitive model (see below) stresses disorders of theory of mind, the emotional schema model stresses disorders of the theory of emotion and mind.

Unlike the schema-focused therapy advanced by Young, Klosko, and Weishaar (2003), emotional schema therapy focuses on *beliefs about emotions* and on *strategies of emotion control*. Schema-focused therapy is not a theory of beliefs about emotions, but rather a theory about *personal attributes* of self and others; it bears some resemblance in this regard to Beck and Freeman's model of personal schemas and personality disorders (Beck et al., 2004). Young et al.'s model proposes that individuals develop concepts of self (e.g., "unlovable," "special," "defective") as a result of early experiences (forming early maladaptive schemas), and these concepts or schemas persist and are maintained through avoidance, compensation, or maintenance. The emotional schema model is not a model of personality per se, but a model of beliefs about and strategies for coping with *emotion*.

Similar to the metacognitive model advanced by Adrian Wells (2009) the emotional schema model proposes that individuals have meta-experiential theories of their emotions. Rather than focusing on the schematic content of intrusive thoughts (e.g., challenging the thought "I am a loser"), the metacognitive approach proposes that evaluation and control of intrusive thoughts result in OCD and other psychological disorders (Salkovskis, 1989; Salkovskis & Campbell, 1994; Wells, 2009). Cognitive appraisals of the nature of thoughts as *only thoughts*, rather than the content of thoughts themselves, underpin OCD. Safety behaviors, thought suppression strategies, self-monitoring, cognitive self-consciousness, and beliefs that thoughts are out of control are often the consequences of problematic appraisals. Psychological disorders are viewed as the results of the *responses* to thoughts, sensations, and emotions that follow from problematic evaluations of the personal relevance of a thought; responsibility for suppressing, neutralizing, or acting on implications of a thought; thought–action fusion; intolerance of uncertainty; and perfectionistic standards (Purdon, Rowa, & Antony, 2005; Rachman, 1997; Wells, 2000; Wilson & Chambless, 1999). The emotional schema model is similar to the metacognitive model in its proposal that appraisals of emotions and strategies of emotion control contribute to the development and maintenance of psychopathology.

Emotional schema therapy also draws on Greenberg's emotion-focused therapy (Greenberg & Paivio, 1997; Greenberg & Watson, 2005) in its emphasis on emotional experience, expression, evaluation of primary and secondary emotions; its viewing of emotions as related to needs and values; and its assertion that emotions may also "contain" meanings (similar to Lazarus's [1999] "core relational themes"). However, emotional schema therapy is specifically meta-emotional (or metacognitive) in that it directly assesses *beliefs about emotions* and how emotions function. Thus the emphasis is not only on Rogerian processes of expression, validation, and unconditional positive regard, but also on the patient's implicit theories of emotion. This is similar to the approach taken by Gottman, Katz, and Hooven (1997). For example, an emotional schema therapist might examine the belief that painful emotions are an opportunity to develop deeper and more meaningful emotions, or the contrary belief that painful emotions are a sign of weakness and inferiority. An emotion-focused therapist utilizes expression and validation as central therapeutic techniques—as would the emotional schema therapist. However, emotional schema therapy views validation as a process that affects other cognitive (or schematic) *evaluations of emotion*. Thus validation leads to a recognition that the patient's emotions are not unique, that expressing emotion need not lead to being overwhelmed, that there is generally less guilt and shame with validation, and that validation assists the patient in "making sense" of feelings. Thus validation leads to changes in *beliefs* about emotion, which can then lead to changes in the emotion itself (Leahy, 2005c).

There are parallels between emotional schema therapy and acceptance and commitment therapy (ACT; Hayes, Luoma, Bond, Masuda, & Lillis, 2006; Hayes, Strosahl, & Wilson, 2012). Similar to ACT, emotional schema therapy stresses the role of avoidance and failed attempts at suppression. The metacognitive emotional schema model, however, provides detailed descriptions of these underlying theories of mind, and proposes specific behavioral experiments to test hypotheses explicitly derived from these propositions about mind and sensations. It is noteworthy that there appears to be convergence between the metacognitive and ACT approaches in the use of mindfulness and utilizing an observing stance toward thoughts and sensations as therapeutic interventions. Similarly, emotional schema therapy also utilizes an observing and detached approach to noticing and accepting an emotion as an "event," rather than attempting to avoid or suppress the emotion. In addition to the use of acceptance and mindfulness, emotional schema therapy emphasizes the important link between emotions and values—encouraging patients to clarify the values and virtues that are important to them, so that difficult emotions may be tolerated.

ACT is a behavioral model of psychopathology, stressing the functionality of behavior and beliefs, experiential avoidance, flexibility, and the contextual nature of personal functioning. While recognizing the immense value of these concepts, the emotional schema model seeks to elucidate an individual's idiosyncratic beliefs or theories of emotions, and in this sense, it does emphasize "content"—that is, *the content of these theories of emotion*. For example, if the patient holds the beliefs that his or her emotions will last a long time, do not make sense, and are shameful, then the therapist will collaborate with the patient to examine the utility and validity of these beliefs. Moreover, experiential avoidance—which is an important component of ACT and behavioral activation models—is understood in emotional schema therapy as maintaining problematic beliefs about emotions (i.e., beliefs that emotions are dangerous, are out of control, and need to be suppressed). Experiences in the emotional schema model affect beliefs about emotions, such as beliefs about durability, need for control, and danger. The ACT model is not specifically concerned with the content of thoughts about emotion and does not explicate the patient's theory of emotion.

The emotional schema therapy approach can be integrated into a wide variety of cognitive-behavioral models, including Beckian therapy, ACT, dialectical behavior therapy (DBT), behavioral activation, and other approaches—with the added emphasis on a patient's specific beliefs about emotions and strategies for coping with emotion. For instance, an emotional schema therapist can use behavioral activation while also investigating the patient's beliefs about what emotions will be activated, their duration, their meaning, and their need to be controlled.

## CENTRAL THEMES OF EMOTIONAL SCHEMA THERAPY

Emotional schema therapy proposes that individuals have implicit theories of emotion and emotion regulation. In emotional schema therapy, the emphasis is on clarifying and modifying a patient's specific theory of emotion, using cognitive or Socratic evaluations, experiential tests, behavioral experiments, and other interventions to assist in normalizing, temporizing, linking emotions to values, and finding adaptive expression and validation. In socializing the patient to the model of therapy, the therapist will stress that emotion itself may not be the problem; rather, the problem may be the evaluation, fear, and need to escape from emotion through problematic strategies of emotion control. Everyone feels sad at times, but only some become depressed. Everyone feels anxious, but only some people develop generalized anxiety disorder. Everyone has irrational fears of contamination or making a mistake, but only some individuals develop OCD.

The emotional schema model stresses the following seven themes:

1. Painful and difficult emotions are universal.
2. These emotions were evolved to warn us of danger and tell us about our needs.
3. Underlying beliefs and strategies (schemas) about emotions determine an emotion's impact on the escalation or maintenance of itself or other emotions.
4. Problematic schemas include catastrophizing an emotion; thinking that one's emotions do not make sense; and viewing an emotion as permanent and out of control, shameful, unique to the self, and needing to be kept to the self.
5. Emotional control strategies such as attempts to suppress, ignore, neutralize, or eliminate emotions through substance abuse and binge eating help confirm negative beliefs of emotions as intolerable experiences.
6. Expression and validation are helpful insofar as they normalize, universalize, improve understanding, differentiate various emotions, reduce guilt and shame, and help increase beliefs in the tolerability of emotional experience (Leahy, 2009b).
7. Learning to acknowledge painful emotions and to develop tolerance for frustration in emotional schema therapy can be understood as part of a model of personal empowerment—that is, increased self-efficacy and more complete meaning in life.

Let us examine each of these general issues.

## Painful and Difficult Emotions Are Universal

Emotional schema therapy views "difficult" emotions—such as sadness, anxiety, anger, jealousy, resentment, and envy—as universal experiences. It is hard to imagine someone going through life without experiencing each of these emotions. The universality of emotion suggests that the patient is not alone (everyone has difficult emotions), and that painful emotions are part of the human condition and part of living a complete life. The goal of therapy is a more complete life—one in which painful emotions have their place, are recognized as part of being human, and as emotions that may reflect the values that are important to the individual. There are no "good" and "bad" emotions, just as there is no "good" and "bad" hunger or arousal. This recognition that emotions are universal serves to normalize, validate, and encourage accepting a wide range of emotions, rather than judging, suppressing, escaping from, or avoiding emotions.

The goal of emotional schema therapy is not for a patient to feel happy or to get rid of sadness or anxiety. This would be like telling a person with generalized anxiety disorder or OCD that the goal of therapy is to eliminate intrusive thoughts. Rather, the goals are for the patient to be able to acknowledge painful and difficult emotions, to accept them as part of the experience of a complete life, to evaluate them in a nonpejorative manner, to avoid catastrophizing emotion, to recognize that emotions are temporary, and to use emotions as a guide to pursuing values and virtues that are important to the individual. Rather than viewing therapy as attempting to "feel good," the emotional schema model helps the patient develop the capacity to feel *everything*.

The recognition that painful emotions are part of life asserts that life can be difficult at times. This may seem trite, or too obvious to need mentioning. But validating that life is difficult, that things may feel impossible, or that hopelessness is an emotion that almost everyone knows also suggests that, since almost everyone will have these feelings, there must be productive ways to cope. If almost everyone has painful emotions, but almost everyone gets past them, there must be a way of going through such an emotion to get past it. If life feels awful at times, it does not follow that life is without meaning and hope.

An advantage of normalizing difficult emotions—and acknowledging that they are part of the human condition—is that patients do not have to believe that painful emotions are a marker of psychopathology or mental disorder. Emotions are not traits; they are experiences that come and go. They are responses to a situation, or evaluations of a situation. Just as hunger is not a permanent trait, an emotion can dissipate if conditions change, perspectives are modified, or attention is directed elsewhere. Moreover, the universal nature of emotions suggests that in many problems of living, a painful emotion is the recognition of the problem. For example, the individual who has a conflict with a good friend may feel angry and sad. These may be human responses to an interruption of a close relationship; it means that something *mattered*. However, the individual may respond to the situation by exaggerating the nature of the conflict—viewing it as awful, permanent, and an indication of failure. But these "magnifying" responses to a response of frustration, anger, and sadness are what lead to more lasting problems. An emotional schema therapist may often say to such a patient, "A lot of us would feel sad (angry, hurt) if this happened. You are human; you have your feelings." But the therapist may also ask, "I can see it makes sense to feel sad, but I am wondering about the intensity of that sadness and what this means to you that it makes you feel so bad." This reframing of sadness as *normal* while examining the *intensity* of the sadness conveys the message that some sadness can be accepted as part of being human, but that the intensity of the sadness may be open to examination and possible modification. There is a difference between "Why do you feel sad?" and "Why do you feel so overwhelmingly sad?"

For example, envy is a common emotion about which people often feel embarrassed or guilty. It is difficult for people to acknowledge their envy;

they would rather focus on the individual about whom they feel envy and that person's shortcomings. Envy is a disparaged emotion and is often associated with rumination, guilt, sadness, and anger. The emotional schema model proposes that envy is a universal emotion and can be used either productively or unproductively. Unproductive use of envy entails avoiding the person about whom one feels envy, criticizing the person, or attempting to undermine him or her. Rumination, complaining, and feeling guilty are also unproductive uses of envy. In contrast, accepting envy as part of being human, and turning envy into admiration and emulation, can be motivating and self-enhancing. The problematic social emotions of jealousy and envy are discussed more fully in Chapters 10 and 11, but for now, envy is neither good nor bad; it is simply part of being human.

Patients can be assisted in universalizing emotions by looking for examples of emotion in the lyrics of songs, poetry, drama, novels, or the stories that they hear from friends and family. For example, jealousy—another disparaged emotion—is the focus of many songs, poems, dramas, and stories, and readers and audiences are attracted to these themes because they resonate with their own experiences. Indeed, the ability to identify with characters in a story makes a story even more appealing. It tells "our story."

## Emotions Were Evolved to Warn Us of Danger and Tell Us about Our Needs

Emotional schema therapy is based on an evolutionary model in which emotions—and the expression of emotions—were evolved because they helped protect members of the species (Cosmides & Tooby, 2002; Ermer, Guerin, Cosmides, Tooby, & Miller, 2006; Tooby & Cosmides, 1992). Emotions are not "psychopathology" or "abnormalities" or signs of "sickness" (Nesse, 1994). Emotions are genetically determined, universal adaptations to challenges in the evolutionarily relevant environment (Nesse & Ellsworth, 2009). For example, fear of open spaces (which is often characteristic of people with agoraphobia) was adaptive in an environment where open spaces invited danger from predators. Potential ancestors who traversed open spaces without consideration of threat from predators were more likely to be seen and attacked, and thereby eliminated from passing on their genes. Anxiety over public speaking was adaptive in a primitive environment where taking a dominant role toward strangers would be seen as insulting and threatening and would lead to retaliation. Sadness was adaptive because it told our ancestors that there was no sense in continuing in a course of action that had met with repeated failure. Anger and aggression were adaptive because they led to protection against conspecifics who might invade one's territory, take food sources, and kill relatives or oneself. Jealousy was adaptive because it protected one's "parental investment" and warded off competitors for sexual access and procreation.

Emotional schema therapy often involves examining how an emotion might make sense from an evolutionary point of view. For example, worry and anxiety about one's children's safety make sense because parents who were more worried about and protective of their children were more likely to have children who survived. One question that helps illustrate this is to ask, "What if our ancestors did not have this emotion? Would there be any negative consequences?" For instance, prehistoric ancestors who did not worry about their children, or who did not respond to the infants' cries, were more likely to have children who wandered off into dangerous forests, who were attacked and killed by predators, and who did not survive to procreate. Ancestors who were incapable of jealousy would have their reproductive partners "stolen," would fail to reproduce, or would end up providing for offspring that were not genetically linked to them, thereby decreasing the survival of their own genes. The emotion of disgust was also adaptive, in that it helped early humans to avoid contamination. Aversion to dirt—so often one of the fears of people with OCD—was an adaptation that led to the avoidance of disease and may be viewed as another form of preparedness (Tybur, Lieberman, Kurzban, & DeScioli, 2013).

Moreover, the evolutionary model emphasizes the automatic and reflexive nature of emotions. The therapist can indicate that it would make sense that a fear of heights would be automatic and immediate, not relying initially on any conscious deliberation. Jumping back from a cliff would be more adaptive than waiting to think about it. Similarly, a fear of snakes, manifested by immediate panic and jumping away, would be more adaptive than a slower, more cognitive deliberation about whether the snake was poisonous. Thus a person's first response may be the "natural" response, regardless of the individual's intelligence and knowledge. Encouraging a quick response is what emotions are good for. They warn, motivate, propel; they are characterized by automaticity and are without conscious awareness (Hassin, Uleman, & Bargh, 2005). If they were slow-acting, they would not have been effective in enabling our ancestors to avoid danger or escape from predators. Emotions are the "first responders"; they rapidly deploy rescue and removal. Emotions are there because they have saved lives. They may be "overreactions" in the current situation, but they have evolved because their rapid and overwhelming nature has been useful in protecting the species.

The message to patients is that their emotions were the emotions that survived millennia of evolution because they were adaptive to the environment that existed. Fear of strangers, fear of open spaces, sadness over loss, hopelessness after failing, loss of interest in sex, anger over being slighted—all of these were emotional responses that were adapted to problems in an evolutionarily relevant environment. For example, consider a woman with bulimia nervosa who claims that she feels she is "starving" when she has not eaten for a few hours. She becomes anxious, panics, and then binges.

How can this sequence of emotions and behavior make sense from an evolutionary perspective? The answer is that until the past century, an overwhelming majority of humans lived close to a subsistence level; hunger and malnutrition were common problems, and binge eating was seldom viewed as an issue, since food was scarce. In such an environment, individuals who would binge after deprivation (and, coincidentally, might also have slower metabolisms) were more likely to avoid starvation. Thus "overreacting" to hunger with panic over "starving" was adaptive for individuals in the evolutionary environment, as was slower metabolism, since calories could be stored and starvation avoided. The question comes back to this: "How would this emotion be adaptive for our ancestors?" In other words, "What is this emotion good for?"

Social emotions—such as humiliation, jealousy, and envy—can also be viewed from an evolutionary perspective. Humiliating a member of a dominance hierarchy would convey the message to other members of the group that this individual no longer could enjoy the privileges of status—or even membership in the group. Thus the fear of humiliation would be a natural fear, since the subsequent exclusion from or loss of status in the group would result in loss of resources and protection (Gilbert, 1992, 2000b, 2003). Envy can also be seen from an evolutionary perspective (Hill & Buss, 2008). Since our ancestors belonged to dominance hierarchies, the loss of status that one would experience in comparison with another member who gained status would reduce the advantages that one might have. Members with higher status would have greater access to potential mates, better access to food, privileges of being groomed by other members of the group, and greater resources for offspring. Status conferred real advantages. Moreover, competing for status (which is characteristic of envious individuals) would also be a natural response, since the ability to move upward would confer the advantages described above. Furthermore, undeserved higher status or privilege might activate natural preferences for fairness or distributive justice, leading to attempts to restore fairness by castigating or rejecting those viewed as attaining unwarranted advantages (Boehm, 2001). Thus, instead of feeling guilty or confused about envy, patients in emotional schema therapy are encouraged to understand the evolutionary value of this emotion, the natural tendencies to engage in competitive dominance behaviors, and the possibility that envy can also motivate them to become more effective and strategic (rather than ruminate, avoid, and complain).

The evolutionary model of emotions addresses a number of problematic beliefs about emotions (i.e., emotional schemas). If emotions have an evolutionary and adaptive origin, then this should help normalize these emotions, reduce guilt, help individuals understand why they feel the way they do, validate that their emotions make sense, and encourage acceptance of what are natural responses. However, the evolutionary model does not imply that individuals cannot change their emotional responses to situations or modify these responses once they have been activated (Pinker, 2002). Rather, the evolutionary model is a first step in helping patients recognize that they are having natural responses (ones that may be prewired), but that by utilizing the many techniques available in emotional schema therapy, they can change their emotional responses.

For example, consider a shy patient's emotional response when meeting strangers for the first time. The patient may report feeling anxious and insecure. An evolutionary interpretation is that these feelings of anxiety and insecurity made sense for our ancestors, when strangers might be homicidal and threatening. The first responses that they might have would be anxiety, hesitancy, and the desire to avoid. Moreover, the social anxiety may be manifested by "appeasement" behaviors, such as lowered voice, downward gaze, changes in posture, apologies, and hesitancy in "taking a stand" (Eibl-Eibesfeldt, 1972). All of these behaviors would communicate to strangers that one is not a threat. This would be the initial, automatic evolutionary response. But the questions in emotional schema therapy are these: How is this automatic, evolutionary response an overreaction to the current situation? Are the members of the group that the patient is going to meet threatening? Are they homicidal? Are they likely to want to humiliate the individual? Emotions are real—but they may be based on false alarms to real dangers that our ancestors faced but that are no longer present. They worked in the past, but they are not working effectively now. They may be the right responses at the wrong time. Although threat-detecting emotions may be based on "better safe than sorry" strategies, their overextension may interfere with productive and meaningful experiences. The patient's knowledge of having an emotion—and of why this emotion has been evoked—need not tether the patient to that emotion.

Throughout this book's discussion of the emotional schema model, the primary focus is on sadness and anxiety. As noted earlier, however, the social emotions—such as shame, guilt, humiliation, jealousy, and envy— are pervasive and troubling experiences. Given the limitations of space, I have chosen to focus Chapters 10 and 11 on jealousy and envy, primarily because they have received less attention in the cognitive-behavioral literature—but also because these are powerful emotions that can lead to abuse, homicide, and suicide, that these are emotions people kill over.

## Beliefs and Strategies about Emotions Determine the Impact of an Emotion

The emotional schema model proposes that one's beliefs about the duration, controllability, tolerance, complexity, comprehensibility, normality, and other dimensions of emotions will affect whether one becomes anxious about having an emotion or is able to tolerate an emotion and experience it as a temporary internal phenomenon. This model assists patients in recognizing how specific interpretations and judgments about emotion may precipitate a sequence of maladaptive coping strategies that, ironically, maintain the negative beliefs about emotion. Each of the categories of emotional schemas will lead to further difficulty in tolerating the experience of emotion. Just as anxious persons may be biased toward threat detection in the external environment (e.g., "The plane will crash," "I will be ridiculed," "My partner will leave me"), there is a similar process of threat detection about one's own emotional experience. For many people with anxiety or depressive disorders, the *experience* of anxiety is threatening. A man with panic disorder believes that his anxious arousal is a sign that he is having a heart attack or will go insane. It must be controlled immediately. A depressed woman who feels sad while alone believes that the sadness is unbearable and an indication that life is not worth living. She believes that she must get rid of this sadness immediately, and thus ruminates to try to figure out what is going on. A woman with OCD believes that her anxious arousal and thoughts while touching a "contaminated" surface are indications of how intolerable the action is. In each case, the experience of anxiety is viewed as threatening, awful, and a sign of increasing danger. In each case, however, the experience is similar to a smoke alarm that is a false alarm: The patient with negative schemas about emotion treats the "smoke alarm" as if it is the "fire" itself. *The alarm is dangerous.* This is a form of thought—action fusion, but a particular kind of fusion; It is a fusion of feeling and reality. "If I feel anxious, then there must be danger."

One can argue that the functionality of anxiety is that it motivates an individual to do something to escape or avoid situations that truly could be dangerous. In the extreme, simply thinking that something is dangerous may not provide the motivation—the necessary discomfort—to do something different. It is like a computer that registers or notices that there is a missile coming at it. Unless there is an instruction in its software to escape, the computer is simply a camera on the world. The dysfunctional emotional schemas—that the emotion of anxiety is escalating out of control and cannot be accepted—were adaptive in that they automatically (without reflection, without delay) activated defensive or offensive responses. Without them, we would not have survived as a species.

Emotions are responses in a *context*. Sadness arises when one experiences a loss; fear is a response to a mortal threat; anxiety is a response to a possible failure; and anger is a response to humiliation and insult. Emotions are linked to the events that trigger them. There is an "about-ness" to emotion—a person is sad *about* being alone, angry *about* being insulted. Clarifying the goals that are blocked or are threatened can help a patient identify the issues that are relevant to an emotion. For example, being angry about traffic may clarify that the patient is overvaluing "getting there on time," while enduring a strong and unpleasant emotional state. Further examination of what the anger is about may lead to other problematic thoughts (e.g., "These people are idiots," or "Why are they blocking me?" or "I can never get what I want"). Emotions have targets, examining the purpose or meaning that underlies an emotion can help modify the emotion.

Sometimes patients may overidentify with an emotion (e.g., "I am an angry person," or "I am sad"), rather than contextualize the occurrence of the emotion (e.g., "I am angry when I think someone has insulted me"). Some individuals view their emotions as traits that are fixed forever in time. This is very similar to how some individuals view ability or performance—either as fixed entities or as capable of incremental change (Chiu, Hong, & Dweck, 1997; Dweck, 2000).

The value of contextualizing an emotion is that it facilitates greater flexibility in appraising and responding to the emotion (Hayes, Jacobson, & Follette, 1994; Hayes et al., 2006, 2012). Since each of us has a wide range of emotions, it would make little sense to identify one's "self" with a single emotion. If emotions are not "self," then there must be something about this situation—or the way in which one evaluates it—that leads to this response. Situations can change, evaluations can change, and emotions can change. This has direct relevance to the evaluation of an emotion, since it raises the question of the consistency of this emotion across time, the emotion's uniqueness to a particular situation or interpretation of a situation, and the degree to which emotions can change. Emotional schema therapy stresses the context of emotion, its variability, the interpretations of context, the interpretations of the emotion, and the emotion regulation strategies that are elicited.

## Emotional Schemas and Emotion Regulation Strategies Are Often the Problems, Not the Solutions

Patients may believe that the problem is either the situation ("reality") or the emotions that they are experiencing. For example, a man sitting at home alone in his apartment may think that "being alone" is the problem, and that "being alone" means that he must feel lonely, sad, empty, and hopeless. As a consequence, he fears that he will have these feelings, and desperately avoids being alone by clinging to self-destructive relationships. Being alone, in his mind, automatically leads to negative thoughts, such as "I must be alone because I am unlovable," "No one cares about me," or "I will be alone forever." In this situation, the reality of being alone "must be depressing." In contrast to the idea that the situation must lead to sadness and loneliness is the view that what he is telling himself about being alone is more of the problem. Thus more traditional cognitive therapy techniques might be helpful through directing him to evaluate the tendency to overgeneralize, catastrophize, label, and engage in fortunetelling. It may be that he does not need to change the situation (or avoid it), but rather to develop more adaptive ways of viewing the situation.

However, once the emotions of sadness, loneliness, emptiness, and hopelessness have been activated, this man may utilize problematic "solutions" to his emotions. These include strategies such as attempts to suppress, ignore, neutralize, or eliminate these emotions through substance abuse and binge eating. Or he may ruminate in order to "figure it out so I can solve this problem for myself." Because he believes that his difficult emotions must be eliminated immediately, he thinks that these solutions may be the only way to cope. However, the solutions have now become problems, along with the problematic schemas.

Since this man's emotion control strategies only temporarily reduce his emotional intensity, the emotions return, thereby "confirming" for him that the problem is worse than he thought it was. He may increase his use of strategies such as rumination or drinking, but the emotions still come back. The idea that emotions come back then makes him even more anxious and more afraid of his feelings, and his sadness, anxiety, and hopelessness escalate.

In contrast to the problematic emotion control strategies used by the lonely man in his apartment, an emotional schema therapist might help him examine a range of other strategies that do not attempt to suppress an emotion, but rather enable him to think and act in adaptive ways while accepting the emotion as a given. For example, the therapist might suggest that this man can accept an emotion as "background noise"—a sound or song that is playing in the background while he is doing other things. Observing the emotion—as he would background noise—allows him to accept an emotion as a temporary experience while he pursues other experiences. Thus the patient can use mindful awareness, detaching from the emotion as he would while following a tune that is played. This detachment can allow the patient to observe the emotion as the emotion comes and goes. In addition, other activities that might be rewarding—such as listening to music, exercising, reading, contacting friends, or making plans—can be pursued while the emotion "plays in the background." Moreover, the patient can recognize that positive and negative emotions may exist in the same "life space." That is, while he is in the apartment with the painful emotions in the background, he can pursue exercises that activate positive emotions, such as gratitude exercises. While focusing on gratitude, he does not need to suppress the emotion of loneliness, but rather to recognize that his life can be large enough to contain all of these emotions.

## Validation Affects Other Emotional Schemas

Emotional schema therapy stresses the importance of validation on the part of the therapist and self-validation on the part of the patient. "Validation" is defined here as acknowledging the element of truth in a person's thoughts and feelings—in other words, "I can understand why you think that and why your feelings make sense." For example, the patient who complains of feeling lonely, sad, and hopeless when alone in his apartment is reporting his thoughts and feelings about that situation. The therapist who validates him can say, "I can understand that you might think that your loneliness will last indefinitely, and that this is very upsetting to you." Validation is not the same as "agreement." The therapist is not saying, "Your loneliness will last forever," but rather, "Your thoughts make sense—and, given these thoughts, it would also make sense that you would feel discouraged." Validation is an attempt to be an accurate mirror of what a patient is thinking and feeling. But just as it provides a mirror as to what is going on inside the patient, it also suggests a window into the possibility of other experiences, other meanings, and other emotions.

Our research (discussed in more detail in Chapter 3) shows that validation is correlated with most of the other dimensions of emotional schemas. Patients who believe that they are validated also believe that they can express their emotions, that their emotions will not last indefinitely, that other people have the same emotions, that their emotions are not out of control, that their emotions make sense, that they can tolerate mixed emotions, and that they can accept the emotions they are experiencing. In addition, validation is related to less rumination and less blame, as well as to lower levels of depression and anxiety. Why should validation be such an important belief about one's emotions? It is not surprising that expression and validation are related, although expression itself is not highly correlated with depression, anxiety, rumination, and most other emotional schemas. Contrary to catharsis-based theories of emotion, it is not simply the *expression* of emotion that counts, but also the cognitive components of validation. For example, an individual who is validated understands that he or she can express emotions, but that they will not go out of control and last indefinitely. This may be because expression without validation only feels more invalidating (and frustrating), leading to increased intensity of expression. If the individual expresses emotion, but others ignore, dismiss, or ridicule this expression, then it can lead to more depression, more anxiety, and more anger. *Expression with validation* helps the individual believe that his or her emotions make sense and that others might feel the same way. Since rumination is often a strategy to make sense of emotion, validation may short-circuit this repetitive fixation on a thought or feeling: "If my emotions make sense to you, then they must make sense." Validation accomplishes important goals. Ironically, some people are reluctant to validate someone who is complaining; they argue that validating will only encourage constant complaining. Although this makes some intuitive sense, the rationale confuses expression with validation. If an individual expresses uncomfortable feelings in the hope of being validated, and validation is accomplished, then further expression will be unnecessary. This is not dissimilar to a tenet of attachment theory: Continued cries by an infant that go unanswered lead to more crying. Comforting the infant when it is crying "completes a system," as Bowlby (1969, 1973, 1980) might have argued. Validation completes a system of seeking a shared meaning.

I examine problematic beliefs about validation in Chapter 6, but emotional schema therapy stresses validation not only as a valuable component of the therapeutic relationship, but also as a powerful tool for modifying emotional schemas and obviating problematic strategies of emotion regulation. An emotional schema therapist will frequently comment that a patient's emotions make sense, that the patient's beliefs (if true) would be troublesome, that others might feel the same way, and that it is important to be heard and understood.

In some cases, patients will invalidate themselves—often saying that they do not have a right to feel the way that they do, that they are "just complaining," or that they are "weak" and "repulsive" for having the emotions that they have (Leahy, 2001, 2009b). This self-invalidation is another emotion control strategy; it is based on the belief that "if I ridicule my feelings, they will go away." This self-invalidation may be reminiscent of the invalidation that they received from their parents who were dismissive ("It's no big deal"), critical ("You are being a baby"), or dysregulated themselves ("I am overwhelmed with my own problems"). Self-invalidation fails to make sense of emotion, fails to normalize emotion, and adds self-criticism and its consequent depression and anxiety to the new mix of emotion problems with which to contend. Individuals who self-invalidate may feel ashamed of disclosing their emotions and thoughts; they may attempt to "get rid" of emotions by keeping them private, fearing that they will be humiliated. An emotional schema therapist is aware of this problem and will address the reluctance that a patient may experience in sharing thoughts and feelings:

> "I can understand that it may feel natural at times to keep your emotions to yourself, hide your thoughts. There could be a lot of reasons why people might keep things to themselves. You may not feel ready; perhaps it takes a while to figure out what you are feeling and thinking; or you might be concerned with how I might react. I wonder if you have had any thoughts about keeping emotions back—keeping things to yourself."

This validation of fear of disclosure allows the patient to recognize that the therapist understands and accepts reluctance, and is open to discussing what that might be like.

## Personal Empowerment Is the Goal of Emotional Schema Therapy

A key element of each of the cognitive-behavioral models is that the patient is directed toward behaviors and experiences that may feel uncomfortable, are feared, or are disturbing. This includes exposure with response prevention in treating OCD, prolonged exposure treatment with posttraumatic stress disorder (PTSD), behavioral activation in the treatment of depression, exposure to interoceptive stimuli in the treatment of panic disorder, and confronting a hierarchy of feared stimuli in the treatment of specific phobia. Discomfort, frustration, and even disgust (in some cases) are the means toward the end. That is, unpleasant emotional experiences are the experiential tools that move a patient forward. Many patients, however, come to therapy with the goal of ridding themselves of discomfort and eliminating frustration; as a result, some either will not comply with consistent exposure exercises or will prematurely drop out. The emotional schema model proposes that therapy can be focused more productively on the goals of personal efficacy, more complete meaning in life, and the achievement of desired purposes. I refer to these goals collectively as "personal empowerment," suggesting that helping patients gain greater control over the ability to engage in difficult tasks will empower them to achieve greater meaning in life. Rather this model suggests that developing the ability to tolerate difficult emotions as a means to an end will be more helpful than focusing on reducing unpleasant emotion. Similar to ACT and DBT, in other words, emotional schema therapy suggests that the willingness to do difficult things in pursuit of valued goals is a more helpful approach for patients.

The model of empowerment advanced here proposes that the patient can ask three questions (Leahy, 2005d, 2013): (1) "What do I want?" (2) "What do I have to do to get it?" (3) "Am I willing to do it?" Thus, a patient who wants to lose 20 pounds (the goal) will have to eat less and exercise more (what has to be done). The question is whether the patient is willing to do what needs to be done. Emotional discomfort, self-discipline, making personal sacrifices, and accepting frustration are all part of the bargain. The emotional schema therapist directly confronts the issue of willingness: "Are you willing to do things that you do not want to do, so that you can get what you want to get?" Indeed, the therapist may say to the patient: "The goal for now is to do something every day that you do not want to do, so that you can develop the self-discipline that you will need to achieve what is important." The model here argues for building resilience rather than aiming for comfort. The therapist can make discomfort tolerance a central goal—a kind of "mental muscle"—so that the patient is urged daily to value thinking that "I am a person who does what is difficult to do." The therapist can suggest that authentic pride comes from overcoming obstacles, not from achieving or having something: "Think about the things that you have done in your life [e.g., having a child, completing college, helping a friend or a sick family member, learning a skill]. Now which of these things involved discomfort and frustration?" It may be that each of them involved significant discomfort. The therapist can continue: "Pride comes from tolerating discomfort—from doing the hard things—to achieve valued purposes." Two concepts are especially helpful here—"constructive discomfort" and "successful imperfection" (Leahy, 2003, 2005d). Constructive discomfort refers to the use of uncomfortable experiences as a means to achieve valued goals. The willingness to experience the discomfort of intensive exercise to get into better shape is an example. Successful imperfection involves the willingness to engage persistently in less than perfect behavior as a means to move toward valued goals. Again, the willingness to exercise on a regular basis—even if this means doing an incomplete workout—can move the patient who wants to lose weight toward the goal of better physical conditioning. Patients are encouraged to monitor their experiences of uncomfortable experiences on a daily basis, and to view these experiences are part of a larger picture of purpose and valued goals. The emphasis is shifted away from feeling good, feeling comfortable, or feeling happy to the ability to use discomfort effectively. The therapist can ask, "If you are going to be uncomfortable anyway, why not achieve something?"

The empowered approach involves developing effective instrumental behavior and self-efficacy. It includes the following aspects: future orientation; goal orientation; problem solving; personal responsibility; personal accountability; investment in discomfort; delay of gratification; persistence; planning; risk taking; productivity; learning and challenge; and pride in performance. Here are definitions of these aspects:

*Future orientation*: Works toward future rewards.

*Goal orientation*: Establishes clear goals and maintains a focus on them.

*Problem solving*: Views frustration as an opportunity to solve a problem.

*Personal responsibility*: Has standards of conduct (i.e., standards of what is right or moral) for the self, and holds the self responsible for performance.

*Personal accountability*: Evaluates the self according to these standards, and holds the self responsible for outcomes where appropriate.

*Investment in discomfort*: Views discomfort as a necessary investment in personal progress.

*Delay of gratification*: Is willing to delay personal gratification in order to achieve rewards later—in other words, is willing to "save" for future.

This model of personal empowerment is shown in Figure 2.1.

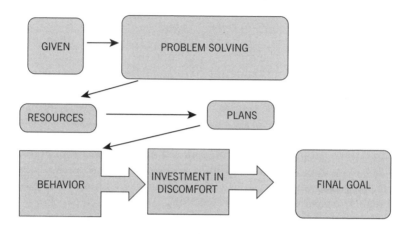

**FIGURE 2.1.** Empowerment and emotion.

## SUMMARY

Emotional schema therapy is not a therapy about feeling good, being happy, or having the ideal life. It recognizes that a complete life carries with it a range of emotional possibilities—some that may be happy, some that may be sad, and some that may simply feel awful. There is no attachment without loss, no meaning without the possibility of disillusionment, no striving without frustration. Emotional schema therapy emphasizes the wisdom of the adage "You need to go through it to get past it." It encourages each patient to view him- or herself as "someone who does the hard things" rather than "someone who looks for the easy way out." The emotional schema model includes concepts such as "constructive discomfort," "successful imperfection," "mental toughness," "keeping your values in front of you," and "witnessing the tragedy" as components of resilience and living a complete life.

If humans could cope only with stress-free environments, there would be no humans alive today. Our ancestors witnessed death on a daily basis, struggled for food, were attacked by predators, and were raped and murdered by neighbors. Resilience must have been a common trait, or early humans would have lain down and died. They did not. They did the hard things, and they survived. This is the message of emotional schema therapy—that life's difficulties are hard to endure, they hurt, they lead to disillusion, and they lead to a full range of emotions. Recognizing that this is part of a meaningful life helps one normalize, validate, and accept the cost of living.

# CHAPTER 3

# A Model of Emotional Schemas

The best and most beautiful things in the world cannot be seen or even touched. They must be felt with the heart.
—HELEN KELLER

This chapter describes how theories of emotion can be augmented by a social-cognitive model of emotions. After briefly reviewing other theories of emotion, I examine the specific dimensions of emotion conceptualization and strategies of emotion regulation, as well as their relationship to psychopathology.

## THE EMOTIONAL SCHEMA MODEL
## VERSUS OTHER THEORIES OF EMOTION

Gross (1998, 2002) has proposed that emotion regulation can occur at several points in a sequence of events. He distinguishes between "antecedent-focused" and "response-focused" emotion regulation strategies—that is, strategies focused on coping with the problem before versus after the emotion has been evoked. Initially, individuals may choose to select situations that are less troublesome—that is, to avoid triggers for problematic emotions. For example, a man going through a breakup may avoid places where he and his ex-partner have gone before. Although avoidance may decrease anxiety or stress, relying on avoidance also decreases the opportunity for rewards or for coping effectively with obstacles. Or people can choose to modify the situation through problem solving or behavioral activation, such as pursuing other rewarding behavior or, in the case of the breakup, dating new people. Indeed, problem solving is a frequently used coping strategy (Aldao & Nolen-Hoeksema, 2010, 2012a, 2012b), but not all stressful situations are amendable to modification or problem solving. Thus unwanted emotions may still arise.

Once these emotions have arisen, individuals can choose to distract themselves from the stimuli that may cause them difficulty. However, distraction is not a generally effective strategy for coping with life's difficulties. Or they can use cognitive restructuring to reappraise the situation. In the breakup example, the man can reassess the advantages of the breakup, evaluate the ex-partner more negatively, or view other alternatives more favorably. Cognitive restructuring is the hallmark of cognitive therapy, and there is considerable evidence that it is effective, although even with rational restructuring difficult emotions may still arise. Finally, individuals can modulate or attempt to control their emotional responses—for example, through suppression. For example, the man undergoing the breakup can suppress his emotions by misusing substances or by trying to "stop feeling so bad." Gross and John (2003) did find that reappraisal was more effective than suppression of emotion; suppression actually led to increased sympathetic nervous system activity.

The stress–appraisal model advanced by Lazarus proposes that individuals experience stress as a result of their evaluations of the external pressures (or stressors) that they confront (Lazarus, 1999; Lazarus & Folkman, 1984). These appraisals of the ability to cope suggest that there is a cognitive component to stress, but the emphasis in Lazarus's model is on *external* sources of difficulty. The emotional schema model proposes that individuals may differ in their evaluations of their own stress experience. For example, they may appraise their stress (anxiety, frustration) along various dimensions, such as duration, comprehensibility, and control. These evaluations—which are emotional schemas or concepts of emotions—may feed back into the stress response, either increasing or decreasing the experience of stress. For example, if I believe that my frustration in coping with a difficult situation is short-lasting, is understandable, and is within my control, I will not become more anxious. In contrast, if I believe that my frustration will go on for weeks, is incomprehensible, and will spiral out of control, then I will experience additional stress. Indeed, I may become even more stressed about this additional stress, setting off a cascade of stressful experiences and evaluations (see Figure 3.1).

The emotional schemas in this model are different from the emotional schemas described by Greenberg and his colleagues in his model of emotion-focused therapy (e.g., Greenberg & Safran, 1987, 1989, 1990). In the Greenberg model, emotions carry in them the cognitive content that may be of value; that is, emotions are activated and tell us something about

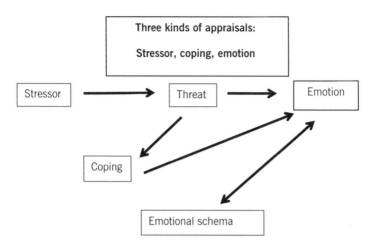

**FIGURE 3.1.** Appraisals of stressor, coping, and emotion.

the meaning of experiences. For example, the emotion of sadness may "contain" the thought "I will always be alone." The emotional schema model draws on the valuable ideas of the Greenberg model, but defines the "schemas" as the concepts, evaluations, and strategies that individuals employ *about* their emotions. While recognizing that inducing an emotion will often activate the thoughts associated with that emotion (which is also consistent with Beck's model), the emotional schema model takes an additional step to inquire what an individual's beliefs are about an emotion itself. The emotional schema model is a social-cognitive model in which emotions are the *objects* of thought, not only the *sources* of thoughts and images. Thus we can inquire what an individual believes will be the duration, controllability, and comprehensibility of an emotion. It is these conceptualizations about emotion that are of particular interest in emotional schema therapy.

Gottman and colleagues' emotion-focused approach identifies meta-emotion "philosophies" that parents may have about their children's emotions (Gottman, Katz, & Hooven, 1996). The most positive such philosophy is that of "emotion coaching," which has five components: awareness of even low-intensity emotion in self and other; viewing a child's negative emotion as an opportunity to get closer and to matter to the child; validation of the child's feelings; assisting in labeling emotion; and problem solving and setting goals with the child (Gottman et al., 1996). Gottman has identified other problematic responses to a child's emotion, such as "dismissive," "contemptuous/critical," and "overwhelmed." The dismissive parent minimizes the child's emotion ("Don't worry. It's no big deal"); the contemptuous or critical parent labels the child as ridiculous or immature ("Stop acting like a baby"); and the overwhelmed parent responds by pointing out his or her own difficulties with emotion ("I can't handle this. I have too many problems of my own"). Research on emotion coaching indicates that it facilitates physiological processes and emotion regulation in the child. A number of studies indicate that parents' beliefs about emotion have a significant effect on childrearing strategies and on outcomes for children (Dunsmore & Halberstadt, 1997; Eisenberg, Cumberland, & Spinrad, 1998; Halberstadt et al., 2013; McGillicuddy-De Lisi & Sigel, 1995). Halberstadt and colleagues (2013) have developed a questionnaire (Parents' Beliefs about Children's Emotions) that consists of seven subscales: Costs of Positivity, Value of Anger, Manipulation, Control, Parent Knowledge, Autonomy, and Stability. These beliefs have been found to be directly related to parental socialization practices. The emotional schema model draws on Gottman's model of meta-emotion philosophies, expanding this model to specific dimensions of explanation, evaluation, and interpretation, and strategies of beliefs about emotion and emotion regulation.

The emotional schema model also draws on "attribution theories"— that is, theories about the causes of events and the stability of emotions (Alloy et al., 1988; Jones & Davis, 1965; Kelley, 1973; Weiner, 1986). Thus several dimensions of interest are whether individuals believe that their emotions are distinctive to them (i.e., exhibit lack of consensus), are caused externally, are invariable (are consistent across situations—i.e., stable traits), or are within effortful control. Other dimensions of evaluations include whether an emotion "makes sense" (i.e., is comprehensible), is dangerous or impairing, is of long duration, or is shameful. In addition, individuals have beliefs about the value of expressions of emotions and whether others will validate them (or dismiss or humiliate them). Some people believe that emotions are a waste of time and that they should be rational all the time—that emotions "get in the way." Others believe that they cannot tolerate mixed feelings and should figure out how they "really feel."

The emotional schema model recognizes that emotions have evolved because they were adaptive throughout the history of the species, providing individuals with threat detection, rapid and intuitive responses, and "modules" for solving problems. For instance, agoraphobia, accompanied by intense anxiety and the tendency to collapse, avoid or escape, is an adaptive module to protect against attacks by predators in spaces where one is vulnerable (open spaces, or closed spaces where exit is blocked). Similarly, the most common fears—of water, dogs, lightning, heights, and spiders— are also adaptive, since they protect against mortal threats. The emotional schema model seeks to normalize a wide range of emotions (including anxiety, sadness, anger, jealousy, envy, and shame) as emotions that have evolved and are automatically activated once a relevant stimulus or situation has emerged for an individual. As described in Chapter 2, this evolutionary model of emotions helps normalize—even universalize—emotions and helps make sense of them, thereby validating individuals' emotional experience, making emotions comprehensible, and reducing guilt and shame over emotions.

Evolutionary or biological models of emotion are sometimes contrasted with social-constructive models of emotion: It is argued that emotions are either biologically determined or cognitively and culturally constructed. The emotional schema model recognizes the value of both approaches. It views the biological predisposition and universality of emotion as information related to the comprehensibility and normality of emotion; it thus addresses the cognitive issues of making sense of, and giving legitimacy to, one's emotions. For example, envy (an often disparaged emotion) is linked in the emotional schema model to biological universals of dominance hierarchy, competition for status and resources, and the insistence on fair distribution. The model also relates the emotion of envy to social constructions that arbitrarily disparage it as a "shameful" emotion. Thus one may have social constructions about biologically predisposed emotions and their elicitors.

Furthermore, many individuals endorse a model of "emotional perfectionism." That is, they believe that their emotions should be clear, under total control, comfortable, "good," and completely comprehensible. This emotional perfectionism is related to a particular theory-of-mind model that I refer to as "pure mind." Individuals endorsing a belief in pure mind believe that they should not have unwanted, intrusive thoughts; "antisocial" feelings; fantasies that seem "impure" or "immoral," or conflicting and confusing sensations, thoughts, or emotions. The emotional schema model proposes that emotions are often chaotic cascades of confusing noise and unpredictable experience, much like a twirling kaleidoscope of perception and sensation, and that attempts to have a pure mind will only lead to failure to suppress and control the unpredictable. Pure mind is often an underlying assumption behind the intolerance of mixed feelings ("Yes, but I don't know how I really feel"), guilt and shame about thoughts and images ("What's wrong with me that I have these feelings?"), and the belief that one's emotions are incomprehensible ("I can't figure out what's wrong with me").

Related to the illusion of pure mind is "existential perfectionism"—that is, the belief that one's life must follow an ideal course, that one should find out "what I should be doing." The underlying assumptions are that there is a given "path" for one to follow, that love and work should be ideal, that conflicts in relationships are always bad, and that choices should provide unambiguous direction. Existential perfectionism is an enduring philosophy about what one's life experience should be. For example, a man faced with a set of somewhat desirable alternatives had great difficulty because he believed that he should find his "true passion," that he should figure out what he "should be doing," and that he should not have to make tradeoffs. He believed that conflicts with his partner meant that the relationship was doomed—as opposed to thinking that conflicts are part of the relationship. He believed that ambivalence is always a bad sign, rather than thinking that ambivalence is often inevitable. Later chapters of this book will show how existential perfectionism, emotional perfectionism, and pure mind contribute to problematic beliefs about specific emotions and lead to unhelpful strategies of emotion regulation.

## EXAMPLES ILLUSTRATING THE MODEL IN ACTION

Consider the following hypothetical situation. John is told that he is being laid off from his job, after less than 1 year. The company is downsizing, but his recent review was mixed and he has not been satisfied with his job for quite some time. John notices a number of physical sensations (rapid breathing, higher pulse rate, a pit in his stomach). He believes that getting fired has triggered a strong emotional response, but he is not quite sure which emotions he is feeling. He feels agitated, as if he wants to throw something or hit something. He wants to contact his now-former boss, but he believes that this would be humiliating, and he realizes he doesn't quite know what to say. He would like to call his friend, Ed, but he feels ashamed and confused and thinks that he would be burdening Ed with his concerns. He notices a number of thoughts that he is having: "I can't believe that I got fired," and "I can't believe that they'd do this without an explanation." He also thinks, "My boss was a narcissist—nothing was ever good enough for her," and "I am better off without this job." But then he notices other thoughts: "I will be out of work and miserable," and "Nothing works out for me." He begins to think, "I am feeling angry, anxious, and sad. I am also feeling confused. And, for some reason, I also feel relieved." These various emotions appear to John to conflict with one another, since he holds to the belief that he should only have one feeling: "I can't figure out how I really feel." So he begins to brood and dwell on his emotions, trying to figure out how he "really feels." He begins to feel ashamed about his anxiety, thinking that being anxious and sad is a sign that he is weak. So he is less inclined to want to discuss this with Ed or his other friends.

John examines his feelings of anxiety and thinks, "I guess I am feeling anxious because I don't know what is going to happen next." But then he wonders if he is feeling anxious because he had too much coffee: "Maybe it's the caffeine." He wonders whether these anxious feelings are caused by these "external events" or by "something about me." He is not sure why he is feeling anxious, sad, angry, confused, and a little relieved: "It doesn't make sense. How can I have so many different feelings? I should feel one way. This is confusing." He begins to ruminate, brooding on his emotions, still trying to figure out how he "really" feels: "Am I relieved to be out of work because I am lazy? Did I *want* to get fired?"

He wonders whether his anxiety is going to last indefinitely. He thinks, "I can't go on each day with this level of anxiety. I won't be able to function." He thinks that his anxiety will prevent him from sleeping, digesting his food, getting his work done, or concentrating on what he has to do. The ideas of danger begin to flood his imagination as he begins to think of going insane, being dragged off in a straitjacket.

John thinks now that he has to get these emotions under control. But he starts weeping. Trying to hold back the tears, he feels even more tense, more afraid, and more out of control. "I can't let this get to me," he says, and then lights himself a joint and says, "This will calm me down." He thinks, "I've got to calm down. I've got to get a handle on things right now, or I will unravel. And who knows what that will lead to?"

As he begins to worry about his anxiety and sadness, he thinks that these feelings could last forever. He fails to realize that many other events can transpire. Perhaps he will wake up tomorrow and be happy not to have to go to work, happy not to have to deal with the drudgery of a dead-end, monotonous job with a critical boss. He doesn't think that he might be relieved to have dinner with Ed or another friend. He fails to recognize that other experiences will have an impact on his feelings. He fails to recall that other unhappy feelings have dissipated with time and experience—that emotions are fleeting, changing, evaporating, constantly coming and going. He focuses on one feeling at one moment and on one detail: getting fired. He has difficulty stepping back and recognizing that many other feelings, other moments, and other communications with other people will eventually eclipse this entire experience. Focused on his emotion right at this moment, he has difficulty anticipating that this too will pass. He begins to panic, feeling a sense of urgency that he has to feel better and get rid of this terrible anxiety immediately. He sees the world through the negative schemas of his anxious feelings—schemas that anchor him to the present moment and prevent him from seeing any possibility for a future.

As this fictional story reveals, poor John has a wide range of negative beliefs, or schemas, about emotions. His emotions do not make sense to him; he does not feel he can express them openly or get validation; he ruminates on his feelings; he feels ashamed; he cannot tolerate his mixed feelings; and he believes that his feelings will go out of control and last indefinitely. John is a good example of how negative evaluations of emotions can lead to problematic coping strategies. Figure 3.2 provides a diagram of the emotional schema model. (In Chapter 5, I discuss how this diagram can be used in socializing a patient to the model.)

Let us examine Figure 3.2, using John as an example. First, he starts with a wide range of emotions—anger, anxiety, sadness, and a feeling of relief. He then notices the emotions and, to some extent, labels them. He then views the emotions as problematic: He believes that it does not make sense to feel some emotions (such as relief); he feels ashamed of his anxiety and sadness; he believes that his emotions will go out of control and last

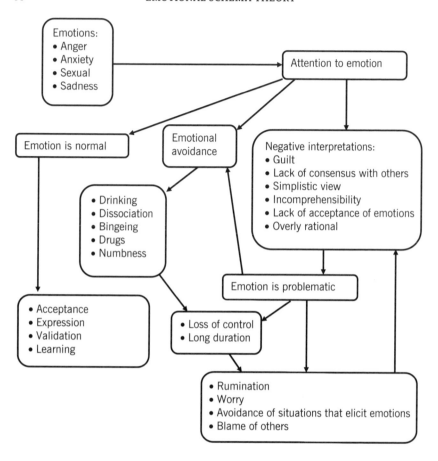

**FIGURE 3.2.** A model of emotional schemas.

indefinitely; and he does not normalize this range of emotions and recognize that a lot of people would have similar feelings. He is intolerant of his mixed feelings, ruminating on why he feels the way he feels, and attempting to identify what he "really feels." With the negative interpretations of his emotions, he attempts to suppress the emotions by smoking marijuana; he avoids people because he is ashamed and believes he is a burden; he blames his former boss and blames himself; he ruminates about what happened in order to "figure it out"; and he worries about the future. John exemplifies the problematic style of responding emotionally to a major life event.

Similarly, imagine Mary, who notices that she is feeling "uncomfortable." It may be that she has a difficult time identifying what the emotion is; at first she only recognizes physiological sensations, such as her fingers tingling, her heart beating rapidly, and her head feeling dizzy. As she reflects on these sensations and what has just happened, she may recognize that she is currently experiencing sadness. The first step in a problematic sequence of emotional schemas is that Mary's sadness is confusing to her; she does not understand what could be making her feel so sad. She engages in negative evaluations of her sadness: "I shouldn't feel sad," "I have no right to be sad," "No one else would feel sad in this situation," and "No one would understand me." She then begins to feel helpless about her sadness, since she cannot point to a reason for it. She then thinks that her sadness will go on indefinitely, it will overwhelm her, she won't be able to function, and she will lose control. She tries to tell herself not to feel sad; she gets angry with herself for feeling sad; and this makes her feel more hopeless and more anxious about her sadness. She then decides that it would be best to avoid other behaviors that she has usually found rewarding, since she is sad and does not have any energy. She worries about being a burden to others, and she thinks that because she feels sad, nothing can help her feel better: "If I feel sad now, then I'll feel sad with my friends." She isolates herself and begins to ruminate about her sadness, which then leads to more sadness. This vicious cycle of emotion–evaluation–problematic coping–emotion (see Figure 3.3) is a common consequence of failed emotion regulation strategies that arise from problematic theories about one's own emotions.

Contrast this scenario for Mary with one illustrating a more adaptive model of emotional schemas and more helpful strategies for coping with sadness. This model is shown in Figure 3.4. In this model, Mary feels the sadness and is able to label the emotion as "sadness." In addition, she is able to normalize it because it makes sense to her; she is able to achieve validation from a friend; and she is able to recognize that her sadness is not

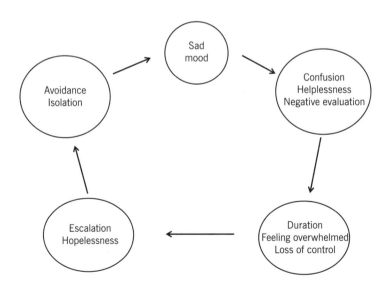

**FIGURE 3.3.** Cycle of emotion and negative emotional schemas for sadness.

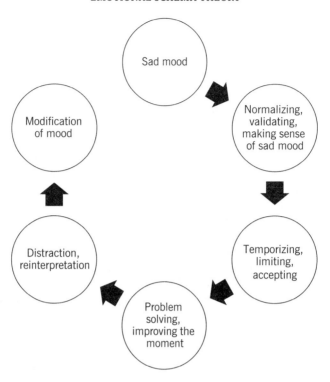

**FIGURE 3.4.** Cycle of coping with sadness, using the adaptive model of emotional schemas.

an unusual response (others would feel the same way). She then believes that her sadness is temporary, has its limits, and will not escalate, and she is able to accept feeling sad for a while. There is no urgency to suppress the sadness or get rid of it. She is not panicking about her sadness. She then activates several emotion regulation strategies that have a good chance of being helpful. She tries to figure out if there is a problem to solve; she considers reinterpreting the situation ("It's not a catastrophe"); she is able to distract herself with other activities; and she is able to improve the moment. As a result of these more adaptive emotional schemas and emotion regulation strategies, her mood improves.

The emotional schema model draws on the view that an emotion follows a sequence of movements, beginning with the appearance of an event, followed by an emotional experience (a perturbation, arousal, or—as Plato observed—a "fluttering of the soul") (Sorabji, 2000). This can then be followed by an evaluation of "what is going on," a consideration of one's relevant goals or values, an examination of alternative actions or interpretations, and a decision to take action. In addition, the *awareness* of an emotion can follow a sequence of movements: The individual recognizes the emotion, interprets the emotion, considers values and goals, and considers alternatives to down-regulate or up-regulate the emotion. For example, consider an alternative version of John's experience of losing his job. He notices that he is feeling angry, sad, anxious, and a bit relieved. He considers what is going on—that the loss of his job has occurred. He identifies his goals—to get a good job, but also to enjoy his life while he is out of work. He considers interpretations ("Whose fault was it?", "Will I be unemployed forever?", "Are there other, better jobs to pursue?", "How should I spend my time?"). He then chooses to spend time with his good friends, give himself time to heal, and keep himself busy, while evaluating the kinds of choices he can make in the future. Similarly, the movements in response to the emotion can include recognizing the arousal and the emotions; normalizing, validating, and acknowledging the duration, comprehensibility, and nature of mixed feelings; identifying his goals and values for meaningful work; taking personal responsibility for his life; acquiring new skills and the enjoyment of life; and activating plans and behaviors that will provide pleasurable and meaningful experiences. The model of movements proposes that we can ask the following: "When an emotion arises, what do you think of or do next?" The emotional schema model proposes that there are two parallel movement patterns: one that focuses on thoughts and actions related to values and goals, and the other that focuses on interpretation, processing, and the use of emotion—also as related to values and goals. A person can move from an emotion to action to values. Thus, for example, a clinician can ask a patient about the emotion of resentment: "Yes, it might make sense that you are feeling resentful at the present moment, but how long do you want to stay with this resentment? Where do you want to go, and what values do you want to pursue?" Emotion is one step—one movement—in this sequence.

## SPECIFIC DIMENSIONS OF EMOTIONAL SCHEMAS

There are 14 dimensions of conceptualization and evaluation of an emotion, and of response to it, in the emotional schema model. I briefly review each dimension here; in later chapters, I discuss how these dimensions are evaluated and the techniques that can be used to address them.

### Duration

How long do emotions last? Some individuals believe that the emotions they experience will last a long time—possibly indefinitely. In clinical practice, my colleagues and I often hear patients with such beliefs say things like "I sometimes fear that if I allowed myself to have a strong feeling, it would not go away." Individuals who believe in long duration of emotions do not view emotions as temporary or situational. In some cases, emotional experiences may be viewed as "traits" (e.g., "I am a sad person"). Rather than viewing emotional experiences as passing phenomena, this dimension leads one to believe that painful emotions may endure and lead to continued suffering.

## Control

Some patients believe that their emotions are out of control and need to be controlled: "If I let myself have some of these feelings, I fear I will lose control," "I worry that I won't be able to control my feelings," and "I worry that if I have certain feelings, I might go crazy." Beliefs in loss of control can be frightening to some people, leading them to believe that they may need to do almost anything to exercise control.

## Comprehensibility

Individuals often believe that their emotions do not make sense. They are confused about their feelings. For example, these individuals may say, "There are things about myself that I just don't understand," "My feelings don't make sense to me," "I think that my feelings are strange or weird," or "My feelings seem to come out of nowhere." The difficulty in making sense of emotion leaves these individuals feeling confused about their experience and feeling helpless about what to do.

## Consensus

Some individuals believe that their emotions are unique to them, resulting in a belief that they are abnormal or even defective. These individuals believe, "I often think that I respond with feelings that others would not have," "I am much more sensitive than other people," or "Others do not have the feelings that I have." Or they may ask, "Do others have the same emotional reactions or experiences I have, or is there something unique or different about my emotions?" Normalizing such individuals' feelings and experiences is an important component of the cognitive treatment of anxiety, PTSD, and OCD. For example, helping a patient with OCD recognize that many people will have similar fantasies or feelings decreases negative labeling of obsessions (Salkovskis & Kirk, 1997). In the emotional schema model, recognizing that others have similar feelings is a form of validation—a process that should reduce depression and anxiety.

## Guilt and Shame

To what degree does one feel shame, guilt, or embarrassment about an emotion? This dimension alludes to the belief that one should not have certain feelings. This is reflected by such comments as "Some feelings are wrong to have," or "I feel ashamed of my feelings." Individuals who feel guilty or ashamed may be inclined to criticize themselves for their emotions, hide their emotions from others, and feel anxious or sad about the emotions that they do have.

## Rationality

Individuals who emphasize rationality rather than emotional experience believe that being logical or rational is a superior way of functioning. They may believe that their emotions must be eliminated or controlled, so that they do not deter them from rational and effective problem solving or functioning. Examples of emphasis on rationality include "I should be rational and logical in everything," and "You can't rely on your feelings to tell you what is good for you."

## Simplistic View of Emotion

Some individuals believe that they should only feel one way about things; they have difficulty with mixed feelings. In some cases, this takes the form of dichotomous thinking about the self ("I am entirely bad") or others ("He is entirely bad"). Differentiated, balanced, and complex views of the self and others include awareness that the same person may have different and conflicting qualities, depending on the situation or time. Thus the self and others are variable. More differentiated thinking allows individuals the opportunity to coordinate apparently conflicting feelings, which are inevitable at times. Examples of simplistic views of self and others include the following: "I can't stand it when I have contradictory feelings—like liking and disliking the same person," "When I have conflicting feelings about someone, I get upset or confused," and "I like being absolutely definite about the way I feel about *myself*." A simplistic view of emotion reflects a dichotomous, all-or-nothing view of experience.

## Values

Individuals who emphasize values believe that their emotions are natural consequences of the values that direct their lives. Thus their goal may not necessarily be "feeling good," but rather "having a meaningful life." The emphasis on values may be derived from an existential cognitive model of emotional processing. Such individuals may believe that anxiety, depression, or anger can help them clarify what "really matters," thereby allowing emotional processing to occur. Emotional schema therapy proposes that values help organize the meaning of action and experience to help individuals clarify what "really matters" to them, so as to give depth and substance to the inevitable difficulties of life. Statements that reflect values include

"There are higher values that I aspire to," and "When I feel down or sad, I question my values."

## Expression

Individuals who believe that they can express their emotions are willing to let their emotions out with others and communicate the range of feelings that they have. The willingness to express feelings reflects an acceptance that emotions are important and can possibly enhance change or understanding. Of course, simply expressing emotions may not reflect a belief that one's style of expression is useful—only that one is willing and able to express emotions. The following items reflect expression of emotion: "I believe it is important to let myself cry in order to get my feelings out," and "I feel I can express my feelings openly."

## Validation

Some people believe that there is a receptive audience for their emotions; that is, others accept, understand, value, and show empathy for them. As I discuss in Chapter 6, validation affects a number of other emotional schema dimensions. Validation normalizes emotion, reduces guilt and shame, helps differentiate emotion, helps the individual realize that the experience of emotion can be accepted and tolerated, and shows that emotions make sense. Examples of varying degrees of belief in (or expectation of) validation include the following: "Others understand and accept my feelings," "I don't want anyone to know about some of my feelings," and "No one really cares about my feelings."

## Acceptance

Some individuals allow themselves to have their feelings; they expend little energy trying to inhibit them. Acceptance is simply the realization that what is, *is*. It allows one to experience the world, including emotions, as a given part of reality. "Ideal acceptance" is without judgment, control, or fear, and marks the starting point from which one can either take action or not take action. Acceptance is like "letting it in" or "letting it be." Examples of comments indicating varying degrees of acceptance are "I accept my feelings," and "I don't want to admit to having certain feelings—but I know that I have them."

## Blame

A common response some individuals have to their negative emotions is to blame other people for their feelings. They may feel provoked, unfairly treated, exploited, ignored, abused, or simply misunderstood—but in each case the "reason" they feel the way they feel is that someone else *caused them to have these feelings*. Items reflecting blame include "If other people changed, I would feel a lot better," and "Other people cause me to have unpleasant feelings."

## Numbness

Some individuals have difficulty experiencing emotions; they often claim that they feel numb, feel nothing, or feel detached from reality. The emotional schema model views numbing as a consequence of emotional avoidance that inhibits any emotional processing of experience. Without access to the direct experience of emotion, these individuals cannot learn that emotions can be tolerated, that emotions do not overwhelm or incapacitate, and that emotions do not last forever. Patients experiencing numbing often say things like "I often feel numb emotionally—like I have no feelings."

## Rumination

Individuals sometimes get "stuck" on an emotion—dwelling on the fact that they are having an unpleasant feeling, asking themselves unanswerable questions (e.g., "What is wrong with me?"), and repeatedly refocusing on their negative experience. Rumination can be viewed as a problematic coping style for unwanted thoughts and emotions. People who ruminate often believe that they cannot let go of an emotion or thought, that they have to figure things out, and that they cannot accept that a thought is simply a thought and an emotion is temporary (Wells, 1995). The emotional schema model argues that rumination is a problematic strategy for coping with unpleasant or unwanted emotion, since it leads an individual to get stuck on an emotional experience or memory, further evoking the negativity of the emotion, and removing one from productive functioning. Examples of comments from ruminating patients include "When I feel down, I sit by myself and think a lot about how bad I feel," "I often say to myself, 'What's wrong with me?'", and "I focus a lot on my feelings or my physical sensations."

## The Dimensions in Relationship to Other Cognitive-Behavioral Models

Many of the foregoing dimensions are relevant to the concerns of other therapeutic models. For example, overemphasis on rationality and logic—or "antiemotionality"—is viewed as problematic by the catharsis and emotion-focused models, but does not have a clear implication for a cognitive model. The emotion-focused model suggests that overrationality may inhibit the expression, validation, acceptance, and self-understanding that follow from allowing emotional experiences. The ACT model (Hayes et al., 2012) views overemphasis on rationality as a form of experiential avoidance—placing language and logic as barriers to the richness and meaning of direct experience. The ability to understand that one can have conflicting and complicated feelings is a sign of higher-level ego functioning, cognitive differentiation, and cognitive complexity in the ego development model (Loevinger, 1976), and is also part of the dialectics of thinking that is a central component of DBT (Linehan, 1993, 2015). Similarly, ACT has proposed that clarification of one's values is an essential component in therapy, especially since valued action may provide the motivation and justification to the individual for difficult emotional experiences. The emphasis is on a purposeful life or a life worth living—a view that has been advanced in DBT as well.

The emphasis on expression of emotion has a long history, going back to the catharsis model advanced by Freud. However, individuals differ considerably in this respect. A cognitive model does not emphasize expression per se as a factor in reducing depression or anxiety, whereas the catharsis and emotion-focused models stress the importance of expression in reducing negative affect and, in the case of emotion-focused theory, increasing comprehension and acceptance. Pennebaker and his colleagues have argued that expressive writing can have significant positive effects on emotion and well-being (e.g., Pennebaker & Chung, 2011). Joiner's interpersonal theory suggests that problematic styles of expression may alienate other people, especially expression of negative affect followed by rejecting advice (e.g., Joiner, Brown, & Kistner, 2006).

ACT stresses the role of acceptance and psychological flexibility in a wide range of psychopathology (Blackledge & Hayes, 2001; Hayes, 2002, 2004; Hayes et al., 2006, 2012), and DBT proposes that radical acceptance is the starting point in many cases for effective change (Linehan, 1993, 2015). Research on crying indicates that people who try to inhibit their crying experience distress (Labott & Teleha, 1996). Similarly, research findings on the ironic effects of thought suppression—that is, attempts to suppress unwanted thoughts and feelings lead to later increases in those experiences—suggest that acceptance of feelings should decrease depression and anxiety (Purdon & Clark, 1994; Wegner & Zanakos, 1994). Emotion-focused and catharsis theories also predict that acceptance of feelings leads to quicker resolution of depression and anxiety.

The emotional schema model views blame as a problematic style of coping with negative emotion, since it takes the responsibility of the emotion and displaces it to someone else over whom one has no control. Thus, blaming others for an emotion would be viewed as rendering oneself helpless in dealing with the emotion. Furthermore, blaming others for emotion can easily lead to other negative schemas, such as rumination, viewing one's emotions as having a long duration, and not feeling understood or validated by others. The emotion-focused model does not suggest that blaming others will be a useful antidote to depression or anxiety, but the catharsis model views blame as a displacement or projection of negative feelings about the self, thereby leading to the prediction of an inverse relationship between depression or anxiety and blame. The cognitive models do not endorse the catharsis model; rather, from the perspective of the cognitive models, one could argue that blaming others is a form of "judgment" focus (in which negative judgments can be applied to both self and others).

Numbness may be the extreme experience of lack of acceptance or "experiential avoidance" of emotion (Hayes et al., 2012). A repressive coping style, sometimes characterized by alexithymia, has been related to dysphoria, eating disorders, and somatization (Taylor, Bagby, & Parker, 1991; Weinberger, 1995). The emotion-focused therapy approach stresses the importance of evoking emotions in order to access an individual's meanings, needs, and problematic coping strategies (Greenberg & Watson, 2005). DBT also recognizes that emotional numbing is the opposite of radical acceptance and is often another form of problematic avoidance. Behavioral models of fear and anxiety argue that activating the "fear schema" is an essential component of modifying fear (e.g., Foa & Kozak, 1986).

Nolen-Hoeksema (2000) and Papageorgiou and Wells (2001a) have shown that rumination is related to greater depression and anxiety, with ruminators often believing that their rumination prepares them for the worst and helps them find a solution to their problems. ACT views rumination as a form of inflexibility and experiential avoidance that leads individuals to get "stuck in their heads" (Hayes et al., 2004, 2012; Hayes, Wilson, Gifford, Follette, & Strosahl, 1996).

As noted both above and in further elaboration of the model, the emotional schema model addresses many of the issues that have been key elements of other theories. For example, experiential or emotional avoidance is a feature of ACT; values are also a major component of ACT; validation is a major element of DBT; and metacognitive awareness of worry bears a resemblance to the beliefs about the nature of emotion. However, the emotional schema model differs from the foregoing models in that it is a social cognitive model about an individual's theory of emotion and emotion regulation; that is, it attempts to outline the content of thinking, the beliefs and assumptions, the schemas and modes that characterize a person's interpretation of emotion and beliefs about its regulation. Indeed, the emotional schema model has some similarity to the general schema model that Beck and his colleagues have advanced, but in this proposed model the schemas are about the nature of emotion. Moreover, the emotional schema model can trace its origins to the model of social-cognitive processes outlined by Heider (1958) in his theory of how individuals explain mental and interpersonal phenomena. As such, the emotional schema model can be viewed as a *social-cognitive* model of emotional experience.

## RESEARCH ON EMOTIONAL SCHEMAS

There is empirical support for the emotional schema model as related to anxiety, depression, and other forms of psychopathology. Of the 14 emotional schema dimensions, 12 are significantly correlated with the Beck Depression Inventory–II (BDI-II) and the Beck Anxiety Inventory (BAI) (Leahy, 2002). In a separate study, a stepwise multiple-regression analysis indicated that guilt/shame, rumination, control, and invalidation were the best predictors of depression on the BDI-II (Leahy, Tirch, & Melwani, 2012). In another study of the relationship among anxiety, psychological flexibility, and emotional schemas, multiple-regression analysis indicated that anxiety was best predicted by beliefs about control, psychological flexibility, and duration (Tirch, Leahy, Silberstein, & Melwani, 2012).

Metacognitive theory proposes that worry is activated and sustained by the "cognitive attentional syndrome," characterized by threat monitoring and problematic mental control strategies (Wells, 2005a, 2005b, 2005c, 2009). Worriers believe that worry prepares them for and prevents negative outcomes; that there must be a continual focus on mental content (cognitive consciousness); and that worry is out of control and must be suppressed. Thus the worriers are locked in a dilemma of positive and negative beliefs about worry. An alternative model of worry is the emotion avoidance theory advanced by Borkovec and colleagues, in which worry as a cognitive strategy temporarily suppresses or avoids the experience of anxious arousal (Borkovec, 1994; Borkovec, Alcaine, & Behar, 2004; Borkovec, Lyonfields, Wiser, & Deihl, 1993). The emotional schema model provides a bridge between the metacognitive and emotion avoidance models, proposing that negative beliefs about emotion may result in the activation of specific metacognitive strategies of worry. In a study of the relationship between a derived measure of negative beliefs about emotion (summing across Leahy Emotional Schema Scale [LESS] dimensions), each of the metacognitive factors in the Wells Metacognitions Questionnaire–30 (MCQ-30) was significantly correlated with negative beliefs about emotions, adding to the construct validity of the LESS (Leahy, 2011b). These findings on the relationship among the LESS, MCQ-30, and depression suggest that metacognitive factors of worry may partly be activated because of negative beliefs about emotion. The pattern of predictors in a stepwise multiple regression on anxiety (as measured by the BAI) also reflect this integrative meta-emotion–metacognition integrative model. Thus the best predictors of anxiety were beliefs about control of emotion (LESS), uncontrollability and danger of worry (MCQ-30), positive worry (MCQ-30) (negative), cognitive self-consciousness (MCQ-30), beliefs that emotions are incomprehensible (LESS), low emotional expression (LESS), and beliefs that emotions are not validated (LESS).

In a study of satisfaction in intimate relationships, a 14-item questionnaire was developed to assess how a participant views his or her partner's *response* to the participant's emotions (the Relationship Emotional Schema Scale or RESS; Leahy, 2010b). In other words, the measure assesses an individual's perception of the partner's emotional beliefs. Every one of the 14 RESS scores was significantly correlated with marital satisfaction (as measured by the Dyadic Adjustment Scale or DAS) (Leahy, 2012a). Again, the multiple-regression analysis reflected intriguing findings, especially about the importance of validation. The stepwise order of LESS predictors of DAS marital satisfaction was as follows: higher validation, less blame, higher values, less simplistic view of emotion, higher comprehensibility, and greater acceptance of feelings (Leahy, 2011a). These data suggest that validation may modify other emotional schemas, thereby assisting in emotional regulation. This may be why patients who are emotionally overwhelmed seek out validation.

Further support for the importance of validation is reflected in the data on the stepwise predictors of the LESS on the scale for alcohol dependence on the Millon Clinical Multiaxial Inventory-III (MCMI-III). The best LESS predictors of alcohol dependence on the MCMI-III were validation, values, simplistic view of emotion, blame, consensus, and numbness (Leahy, 2010a). These findings suggest that individuals with a history of alcohol dependence believe that their emotions are not validated; their emotions are not related to their values; they have difficulty tolerating mixed feelings; they blame others; they believe that others do not feel the same way as they do; and they often experience emotional numbness. Perhaps such individuals may derive validation, relationship to values, differentiation of complex emotions, reduced blame, and consensus from group meetings such as Alcoholics Anonymous.

An examination of the predictors of higher scores on the borderline personality dimension of the MCMI-III revealed the following predictors: comprehensibility, rumination, validation, numbness, blame, simplistic view of emotion, control, values, and rationality (lower). Thus individuals who scored higher on borderline personality believed that their emotions did not make sense; they ruminated; they experienced less validation; they felt numb; they blamed others for their feelings; they had difficulty tolerating mixed feelings; they believed that their emotions were out of control; they believed that their emotions were not related to their values; and they placed less emphasis on rationality. These data are largely consistent with the DBT model of borderline personality disorder, which suggests that "myths about emotion" constitute a central feature of this disorder, that invalidation is a core vulnerability, and that emotion dysregulation is paramount. Moreover, the emotional schema data provide more specific descriptions of these "myths."

Emotional schemas are differentially related to a wide range of personality disorders. Adult patients completed the LESS and the personality disorder dimensions of the MCMI-III (Leahy, 2011a). Individuals scoring higher on avoidant, dependent, and borderline personality had overly negative views of their emotions, while individuals scoring higher on narcissistic and histrionic personality had overly positive views of their emotions. Unexpectedly, individuals scoring higher on compulsive personality also had positive views of their emotions. The latter finding may reflect the possibility that compulsive individuals do not distinguish between thoughts and emotions on this measure, believing that what they think or feel makes sense to them. Contrast these results with the multiple-regression findings for individuals scoring higher on narcissistic personality: lower guilt/shame, expression, and rumination, and higher values. These data suggest that narcissistic individuals have less guilt about their emotions, believe that they can express their feelings, ruminate less about how they feel, and believe that their emotions are related to their values. Just as narcissistic individuals may idealize their own identities, they also seem to idealize their own emotions.

## THE ROLE OF EMOTIONAL SCHEMAS IN PSYCHOPATHOLOGY

The research described above indicates that emotional schemas are correlated with a wide range of disorders—depression, anxiety, chronic worry, substance dependence, relationship dysfunction, and personality disorders. The emotional schema model proposes that once an emotion is aroused or elicited, the interpretations, reactions, and emotion regulation strategies will determine whether the emotion will be maintained, escalate, or decrease. Of course, correlational analyses cannot definitively answer the question of causal direction, but the large number of significant findings suggests that emotional schemas are an important part of the experience of processing emotion.

Certain emotional schemas appear to be more predictive than others of certain disorders. For example, guilt/shame, rumination, control, and validation were the best predictors of depression on the BDI-II (Leahy, Tirch, & Melwani, 2012). It is not surprising that guilt would predict depression on the BDI-II, since the BDI-II contains a number of items reflecting self-critical and regretful thinking. Consistent with the work of other researchers, rumination was highly correlated with depression, since rumination is often a coping strategy for depression (Nolen-Hoeksema, 1991, 2000; Papageorgiou & Wells, 2004, 2009; Wells & Papageorgiou, 2004). Control was a major predictor of depression, suggesting that individuals who feel helpless about modifying their negative mood are more likely to be depressed. This is consistent with helplessness and hopelessness theories of depression, which suggest that beliefs about effectiveness in producing desirable outcomes and avoiding negative outcomes are significant determinants of the onset and maintenance of depression (Abramson, Metalsky, & Alloy, 1989; Alloy et al., 1988; Panzarella, Alloy, & Whitehouse, 2006). In the Leahy, Tirch, and Melwani (2012) study, negative beliefs about control of emotions were highly correlated with both risk aversion and psychological flexibility, suggesting that individuals are less likely to risk change if they believe that their emotions cannot be regulated, and less likely to respond flexibly in different contexts if they believe that they cannot control their emotions.

The finding that validation is a major predictor of depression supports the view that depression encompasses an interpersonal component of lack of support and connectedness. This is consistent with several theories of depression, including the theory underlying interpersonal psychotherapy (Klerman, Weissman, Rounsaville, & Chevron, 1984), Joiner's interpersonal theory of depression (Joiner et al., 2006; Joiner, Van Orden, Witte, & Rudd, 2009), attachment theory (Bowlby, 1969, 1973, 1980), mentalization theory (Bateman & Fonagy, 2006; Fonagy & Target, 2006), object relations theory (Kohut, 1971/2009, 1977), and the theories behind client-centered therapy (Rogers, 1951; Rogers & American Psychological Association, 1985) and DBT (Linehan, 1993, 2015). But how does validation work? Validation scores on the LESS were significantly correlated with scores on each of the other 13 emotional schemas except rationality (Leahy, unpublished study, 2013). A stepwise multiple-regression analysis indicated that the best predictors of invalidation were blame, higher duration, and lower comprehensibility. Thus patients who felt validated were less likely to blame others, believed that their emotions would not last indefinitely, and believed that their emotions made sense. It is instructive that validation is such a central emotional schema, related to almost all of the other schemas, and so highly predictive of depression, blame, duration, and comprehensibility. In the chapters to follow, I emphasize the importance of validation and self-invalidation in the practice of emotional schema therapy.

Similarly, the multiple regressions of emotional schemas for anxiety (on the BAI) also indicated that control, psychological flexibility, and beliefs about duration were the best predictors of anxiety (Tirch et al., 2012). Anxiety is often experienced as an unraveling or loss of control over the danger of a situation, or over the danger of the emotions that one experiences (Barlow, 2002; D. M. Clark, 1999; Hayes, 2002; Heimberg, Turk, & Mennin, 2004; Hofmann, Alpers, & Pauli, 2009; Mennin, Heimberg, Turk, & Fresco, 2002; Rapee & Heimberg, 1997; Wells, 2009; Wells & Papageorgiou, 2001). For example, panic disorder reflects a belief that one's experience of anxiety will unravel, leading to insanity or medical danger; social anxiety disorder (formerly social phobia) reflects the belief that one will lose control of anxious sensations and be humiliated; and PTSD (which was classified as an anxiety disorder until recently) reflects the belief that an uncontrollable danger is happening now. Moreover, beliefs that control is necessary, since loss of control will lead to further catastrophe, underlies the paradox of most anxiety disorders: that one needs to be in control of sensations and emotions, that one cannot control them, and that further control is therefore necessary. Individuals become more anxious because they believe that loss of control is necessarily dangerous. Indeed, mindfulness and acceptance approaches target these concerns by having patients relinquish attempts to control anxious thoughts, sensations, and emotions, and instead take a nonjudgmental and observing stance toward these phenomenological experiences (Hayes et al., 2006, 2012; Roemer & Orsillo, 2009).

Given the multifaceted contributions of negative beliefs about emotions and specific emotional schemas to a range of presenting psychological problems, the goal of emotional schema therapy is to assess patients' idiosyncratic theories of their own emotions and the emotions of others, and to examine how possible modification of these "naive theories" can affect functioning. Emotional schema therapy utilizes a wide range of techniques and conceptualizations to address patients' negative appraisals of emotion and problematic strategies of regulation (e.g., avoidance, suppression, substance misuse, numbing, escalation, angry retaliation).

## SUMMARY

The emotional schema model is a cognitive model of the appraisal of emotions in self and others. In this model, "schemas" represent interpretations, evaluations, attributions, and other cognitive assessments of emotion, as well as emotion regulation strategies that may prove to be helpful or unhelpful. This model reflects multiple influences: Beck's cognitive theory, Wells's metacognitive theory, Greenberg's emotion-focused theory, models of mindfulness, Gottman's model, ACT, and DBT. However, unlike these other models, the emotional schema model is a *social-cognitive* model of appraisals of emotion (rather than thoughts or behavior). It is a model of the theory of emotion that characterizes how individuals respond when they (or others) experience or express an emotion. Emotional schema therapists assess patients' emotional schemas by using the LESS or its successor, the LESS II (see Chapter 4). Each scale consists of 14 dimensions reflecting beliefs about duration, control, comprehensibility, consensus, guilt/shame, and other evaluations and interpretations, as well as strategies such as acceptance, rumination, and blame. Research on emotional schemas supports the view that these beliefs are related to a wide range of psychopathology, including depression, anxiety, substance misuse, relationship discord, and personality disorders.

# PART II

## BEGINNING TREATMENT

# CHAPTER 4

# Initial Assessment and Interview

All the knowledge I possess everyone else can acquire,
but my heart is all my own.
—JOHANN WOLFGANG VON GOETHE

The first sessions with a patient can provide the therapist with significant information about the specific emotions that are troubling the patient; the patient's beliefs about these emotions; the history of how emotions have been handled in the family of origin; the ways the patient's current relationships with people function emotionally; problematic strategies for dealing with emotion; and past attempts to cope with troubling emotions. In addition to this information, the therapist should note how emotional topics are discussed; what the intonation and the nonverbal nature of this expression are like; how the patient may shift from an emotional topic to an unrelated topic; and whether (and, if so, how) the patient attempts to suppress emotion or, conversely, to escalate an emotion once it is activated. Sometimes implicit beliefs about emotion are reflected in what the patient seeks in therapy: "I want to stop feeling sad," "I can't stand how my wife treats me," or "I understand that this is short-term therapy." Emotional goals that reflect beliefs about emotion and "feeling good" may be desirable, but may also mask intolerance of emotional experience. As with any psychological or psychiatric intake, the therapist will be concerned with determining the nature of psychiatric diagnosis (currently and in the past), and will assess cognitive styles and biases, behavioral deficits and excesses, interpersonal losses and conflicts, personal strengths and skills, and motivation for change (Morrison, 2014).

Emotional schema therapy begins in the first session or, in the case of patients who complete forms before coming into therapy, in the initial assessments with self-report forms. At the American Institute for Cognitive Therapy, we require patients to complete a comprehensive self-report packet that includes general information (e.g., history of therapy, substance use history, current and past medications, presenting complaints), as well as a wide range of self-report questionnaires. Patients complete the following forms:

1. Beck Depression Inventory–II (BDI-II; Beck, Steer, & Brown, 1996)
2. Beck Anxiety Inventory (BAI; Beck & Steer, 1993)
3. Leahy Emotional Schema Scale II (LESS II; Leahy, 2012b)
4. Positive and Negative Affect Schedule (PANAS; Watson, Clark, & Tellegen, 1988)
5. Metacognitions Questionnaire 30 (MCQ-30; Wells & Cartwright-Hatton, 2004)
6. Emotion Regulation Strategies Questionnaire (ERSQ; Aldao & Nolen-Hoeksema, 2012a)
7. Acceptance and Action Questionnaire–II (AAQ-II; Bond et al., 2011)
8. Dyadic Adjustment Scale (DAS; Spanier, 1976)
9. Relationship Emotional Schema Scale (RESS; Leahy, 2010b)
10. Measure of Parental Styles (MOPS; Parker et al., 1997)
11. Experiences in Close Relationships—Revised (ECR-R; Fraley, Waller, & Brennan, 2000)
12. Self-Compassion Scale—Short Form (SCS-SF; Raes, Pommier, Neff, & Van Gucht, 2011)
13. Millon Clinical Multiaxial Inventory–II (MCMI-III; Millon, Millon, Davis, & Grossman, 1994)

The battery of self-report forms is emailed to the patient before the first meeting, so that the clinician can have access to a wide variety of information about psychiatric disorders (including personality disorders), severity of symptoms, relationship satisfaction, emotion regulation strategies, metacognitive factors in worry, attachment issues, socialization experiences, psychological flexibility, and other issues. Of particular interest in emotional schema therapy are problematic emotion regulation strategies, the patient's conceptualization of emotion, the history of emotional socialization, and the effects of these processes on psychological well-being. In this chapter, I first review the specific content of most of these self-report forms, and then describe the goals of an emotional schema interview during initial assessment. Finally, the information gained in the interview is linked to establishing goals in therapy and developing a case conceptualization that can guide treatment.

## SELF-REPORT EVALUATION

Initially, the LESS II—a 28-item questionnaire that measures 14 dimensions of emotional schemas—is given. This questionnaire assesses how the patient thinks and responds when feeling "down." However, additional questionnaires based on the LESS II can be given, depending on the emotion of interest. For example, the LESS–Anxiety and the LESS–Anger cover the same 14 dimensions as the LESS II, but are focused on how the patient thinks about and responds to these particular emotions. Some patients may have problematic schemas about sadness or anxiety, but they may believe that their anger is justified, that it makes sense, and that they are in control. Even though one might interpret this as a sign that they do not have a problematic view of anger, the clinician will want to assess whether such a patient's positive view of their emotion is dysfunctional for interpersonal relationships. This is not uncommon with patients whose anger has interfered with relationships or work; their emotional schemas may be overly positive. As indicated in Chapter 3, our research demonstrates that individuals who score higher on narcissistic and histrionic traits have especially positive views of their emotions. The 14 dimensions of the LESS II are shown in Figure 4.1. (Note that some of these are actually reversed versions of the dimensions as described in Chapter 3.)

Let's look more carefully at each dimension of the LESS II. The first dimension, Invalidation, refers to the belief that others do not understand or care about the individual's emotions. This is a central component of DBT and is a major factor in how people learn that their emotions matter, make sense, and are valued by others. The second dimension, Incomprehensibility, refers to the idea that one's emotions make sense—that emotions are not meaningless or chaotic, or come out of nowhere. Indeed, a central feature of the emotional schema model is psychoeducation of the patient, which helps the individual make sense of his or her panic, depression, social anxiety, or other problems. The third dimension, Guilt and Shame, refers to the belief that one should not have the emotions that one is having—that these are reflective of a character flaw, weakness, or undesirable personal qualities. For instance, an individual may become self-critical for being anxious or depressed, which only exacerbates the problem. The fourth dimension is Simplistic View of Emotion, which refers to intolerance of mixed feelings or of emotional ambivalence. The fifth dimension, Devalued, reflects the belief that one's emotions are not related to one's values. For example, a man who claims that he feels sad because he misses his

*Note:* **R = Reversed score** (1 = 6; 2 = 5; 3 = 4; 4 = 3; 5 = 2; 6 = 1)

**Invalidation** = (Item 06**R** + Item 12) / 2

    Item 6.   Others understand and accept my feelings. **(Reversed score)**

    Item 12.  No one really cares about my feelings.

**Incomprehensibility** = (Item 03 + Item 07) / 2

    Item 3.   There are things about myself that I just don't understand.

    Item 7.   My feelings don't make sense to me.

**Guilt** = (Item 02 + Item 10) / 2

    Item 2.   Some feelings are wrong to have.

    Item 10. I feel ashamed of my feelings.

**Simplistic View of Emotion** = (Item 23 + Item 28) / 2

    Item 23. I like being absolutely definite about the way I feel about someone else.

    Item 28. I like being absolutely definite about the way I feel about myself.

**Devalued** = (Item 14**R** + Item 26**R**) / 2

    Item 14. When I feel down, I try to think of the more important things in life—what I value. **(Reversed score)**

    Item 26. There are higher values that I aspire to. **(Reversed score)**

**Loss of Control** = (Item 05 + Item 17) / 2

    Item 5.   If I let myself have some of these feelings, I fear I will lose control.

    Item 17. I worry that I won't be able to control my feelings.

**Numbness** = (Item 11 + Item 20) / 2

    Item 11. Things that bother other people don't bother me.

    Item 20. I often feel "numb" emotionally—like I have no feelings.

**Overly Rational** = (Item 13 + Item 27) / 2

    Item 13. It is important for me to be reasonable and practical rather than sensitive and open to my feelings.

    Item 27. I think it is important to be rational and logical in almost everything.

**Duration** = (Item 09 + Item 19**R**) / 2

    Item 9.   I sometimes fear that if I allowed myself to have a strong feeling, it would not go away.

    Item 19. Strong feelings only last a short period of time. **(Reversed score)**

*(continued)*

**FIGURE 4.1.** Fourteen dimensions of the Leahy Emotional Schema Scale II (LESS II). From Leahy (2012a). Copyright 2012 by Robert L. Leahy. All rights reserved. (Do not reproduce.)

**Low Consensus** = (Item 01 + Item 25**R**) / 2

    Item 1.   I often think that I respond with feelings that others would not have.

    Item 25.  I think that I have the same feelings that other people have. **(Reversed score)**

**Nonacceptance of Feelings** = (Item 24**R** + Item 18) / 2

    Item 24.  I accept my feelings. **(Reversed score)**

    Item 18.  You have to guard against having certain feelings.

**Rumination** = (Item 22 + Item 16) / 2

    Item 22.  When I feel down, I sit by myself and think a lot about how bad I feel.

    Item 16.  I often say to myself, "What's wrong with me?"

**Low Expression** = (Item 04**R** + Item 15**R**) / 2

    Item 4.   I believe that it is important to let myself cry in order to get my feelings "out." **(Reversed score)**

    Item 15.  I feel that I can express my feelings openly. **(Reversed score)**

**Blame** = (Item 08 + Item 21) / 2

    Item 8.   If other people changed, I would feel a lot better.

    Item 21.  Other people cause me to have unpleasant feelings.

**FIGURE 4.1.** *(continued)*

partner may not accept the emotion of sadness as a necessary component of valuing intimacy and commitment. It is possible that one can tolerate and accept difficult emotions if they are part of a valued life.

The sixth LESS II dimension, Loss of Control, refers to the belief that one's emotions need to be controlled—in some cases, suppressed—and that allowing oneself to feel anxious or sad will lead to unraveling of emotion. The seventh dimension is Numbness, which refers to the belief that one does not experience intense or strong emotions (or any emotion), and that one's emotional experience lacks strength or impact. The eighth dimension is Overly Rational, which reflects the belief that one should be rational, not emotional, and that emotionality is something to be avoided and replaced by rational or logical thinking. The ninth dimension, Duration, reflects the belief that one's emotions will last indefinitely and that they will go on and on in a way that might not be tolerable. For instance, a woman who feels sad may believe that her sadness will continue for a long period or perhaps forever, and this may add to her feelings of hopelessness.

The 10th LESS II dimension, Low Consensus, reflects the belief that other people do not share one's emotions, or that there is something unique or different about one's emotional experiences; as a result, one may feel alone in the world and defective in having these experiences. The 11th dimension is Rumination, which reflects the belief that one must dwell on negative feelings and focus on their meaning or lack of meaning, often in a repetitive and endless fashion. For example, a person who feels sad focuses on the experience of sadness, asking, "What's wrong with me?" or "Why is this happening?" in a repetitive way where no answer to these questions seems sufficient. Nonacceptance of Feelings is the 12th dimension, which reflects the belief that one cannot allow emotions of certain kinds to be experienced and that they need to be avoided or eliminated. The 13th dimension, Low Expression, reflects the belief that one cannot openly express emotions, such as by talking about emotions, sharing them, or nonverbally displaying them (e.g., crying). This is different from the Invalidation dimension, which refers to the belief that others do not understand and care about emotion. One can express emotion but feel invalidated. The 14th dimension is Blame, or the belief that the emotions one is having are due to the action or inaction of other people. For instance, a man may say that his anger is due to the behavior of his wife, rather than reflecting that his anger may also be partly due to the way he views things.

In addition, we utilize a self-report form that assesses how a patient views his or her partner's response to the patient's emotions—the RESS, subtitled "How My Partner Handles My Emotions" for patient use. The RESS is shown in Figure 4.2.

The therapist can also derive other emotional schema scales to "fit" a patient's central emotional concern. For example, the LESS II can be modified to assess schemas about loneliness, envy, jealousy, hopelessness, or any other emotion. The therapist can also assess emotional schemas about urges, such as binge eating, purging, checking, or other compulsive behavior. Although there are no norms for the general population, higher scores on the original LESS are related to depression, anxiety, substance dependence, and personality disorders. The 11 other self-report forms we use are listed above, and descriptions of most of these scales can be found in Appendix 4.1.

Of course, clinicians may decide to use only some (or none) of these forms, but our experience is that this comprehensive initial assessment provides both the patient and clinician with significant information that is relevant to developing a case conceptualization and treatment plan. For example, the LESS II provides information about specific problematic beliefs about emotions, the ERSQ provides information about preferred strategies of emotional regulation; the PANAS indicates the balance or ratio of positive and negative emotions; the AAQ-II provides information about psychological flexibility that may be related to responses to troublesome emotions; the MCQ-30 provides information about beliefs about intrusive thoughts that will be directly relevant to beliefs about problematic emotions; the DAS indicates which areas of the primary intimate relationship are troublesome; the RESS identifies how the patient thinks his or

## HOW MY PARTNER HANDLES MY EMOTIONS

We are interested in how you think your partner responds to you when you have painful and difficult emotions. Use the following scale and place the number that best describes how you view your partner's response to your emotions next to the statement. Complete this questionnaire only if you have a partner.

1 = Very untrue      2 = Somewhat untrue      3 = Slightly untrue
4 = Slightly true      5 = Somewhat true      6 = Very true

1. Comprehensibility  My partner helps me make sense of my emotions. _____

2. Validation  My partner helps me feel understood and cared for when I talk about my feelings. _____

3. Guilt/Shame  My partner criticizes me and tries to make me feel ashamed and guilty about the way I feel. _____

4. Differentiation  My partner helps me understand that it is OK to have mixed feelings. _____

5. Values  My partner relates my painful feelings to important values. _____

6. Control  My partner thinks that I am out of control with my feelings. _____

7. Numbness  My partner seems to be numb and indifferent when I talk about my feelings. _____

8. Rationality  My partner thinks I am irrational a lot of the time. _____

9. Duration  My partner thinks that my painful feelings just go on and on. _____

10. Consensus  My partner helps me realize that many people also feel the way I feel. _____

11. Acceptance  My partner accepts and tolerates my painful feelings and doesn't try to force me to change. _____

12. Rumination  My partner seems to think over and over and seems to dwell on why I feel the way I feel. _____

13. Expression  My partner encourages me to express my feelings and talk about the way I feel. _____

14. Blame  My partner blames me for feeling so upset. _____

Now, look back at these 14 statements, and please answer the following:

What are the three worst ways that your partner responds to you?   ____ ____ ____

What are the three best responses that your partner gives you?   ____ ____ ____

**FIGURE 4.2.** Relationship Emotional Schema Scale (RESS). Copyright 2010 by Robert L. Leahy. All rights reserved. (Do not reproduce.)

her intimate partner responds to the patient's emotion; the MOPS provides information on problematic experiences with parents during childhood; the ECR-R provides information about anxiety and avoidance in intimate relationships; and the MCMI-III provides a wide range of normalized scores for personality disorders and other dimensions of psychopathology. With this comprehensive initial assessment, the clinician will have an excellent start on understanding the patient's specific problem areas, emotion beliefs, socialization experience, and emotion regulation.

## INITIAL INTERVIEW

The initial interview may take two or more sessions, and, preferably, the clinician will have access to all the intake forms. Along with evaluating the presence of mood and anxiety disorders, substance use disorder, personality disorders, and other diagnostic categories, the emotional schema therapist will be particularly interested in which emotions the patient is most concerned with, the ways in which these emotions are currently expressed in the interaction with the therapist, the patient's beliefs about emotion, the current and past history of attempts at emotion regulation, the nature of emotional socialization in the patient's childhood history, and the specific dimensions of emotional schemas the patient exhibits.

## Primary Emotional Concern

Patients often come to therapy focusing on a single emotion—or only a few emotions. For example, a married woman described her primary concern as her anxiety about having panic attacks, and her fear of loss of control and humiliation due to these attacks. In the course of the initial interview, she described her husband in ideal terms—"perfectly understanding" and "wonderful." The initial diagnosis was panic disorder with agoraphobia. However, subsequent sessions with her revealed a considerable amount of anger toward her husband, whom she viewed as dismissive and unavailable. Thus she appeared to want to project a harmonious relationship with her husband, while criticizing her own "weakness" in having panic disorder. Another patient, a married man, initially complained of fear of panic attacks in traveling through tunnels. He only briefly described his conflicts with his wife and two daughters. On further inquiry, the emotion that was influencing him the most was his considerable anger—even contempt— toward his wife and, secondarily, his older daughter; he believed that they were not showing him sufficient respect. The presenting emotion may therefore not be the only important emotion for the patient and therapist to address. When the presenting complaint and the underlying emotional dysregulation issues are incongruent, as in the two examples above, the clinician will be interested in why certain emotions are viewed as of more concern than others. For example, it may be less ego-dystonic for a man who has difficulty controlling his anger to focus on his wife's "illegitimate" concern about his anger than to focus on his anxieties about being "humiliated" or "controlled."

## Expression of Emotion

Patients differ in their expression of emotion in the initial and subsequent sessions. Some patients are openly expressive (crying, showing a sad face, lowering their eyes), whereas others may come across as bland, indifferent, or aloof. In some cases, a patient may nonverbally display emotions that are inconsistent with the content of what is being said. The therapist should observe vocal intonation, facial expression, eye contact, body posture, hesitations in speaking, attempts to keep from crying, changing the subject when discussing difficult topics, gesticulation with the hands, movements of the body, and other nonverbal signs of emotion. Is the content of what is being said congruent with the nonverbal expression that is being observed?

A young woman told the therapist that the reason that she was seeking out cognitive-behavioral therapy was that she had difficulty falling asleep: "If you can teach me a few tricks, it would be helpful to me." However, her history was one of significant psychopathology, including major depressive episodes, eating disorders, self-cutting, a suicide attempt, multiple-substance abuse (current and past), self-defeating relationships with men, and generalized anxiety. As she described her history, she had an inappropriate smile on her face, often joking and minimizing what she was saying (e.g., "That was funny then"). The following exchange ensued:

THERAPIST: You are describing some real difficulties and tragedies in your life, but you are talking as if it is all a joke—something that we shouldn't take seriously. I wonder why you would come across in this way—making believe that your emotions and experiences are simply a superficial joke.

PATIENT: I don't want to sound like a whiner. I don't want to make a big deal out of things that happened to me. All I want is a few tricks to help me sleep.

THERAPIST: It sounds like we shouldn't take your emotions seriously. Is that how you relate to people—someone not to take seriously?

PATIENT: I'm the party girl. I'm the one who gets up on the bar and dances. I'm the one who people laugh at.

THERAPIST: What if they took you seriously and got to know you?

PATIENT: I don't let anyone know me.

This led to a discussion of how her parents responded to her emotion when she was younger.

> PATIENT: I remember when I was 16 and I was on a trip to Europe, and my boyfriend told me he was breaking up with me. When I got home, I tried to overdose. My mother took me to the hospital and she told me, "This must be jet lag." She didn't think I needed therapy. We are the family that looks good; we belong to the country club. We don't talk about problems.

While this patient attempted to cope by projecting an image of being shallow, superficial, and the "party girl," her suffering was experienced as incomprehensible and uncontrollable. Having been marginalized and invalidated by her parents, she relied on self-invalidation and attempts to minimizing her problems. Moreover, having "difficult emotions" was viewed as "failing the family," thereby leading her to distrust herself—and the therapist: "I won't let you see me cry."

Other nonverbal expressions of emotion include the patient's general appearance and movements. For example, is the patient attired in anhedonic or provocative clothing? Are the patient's movements slow and measured? Is the patient physically agitated (e.g., gesticulating when feeling emotional)? Does the patient maintain eye contact? Is the intonation of the voice low, a monotone, unemotional? Does the patient smile inappropriately? Are there other nonverbal factors? Especially relevant is whether the nonverbal expression is congruent with the verbal content of what is being said. Is the patient describing disturbing or even traumatic events in a monotone, with no emotion, or even with an incongruous smile? How do the emotions that underlie the history and experience express themselves in the patient's presentation?

## Beliefs about Emotion

The emotional schema therapist is particularly interested in the patient's beliefs about emotion. These include beliefs about "good" and "bad" emotions; shame over other people's knowing about the patient's emotions; beliefs about duration and need for control; tolerance for mixed feelings; beliefs about whether other people have the same emotions; and beliefs about the need to express emotions. I discuss each of these dimensions in considerable detail throughout this book, but in the initial interview the therapist can begin to collect information about these emotional schemas. The LESS II can help identify some of these beliefs, and the therapist can use the LESS II results as the basis for further inquiry.

THERAPIST: I noticed on the [LESS II] questionnaire that you thought that other people could not understand your emotions. Which emotions do you think other people would not understand?

PATIENT: Well, the fact that I am depressed. I don't understand it. After all, I have a nice home; my husband is very supportive; what do I have to be depressed about? I should feel happy.

THERAPIST: When you do talk about your depression, what does your husband say?

PATIENT: He tells me that I don't have anything to feel bad about. He tells me there are a lot of people who have real difficulties, and they aren't depressed. He tells me I should feel grateful.

THERAPIST: It sounds like he is saying that you do not have a right to be depressed. How does it make you feel when he says this?

PATIENT: It makes me more depressed because I feel—well—I don't even have a right to these feelings, and I think I must be selfish. And then I wonder if I am failing him because I am depressed.

THERAPIST: Are there any other feelings that you have when he says this?

PATIENT: I guess I feel angry. I know I shouldn't. He's only trying to be helpful.

THERAPIST: So it sounds like you think your depression and your anger don't make sense to you, and that you don't have a right to these feelings and that no one—including you—understands this. So that must be hard for you—having feelings that don't make sense, no one understands, and you feel guilty about this.

PATIENT: Yeah, it's like a vicious circle.

Another patient indicated that the reason he was seeking therapy was that his wife thought he had an "anger problem." He acknowledged that he sometimes lost his temper, but that he had been improving in recent weeks. He observed that his wife would not pay attention to what he was saying, that she often forgot what he had requested, and that she was not as practical as she should be in solving problems. "I can't stand it when people say, 'I can't.' That's not in my vocabulary. That's a cop-out." He indicated that his anger made sense, that it was his wife who was making him angry, and that he worked hard to support his family and did not feel appreciated. "If she would only listen to what I say, we wouldn't have any problems." In his case, he had problematic beliefs about his wife's emotions and needs. He thought that she should be tuned in to everything he said, do everything on his terms, not oppose him, and appreciate all the good things he did. However, he did observe that he could not understand why he was so enraged when she did not "hear" him. This led to a discussion of how his parents had responded to his emotions when he was growing up. He described his mother as intimidated by his angry and controlling father, and noted that she often tried to "make peace," or at least stay out of his way. He also described how his father would "be supportive."

> THERAPIST: So how would your father respond to your emotions when you were a kid?
>
> PATIENT: Let me give you an example from a few years ago. I called him up and he asked me, "How are things going?" and I told him, "Great." And he said, "That's what I want to hear—'Great.' That's what I want to hear." But you know, that's exactly it. He doesn't want to hear anything else. Just that things are fine. When I was a kid, and this other kid bullied me, he said, "Things will be OK. Don't worry. Just get on with it." He never had any time for me.
>
> THERAPIST: It sounds like he was dismissive of your feelings, and you felt obligated to tell him you were OK all the time.
>
> PATIENT: Oh, he was a good father. (*Hesitating.*) I don't want to speak badly of him.
>
> THERAPIST: Do you think you are being disloyal in talking about this?
>
> PATIENT: Maybe. A little. He tried.

In this particular case, the patient was sensitized to invalidation from his wife, based on his prior history of invalidation by and dismissiveness from his father. Moreover, he believed that his wife should acquiesce to him in the same manner that his mother did toward his father. On further inquiry, the patient described several periods of major depression, when he had no idea why he was depressed and had to take time off from work. He believed that no one understood him, including himself: "I had no idea why I felt so depressed." Problematic emotional schemas—especially those related to invalidation and self-invalidation—often reflect lack of insight. In this particular case, the individual reported that he did not understand why he felt the way he did, as he continued to defend his father as a "good guy." In fact, to him, his emotions were both a sign that he was failing his father and a badge of dishonor. Ironically, he viewed his wife's emotions in similar terms—as unjustified complaining and lack of gratitude.

This patient had specific beliefs about expression and validation of his emotion. He believed that he needed to express his anger directly and forcefully, and that he was entitled to do so in a hostile manner. He also believed that his wife should validate his feelings and desires by immediately complying, and that if she did forget, it was a sign that she did not respect him. The invalidating environment of his childhood—and his current situation of feeling invalidated by his father—contributed to his belief that no one really cared about his feelings, and that he needed either to keep his feelings to himself with his father or to express them dramatically with his wife and daughter.

A woman whose husband had died several years prior to therapy described herself as leaving her office, walking home while sipping whiskey from a bottle in a bag, and arriving at home intoxicated. On the LESS II, she indicated that her emotions did not make sense; that she should not have the feelings she had; that no one could understand her feelings; that if she allowed herself to express herself, she would lose control; and that she felt guilty and ashamed about her emotions.

> THERAPIST: What would happen if you arrived home in your apartment and had nothing to drink? What if you were not high? How would you feel, and what would you think?
>
> PATIENT: I'd feel really lonely, sad. There is no one there for me, no one to come home to. I'd feel empty. I don't know; it would be hard. (*Crying*)
>
> THERAPIST: So you would have feelings of sadness, loneliness, and emptiness. You indicated on the questionnaire that your feelings don't make sense to you. Which feelings don't make sense?
>
> PATIENT: All of these feelings. I mean, I have a good job. Why should I feel so sad at times? I don't know what's wrong with me.
>
> THERAPIST: Could it be that you feel sad and lonely because you miss your husband who died?
>
> PATIENT: I know I do. But why can't I get over it?
>
> THERAPIST: So you are still missing him, and you wonder what's wrong with you that you have these feelings. And you seem to think that you can't tolerate those feelings when you get home, so you try to get rid of them before you arrive.
>
> PATIENT: Yes. I find it so painful.
>
> THERAPIST: And you also said that you don't think anyone could understand the way you feel. So do you tell anyone?
>
> PATIENT: Only you, for now.

## Emotional Socialization

Beliefs about one's own emotions and those of others are often established in childhood through the responses of parents to emotional expression.

The therapist can ask the patient, "When you were a child, who would you turn to if you were upset, and how would the other person respond?" Drawing on Gottman's model of emotional socialization in the family, the therapist will note whether the parent (or other person) was dismissive, dysregulated, overwhelmed, or contemptuous—or, alternatively, engaged in "emotion coaching" by inquiring, validating, expanding and helping with problem solving (Gottman et al., 1996, 1997; Katz, Gottman, & Hooven, 1996). Often individuals who have experienced dismissive responses from their parents (e.g., "It's no big deal. Things will get better") will say, "My mother [or father] was supportive," rather than characterizing the response as minimization and dismissal. However, with further inquiry the therapist can determine precisely what was said and ask the patient, "If you were going through a difficult time now, would such a response seem supportive or curt and dismissive?" Other areas can then be explored: Did the parents have enough time for emotions? Was emotion even discussed in the home? Were certain emotions or feelings viewed as problematic, immature, or bad? Were the parents dysregulated and overwhelmed with their own emotions? Was there a sibling who was so distraught that the family had no time for the patient's emotions? Consider the following examples of problematic emotional socialization:

> A woman described how her mother would ridicule her when she would cry, and tell her that she was "just spoiled." She tried to get her mother's approval by being "pretty" and "dressing nicely," but nothing seemed good enough. As an adult, she believed that her emotions did not make sense, and that the only way she could be heard by someone was to treat all negative events as crises and cry intensely.

> An alexithymic man indicated that his highly educated and achievement-oriented family would have "rational" and "informative" discussions about politics and business, and that emotions were viewed as getting in the way of being productive and mature. As an adult, he had great difficulty identifying his emotions or recalling how he felt, as well as considerable difficulty making decisions. He believed that it would be unwise to disclose emotions to friends, family members, or his current girlfriend, lest they use his "weakness" against him.

> A rather "macho" young man, with cut-off sleeves and bulging muscles, took a hostile and provocative stance toward the therapist (male) in the first session. Although the patient came from an upper-middle-class background, he tried to sound like a tough gangster. The competitive environment of achievement and status that he had experienced while growing up had made him feel anxious and sad, but these "effeminate" emotions were disparaged. His father alternated between criticism of him and vain attempts to rescue him, while the patient carried on his masquerade of being provocative and tough.

A woman described how she wanted her mother's support when she was a child, but could not trust her mother. She would pout, cry, and eventually scream to get her mother's attention, but her mother would vacillate among indifference, contempt, and faked attempts to get close. She recalled an occasion when her mother opened her arms and offered to forgive her, and she went to be hugged by her mother, who then slapped her. As an adult, she had bulimia nervosa, was often afraid of her emotions, and thought that no one could be trusted.

Of course, emotional socialization includes behavior in addition to emotion. It includes touching, hugging, caressing, and holding. Did parents and other members of the family touch or caress the child, play with the child physically? What was the child's response to that? How does the adult patient respond to touch? Does the patient feel comfortable touching people? A young man with social anxiety described his feeling awkward about touching a woman on a date: "Isn't it a little pushy to touch her or to kiss her? Won't she be offended?" He presented in therapy in an overly formal, intellectualized manner, exceptionally polite and respectful. The therapist asked him how he felt when friends might touch him, and he said, "People see me as untouchable. When I was in college, my girlfriend broke up with me—I guess I wasn't affectionate and warm enough. I was telling my roommate, and I said to him I needed a hug, and he told me, 'But I thought you were untouchable.' "

Another young man indicated that his father had been cold and aloof, often condescending and critical of him. His father, a highly intellectualized man, had exercised power over the patient when he was a child and still did so. The mother was deferent toward the father, whose narcissism seemed to rule the family. The patient indicated that as a kid, the most affection he had received was from a nanny who would play with him, hold him, and touch him. As an adult, he felt undeserving of intimacy and love from any woman who was intelligent and successful, and often sought out prostitutes who he knew would never reject him. He reported a revulsion toward his body, which eventually developed into body dysmorphic disorder. Neither parent was viewed as a source of emotional comfort during childhood, and the patient acknowledged that his temper tantrums were the only way he could get any attention.

## Problematic Emotion Regulation Strategies

In the initial interview—and throughout therapy—the clinician should evaluate how the patient responded to his or her emotions from childhood onward, and what regulation strategies the patient used. Which emotions were difficult to tolerate? What thoughts arose when these emotions occurred? How did the patient as a child or adolescent cope with these emotions? The therapist should inquire directly about specific strategies, including avoiding situations that elicited emotions ("Were there things that you avoided doing because they led to certain emotions?"), sexual acting out, escalating intensity of complaining, screaming, tantrums, substance misuse, food restriction, binge eating, or reassurance seeking.

THERAPIST: So when you were a kid and you felt upset, what would you do to handle those emotions?

PATIENT: Going to my parents was a waste of time. Dad was usually high on weed or high on drinking, and Mom would have a few drinks and she was just not there. And, you know, we didn't talk about emotions. I was alone with what I felt.

THERAPIST: So what did you do to calm your emotions?

PATIENT: I smoked a lot of weed. Just spaced out. It calmed me down. I could forget.

THERAPIST: Anything else?

PATIENT: I found out I was attractive when some of the boys would come up to me. So they would want to have sex, and to fit in, I was willing. It made me feel like I was good-looking. My looks had changed, so now I was what they wanted, and I gave it to them.

THERAPIST: How about now? How do you deal with your feelings?

PATIENT: I just try to have a good time, smoke some weed—I get high every night. And drinking. I did cocaine for a while. It got out of hand. And if a guy wants me, I figure, why not? At least I can do that.

THERAPIST: Do you ever share how you really feel?

PATIENT: No, that's not me. I'm not weak. That's what you psychologists want me to do, but what's the use? No one cares anyway. No one really knows who I am.

THERAPIST: If I got to know who you are, what would happen?

PATIENT: You wouldn't like me.

Another young woman described her adolescence as a time when she could not get her mother to pay attention to the way she felt. She had felt depressed, anxious, and unloved; she was ashamed of her appearance; and she sought out support from her mother. Her mother was a pediatrician who told her, "You think you have problems? I deal with children who are sick and dying. You're just spoiled." The patient continued, "When I was 13 I became anorexic, starving myself, refusing to eat, losing weight. I thought that I could get my mother's attention. But nothing worked." This patient complained that her estranged husband never seemed to connect with her emotionally, but that she had a lover (a married man) who was someone she could talk to. In her first few sessions in therapy, she wondered out loud if she was too needy, too emotional—echoing the voice of her critical mother, who had dismissed her emotionally.

A man reported that when he was an adolescent, he was often bullied by other children; they would call him names and ridicule his comparatively short stature. He indicated that he had decided that he would not show any feeling and that he would simply treat them in a "logical" manner, recognizing that this was "about them," not "about me." This sounded exceptionally rational and stoic for an adolescent. He also described how he had always wanted to become a scientist, since he was attracted by the rigor and precision of science and math. He noted that his mother was somewhat inarticulate about emotion, and that his father, an amateur scientist, was preoccupied with his "inventions." The reason he was seeking therapy was that his wife had just told him that he was insensitive and condescending, and did not connect with her emotionally.

THERAPIST: What does she mean by the idea that you are insensitive?

PATIENT: I guess I say things that hurt her feelings. But I'm not really aware of it at the time. [Patient then describes an example of a condescending and patronizing remark he made to his wife.]

THERAPIST: How do you think she felt when you said that?

PATIENT: I guess she was angry. She told me she was angry.

THERAPIST: What was your intention in saying that?

PATIENT: I just wanted to give her the correct information. But, you know, I often say things like that—correcting people, telling people what the facts are.

THERAPIST: It sounds like you often think that facts are more important than feelings.

PATIENT: I do care about her feelings, when I think about it. I feel a little guilty. But I guess I am not thinking about her feelings when I say these things.

This particular individual had been coping with emotions through intellectualizing about the bullying when he was an adolescent, believing that he could "outthink" his hurt feelings. As a result, he had become less aware of his own feelings and unconcerned with the feelings and intentions of others. As a scientist, he was successful in his work, but he had difficulty reading his own and others' emotions. His intentions were not nefarious, as his wife supposed; rather, he was unintentionally unaware and had used facts and logic as a way of gaining some "control" over the threatening environment of his adolescence. Since he was quite intelligent, he received considerable reinforcement for this in his professional life, but the quality of his relationship with his wife was deteriorating.

Some patients turn to others to regulate their emotions, rather than relying on their own ability to soothe or calm themselves. For example, a patient with borderline personality disorder indicated that when she felt emotionally uncomfortable she would call her mother (regardless of the time of day or night), cry on the phone, and complain about how terrible her life was. When her mother would suggest that she use the techniques she had learned in DBT, she would scream at her, "Don't try to be my therapist!" She and her mother shared a similar belief about the young woman's emotions—that she was incapable of regulating her emotions on her own, and that the mother was responsible for making her feel better. This dual dependency on reassurance seeking, coupled with help rejection, led to further conflicts between mother and daughter, which helped confirm their jointly held belief that the daughter was incapable of regulating her own emotion. The therapist may recognize the value of social support and validation, but can inquire about such patients' beliefs that others are needed to regulate their feelings.

THERAPIST: How does that work out for you when you turn to your mother to soothe your feelings?

PATIENT: I know she loves me, but we get into arguments.

THERAPIST: Maybe you are asking her to do something that she is not capable of doing—to regulate the way you feel.

PATIENT: If she cared about me, she'd help me.

THERAPIST: But that seems to imply that you don't have any tools to use for your emotions. You told me that you have been going to a DBT group for a couple of months. Aren't there some tools there?

PATIENT: Yeah, but I just don't feel I can use them when I am upset.

THERAPIST: If you don't try to use them when you are upset, and you try to get your mother to soothe you—and she isn't capable—that must be frightening and even more upsetting.

PATIENT: It is.

THERAPIST: But maybe if you own the emotion (it's your emotion), you also own the solution—the tools that you have.

PATIENT: I know you're right. But it's hard.

THERAPIST: Yes, it's hard. But you have done a lot of things that are hard. And you might find that the tools are useful if you use them. Maybe we can anticipate that you will feel really bad sometime this week and make a plan about the tools that you might use.

## Specific Dimensions of Emotional Schemas

The emotional schema therapist is interested in the patient's specific beliefs about duration, control, acceptance, and other emotional schema dimensions introduced in Chapter 3 and assessed (some in reversed form) by the LESS II. Later chapters discuss in more detail how the clinician can address these beliefs by using a wide variety of techniques, but in the initial interview the therapist can ask questions directed at these dimensions.

- *Validation.* "Do you think other people understand and care about your feelings?" For example, a young woman with borderline personality disorder indicated that her parents did not understand her and that she couldn't get them to see things her way. She believed that when they gave her advice or tried to put things in perspective, they did not care about her feelings and only wanted things their way.

- *Duration.* "When you feel upset, how long does it feel it will last at the time that you are upset? Does it feel like a fleeting feeling, or something that will go on and on?" For example, a woman feared that her sadness would go on indefinitely and that she would always be depressed. Similar to many patients with emotional schemas about duration, she viewed an emotion as a trait that was lasting rather than a feeling that was temporary.

- *Control.* "Do you fear that your emotion will go out of control? Specifically, what do you fear will happen if it goes out of control? Can you tell me the worst possible outcome that you envisage? Is there a visual image that you could provide about what it looks like to be out of control with that feeling?" For example, a patient believed that his anxiety would escalate and go out of control when he was traveling by air, and he feared he would stand up, shout, run to the door, and bang on the door. None of this ever happened, but he regarded his imagining of losing control as the sign that he *was* losing control.

- *Guilt/shame.* "Are there some emotions that you feel guilty about? What is the reason that you think you should not have an emotion?" For example, a married man felt guilty that he found other women sexually appealing, and he feared that his fantasy about them would lead to loss of control and the destruction of his marriage. "Are there some emotions that you are embarrassed about? Would you be afraid that some people might find out? What would it mean to you if they found out that you felt this way? Do you fear that there are things about you that I might learn that would embarrass you?" For example, a religious man described how he had feelings of sexual arousal toward other young men in Hebrew class, and said that this desire on his part would be humiliating if other people found out. He also feared that if he confided in the therapist, there was a risk that others in his community might find out he was in therapy, and that he would be ostracized as a result.

• *Simplistic view of emotion.* "When you have mixed feelings about someone—including yourself—is that difficult for you? How do you handle those mixed feelings [e.g., reassurance seeking, collecting information, indecisiveness, rumination, procrastination, criticism]? Why does it bother you that you have mixed feelings?" For example, a man described his mixed feelings for his girlfriend and was reluctant to tell her that he loved her and was willing to make a commitment. He would seek reassurance from male friends; try to prove to himself that marriage was a bad situation, regardless of the partner; and ruminate about his indecisiveness. He believed that his feelings should be pure and total.

• *Expression.* "Are there feelings that are hard to express? What are they? What do you fear might happen if you expressed those feelings? If you are concerned about expressing a feeling, how do you handle that?" For example, a woman who had recently struggled as a single person to get pregnant feared that her emotions would "spill out" at "inappropriate times" (in church, at a wedding ceremony, while reading a sensitive story during a plane ride). She indicated that she was afraid that if she started to express her feelings, she would cry, and this would be humiliating in therapy.

• *Comprehensibility.* "Are there feelings that don't make sense to you? Which feelings? When your feeling doesn't make sense, what do you think or do next?" For example, the widow described earlier in this chapter indicated that she could not understand why she felt so upset when she returned to her empty apartment after a long day at work. Anticipating that she would feel upset, she would drink while walking home.

• *Values.* "Are your feelings of sadness, anxiety, anger, or loneliness related to things that you value?" For example, a single woman, after a breakup, cried as she described how lonesome she was feeling since the breakup. Initially wondering why she "should feel so badly," she observed that she valued intimacy, love, and commitment, and so her sad and lonely feelings were consequences of those values.

• *Numbness.* "Are there times when you feel numb? Are there times when you notice that things that bother other people don't bother you? How do you think or feel about this numbness?" For example, an alexithymic man observed that he often felt nothing when he saw or heard things that might upset other people. When his girlfriend cried, he vacillated between indifference and minor frustration. He indicated, in a dismissive fashion, "I'm not emotional. I think emotions are a waste of time. Anyway, people will use your emotions against you."

• *Consensus (similarity to others).* "Are your feelings different from those of other people? Which feelings do you have that seem out of the ordinary? What does it mean to you that you have feelings that you think other people don't have?" For example, the woman described earlier who drank as she walked home from work indicated that her feelings of sadness, emptiness, and loneliness were different from the feelings that other people had. She felt confused, embarrassed, and worried that she had a range of feelings that seemed distinct to her. As a result of her belief that she was "uniquely disturbed," she was reluctant to share her feelings with others.

• *Rationality.* "Do you think you should be rational and logical in almost everything? Do you think that emotions get in the way?" For example, the alexithymic man described above was especially focused on rationality; he viewed emotions as a waste of time and as interfering with rational, effective thinking. He would criticize himself for being emotional, and believed that his family would view him as out of control if he described his depression to them.

• *Acceptance.* "Is it difficult simply to accept that you have a feeling when you have it? Which feelings are harder to accept? Why? What would you fear would happen if you simply accepted a feeling for now?" For example, a man who suffered from panic disorder believed that he could not accept the sensations of anxiety or his worry about anxiety; he believed that if he accepted his anxiety, he would let his guard down and go out of control.

• *Rumination.* "Do you often dwell on your negative feelings and become preoccupied with your thoughts and emotions?" For example, a single man described his feelings of emptiness and lack of purpose, and could not understand why he was unhappy, given the objective signs of his success. He ruminated about these feelings and thought that he had some deep-seated problem that no one could help him with.

• *Blame.* "Do you blame people for your feelings and think that you would feel a lot better if other people changed?" For example, the married man described earlier whose wife insisted that he see a therapist for his anger indicated that the reason he felt angry was that his wife would not listen to him or do what he wanted her to do.

In addition to these 14 dimensions, the clinician can inquire about the patient's sense of *time urgency* when emotions arise: "When you have an emotion, is there a sense that you need to do something immediately to 'handle it'?" Some individuals believe that an intense emotion will escalate unless quick action is taken; this belief may lead to impulsive behavior that serves the function of immediate gratification through the temporary reduction of emotion. For example, a woman who had feelings of sadness and emptiness related to her conflicted relationship with her partner believed that she needed to get rid of those feelings immediately, leading her to binge-eat. This resulted in immediate feelings of some gratification, but later resulted in self-critical thoughts and the belief that she was out of control. Other emotional beliefs that can be assessed include beliefs about the changeability of an emotion—for instance, "What could be some factors that might lead you to feel a different and more desirable emotion?" As indicated in Chapter 3, predictions about future emotions based on current emotions often ignore intervening events or coping strategies that might change an emotion. Does the patient believe in the evanescence or transience of emotions, or is the current emotion viewed as a fixed trait that is independent of events and other behavior? Finally, emotional goals can be explored, such as the desire for serenity, satisfaction, love, appreciation, and compassion. It may be necessary for the therapist to introduce the idea that emotions can also be goals as well as current feelings, and that the patient can imagine developing a plan for living and a practice of behavior, thinking, taking risks, and relating that might engender a new and "more desirable" set of emotions. Rather than thinking of emotions as "just happening to me," the patient can examine which emotions he or she would like to grow with. Some of these ideas about emotional goals are discussed in Chapter 9.

## DEVELOPING A CASE CONCEPTUALIZATION

After the initial assessment and interview, the clinician can begin to work with the patient to develop a case conceptualization from the perspective of emotional schema therapy. Although recognizing the importance of a standard diagnostic workup, the clinician will want to evaluate how beliefs and problematic emotion regulation strategies contribute to these standard diagnostic categories. For example, how do beliefs about the duration and control of emotion contribute to a substance use disorder? How do beliefs about the inability to obtain validation, the uncontrollability of emotion, and the intolerance of mixed feelings contribute to borderline personality disorder? In order to illustrate how a case conceptualization can be developed, let us begin with the case of the "party girl" described earlier in this chapter—a young woman who presented with cannabis abuse, alcohol abuse, history of cocaine abuse, current bulimia nervosa, major depressive disorder, generalized anxiety disorder, insomnia, past history of cutting, past suicide attempt, borderline personality disorder, and self-defeating relationships with men. The general outline below can be used in developing a case conceptualization for this individual, and Figure 4.3 can be used as a general guide.

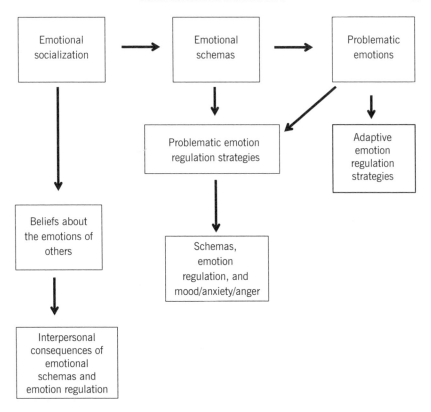

**FIGURE 4.3.** Case conceptualization model.

1. *Which emotions are problematic from the patient's perspective?* Anger, anxiety, loneliness, sadness.

2. *Predominant emotional schemas.* Emotions are incomprehensible, last indefinitely, are different from the emotions of others, need to be suppressed or eliminated immediately, are different from those of others, are signs of weakness, are shameful, and cannot be expressed or validated.

3. *Emotional socialization.* Early and current history of invalidation by both mother and father; humiliated and dismissed because of her feelings of sadness and loneliness; made to feel disloyal to the family because she is "selfish" with her emotions; role models of parents "handling" their emotions through drug and alcohol abuse; emphasis on putting on a good image rather than being authentic; emphasis on physical appearance rather than personality and character.

4. *Problematic emotion regulation strategies.* Avoidance; trying to appear cheerful; deferring to the needs of others; cannabis, alcohol, and

cocaine abuse; acting-out sexual behavior; self-cutting; rumination, worry, and dismissing her need for help.

5. *Adaptive strategies of emotion regulation*. Able to use problem solving and to form alliances with mental health workers; seeking out therapy and medication.

6. *Beliefs about emotions in other people*. Idealizing the capabilities of others (they are viewed as "having it all together," not needing help, happy with their lives); belief that she should soothe and calm the emotions of her mother and father; belief that she is obligated to please a man so that he feels good, to prevent rejection. She focuses less on the vulnerabilities that others might have, either expecting them to be strong and perfect or dismissing them as weak and inferior. She views herself as a "people pleaser"; she is especially focused on being sexually provocative with men who are strangers, to "prove that I can get them." She has little insight into the emotions of her mother and father or the men she dates.

7. *Relationship of emotional schemas, emotion regulation and depression, anxiety, anger*. Since she believes that her emotions will last indefinitely and escalate, she seeks out cannabis, alcohol, cocaine, and purging to eliminate uncomfortable feelings and thoughts. Believing that her emotions do not make sense, are shameful, and are signs of weakness, and that others do not share her feelings, she is reluctant to express emotion, show emotion nonverbally, or seek out validation. She views validation as a pathetic weakness. She fears expressing anger because she does not feel entitled to angry feelings, and she fears that expressing anger will lead to complete rejection. Isolated from others with her emotional difficulties, she either ruminates about what is wrong with her or self-medicates with drugs and alcohol.

8. *Interpersonal consequences of emotional schemas and emotion regulation*. Since she believes that she is fundamentally flawed and unlovable, she does not share her feelings with others. Fearing that she might become attached and trusting if she were with a "good guy," she views "nice guys" as "losers"—but her fear is acknowledged to be that she knows that the "bad guys" would never work out, so she has already discounted the rejection and abandonment. Becoming emotionally close to a "nice guy" is frightening, since rejection by him would be more painful. Therefore, she either avoids these men or provokes them to reject her. Attempts to maintain relationships on a superficial level, since she views herself as a "party girl" who feels "nothing serious." She claims to be afraid to "open a can of worms" with other people—or with her own emotions. Views close relationships as "dangerous" because "people can get to know what you are really like."

## SUMMARY

The objectives in the initial meetings with a patient are to elaborate his or her theory of emotion and emotion regulation; link this to the patient's history of emotional socialization; examine how these beliefs are sustained in current interpersonal relationships; evaluate the consequences of problematic emotion regulation or avoidance strategies; and develop an understanding of how the patient's beliefs and strategies of emotion maintain or exacerbate depression, anxiety, substance misuse, and relationship difficulties. Sharing the case conceptualization—indeed, using the diagram in Figure 4.3—may provide the patient for the first time with an understanding of how his or her beliefs about emotions have developed, and how these beliefs may be at the core of the patient's reliance on avoidance, low frustration tolerance, and other unhelpful strategies.

The treatment plan for the patient has already begun with the assessment (and will continue with ongoing assessment). It will also include socializing the patient to the treatment model; identifying specific problematic dimensions of emotional schemas; identifying the triggers for emotion; examining the helpful and unhelpful emotion regulation strategies that the patient has used; clarifying the patient's values and determining goals that the patient would like to achieve; reviewing the role of passivity and isolation; engaging the patient in behavioral activation and exposure as indicated; and assisting the patient in developing a wide range of skills for emotion regulation (e.g., cognitive restructuring, building tolerance for discomfort, overcoming experiential avoidance, practicing the fear, and mindful detachment). The forthcoming chapters present specific interventions that address a wide range of issues related to problematic beliefs about emotions in self and others, and describe how the clinician can assist the patient in pursuing valued goals.

## APPENDIX 4.1. DESCRIPTION OF INTAKE MEASURES

The Positive and Negative Affect Schedule (PANAS) yields two general factors, Positive and Negative Affect. Individuals can score high or low on either factor. Scores on the PANAS are stable over a 2-month period and are related to other measures of emotionality and personality. The clinician should note which positive and negative emotions are most commonly experienced, as well as the ratio between positive and negative emotions. Of particular interest is whether the patient reports an absence of positive emotions, but a high endorsement of negative emotions. Therapy can focus on increasing the frequency of positive emotions. Some patients may report low frequency of either kind of emotions, suggesting anhedonia or alexithymia. For a patient who scores high on Negative Affect, the specific emotions can be identified, along with the beliefs about these emotions and the strategies of emotion regulation that are elicited.

The Emotion Regulation Strategies Questionnaire (ERSQ) assesses 10 different responses to emotions, some of which may be problematic (e.g., push down feelings, hide feelings, worry, criticize oneself) and others may be helpful (e.g., try to think of things differently, accept, solve problems). This questionnaire will be helpful in assessing how the patient's negative emotional schemas are related to specific problematic strategies for coping with emotion, and its results may be helpful in explaining these relationships to the patient, as described in Chapter 5. This scale is presented in Figure 5.1 of Chapter 5.

The Metacognitions Questionnaire–30 (MCQ-30) assesses five factors that underlie worry, based on Wells's metacognitive model: Positive Beliefs about Worry, Negative Beliefs about Worry, Cognitive Confidence, Need for Control, and Cognitive Self-Consciousness. These factors are not only relevant to how individuals think about or respond to their intrusive thoughts (i.e., worry), but also indicative of how individuals think about their emotion. For example, negative beliefs about emotion and need for control of emotion have direct parallels in two of the MCQ-30 factors. Moreover, individuals who are continually focused on their emotion are likely to show higher scores on Cognitive Self-Consciousness. These individuals are presumed to have difficulty "getting outside of their heads." These metacognitive factors are in fact related to problematic emotional schemas, with individuals who endorse negative beliefs about their emotions more likely to endorse positive beliefs about the function of worry while simultaneously believing that worry needs to be controlled.

The Acceptance and Action Questionnaire–II (AAQ-II) is based on the model of psychological flexibility, mindfulness, and acceptance advanced by Hayes and his colleagues. Individuals with negative emotional schemas are more likely to be low in psychological flexibility, to have difficulty accepting their thoughts and emotions, and to have trouble obtaining detachment from them. ACT concepts and techniques may be quite helpful in facilitating greater acceptance and less entanglement with momentary emotions while focusing on valued goals.

The Dyadic Adjustment Scale (DAS) is a widely used measure of relationship satisfaction, assessing areas of conflict between partners. Higher scores are associated with greater relationship satisfaction. Our research indicates a strong relationship between scores on the DAS and a patient's perception of how his or her partner views the patient's emotions.

The Measure of Parental Styles (MOPS) comprises three dimensions for recollections of how the mother and father responded to the patient when the patient was a child: Indifference, Abuse, and Overcontrol. Individuals who have experienced indifference, abuse, or overcontrol from either parent would be expected to have negative beliefs about their own emotions, difficulty trusting others, and difficulty experiencing validation.

Responses on the Experiences in Close Relationships—Revised (ECR-R) scale are of interest for emotional schema therapy, in that some individuals may become dysregulated in close relationships because of their anxious attachment, or may become detached because of their fears of engulfment, control, or fears of rejection. This scale measures both anxious and avoidant attachment styles in adult close relationships. Examination of individual items may provide the clinician with information about the triggers in close relationships that might elicit anxiety, jealousy, anger, or sadness.

The Self-Compassion Scale—Short Form (SCS–SF) is a 12-item questionnaire that assesses how the individual responds to negative emotions. The scale assesses six dimensions (Self-Kindness, Self-Judgment, Common Humanity, Isolation, Mindfulness, and Overidentified). Self-compassion is related to a wide range of measures of psychopathology (Neff, 2012). The SCS-SF provides the clinician with information as to how the patient may self-soothe or regulate emotions—either relying on showing kindness toward the self, normalizing emotion by finding common humanity, or (alternatively) criticizing the self or becoming overidentified with an emotion.

Finally, the Millon Clinical Multiaxial Inventory–III (MCMI-III) is a widely used, standardized self-report form that yields factor scores on 10 clinical syndromes and 14 personality disorders. The MCMI-III is of particular value for evaluating such areas of functioning as depression, anxiety, PTSD, substance abuse, and a wide range of personality disorder dimensions based on Millon's model.

# CHAPTER 5

# Socialization to the Emotional Schema Model

One ought to hold on to one's heart; for if one lets it go,
one soon loses control of the head too.
—FRIEDRICH NIETZSCHE

After the initial assessment and interview have been completed, the first stage of therapy proper focuses on helping the patient understand what emotional schemas are; how they affect the maintenance of anxiety, and depression, or other psychiatric disorders; how beliefs about emotion lead to problematic coping strategies; how these beliefs about emotion were learned; and how changing these beliefs and strategies may positively affect the patient's functioning. The patient's understanding of his or her theory of emotion is an essential component of emotional schema therapy. By recognizing emotional schemas as "theories" or "individual constructions," the patient may come to understand that some theories do not necessarily fit reality and that new theories may be more adaptive.

## TEACHING THE PATIENT ABOUT EMOTIONS AND EMOTIONAL SCHEMAS

The first step in socializing the patient to the emotional schema model is to help identify what emotions are and how they are different from thoughts, behaviors, and reality.

THERAPIST: We are going to be talking a lot about your thoughts, your emotions, and your behavior. They are all linked together, but they are different. For example, let's imagine that you think that you have too much work to do, and that your boss is going to really get angry with you. Those are your thoughts about what is going to happen. But then you notice that your heart is beating rapidly; you are feeling anxious and a little angry at your boss; and you are thinking that your boss is unfair with you. Now your sensations—your heart beating rapidly and your feeling anxious—are your emotions. But you can also see that your emotions can involve thoughts about your boss. And you might behave differently. You might work extra hard or complain to your coworkers. So emotions have sensations, an awareness of how you are feeling; you may have thoughts about something; and you might relate to people differently. Your emotion is anxiety, and it involves your sensations, your awareness of how you are feeling, your thoughts that your boss might be upset, and how you relate to people when you are anxious. Does this make sense?

PATIENT: How are emotions different from thoughts?

THERAPIST: Well, thoughts are statements like "My boss is always difficult" or "I will never get this done." The interesting thing about these thoughts is that we can test them out against the evidence. We can collect evidence about whether your boss is always difficult, or whether you will get the job done. In a sense, thoughts can be true or false or somewhere in between. But if you say you are feeling anxious and your heart is beating, we don't ask if that is true. We assume you are right about that—you know your emotions when you are experiencing them. But we might ask you what you are anxious *about*.

PATIENT: How is this going to help me?

THERAPIST: Good question. We could look at your thoughts or look into changing your behavior. That would be helpful. But we also know that you may have difficulty at times with your emotions. So we might want to see what you do or what you think when you are feeling anxious or sad.

PATIENT: What could I be thinking?

THERAPIST: You might have thoughts about your anxiety. For example, you might think that it doesn't make sense, or that it might last a long time, or that it is dangerous. And those thoughts about your anxiety might make you more anxious.

PATIENT: So I might get anxious about being anxious?

THERAPIST: Possibly. That might be true. We will have to see.

Following this introduction to what an emotion is, the therapist provides the patient with an overview of the principles of emotional schema therapy. The LESS II results from the assessment (see Chapter 4) provide the therapist with targets for discussion—that is, the patient's specific beliefs about durability, control, comprehensibility, and other dimensions of emotional schemas.

THERAPIST: I noticed on the [LESS II] form that you believe that your emotions will last a long time. Which emotions do you think will last a long time?

PATIENT: I guess my sadness. When I am feeling down, I think that it's going to go on forever. I just won't get out of it.

THERAPIST: So you have a belief about the duration of your sadness— that it will be long lasting. Does that make you feel hopeless at times?

PATIENT: Yes, I guess it does. I think I won't get out of that mood.

THERAPIST: So when you feel it's hopeless and your sadness will last forever, what do you do next?

PATIENT: I guess I sit and wonder about it. I just keep thinking about it: "Why do I feel this way? What's wrong with me?"

THERAPIST: So we can see here that you feel sad; then you think it will last forever, which makes you feel hopeless; you then ruminate and dwell on this. Then how do you feel when you are ruminating?

PATIENT: Sad.

In this example, the therapist is able to link a belief about durability to another emotion (hopelessness), and then link this to rumination, which then maintains the sadness. This illustration of a self-fulfilling, self-confirming emotional schema process is the first step in linking beliefs about emotion to problematic coping and depression. The inquiry begins with a focus on the emotion, what the individual thinks about the emotion, and the problematic coping strategy that is activated. Beliefs about emotion are linked to coping with emotion.

THERAPIST: Let's take another look at what you say about your emotions. On one of the items, you said that your emotions don't make sense to you. In other words, they seem incomprehensible. Which emotion seems incomprehensible?

PATIENT: Well, I don't understand why I feel so sad. I have a good job and a good marriage, and I am healthy. What could be a reason to be so sad?

THERAPIST: OK, when you think that your feelings are incomprehensible, what do you do next?

PATIENT: I keep asking my wife if I am going to be OK. She's supportive at times, but I can see that it might be alienating her. And that upsets me, too.

THERAPIST: So it sounds like you think your feelings don't make sense, and then you repeatedly ask for reassurance, and then you worry about alienating your wife?

PATIENT: Yes, that makes me sad, too.

THERAPIST: So, what we have been looking at is that you have beliefs about your emotions—that they will last forever, and that they don't make sense—and these beliefs make you feel more sad and more hopeless, and then you ruminate and seek reassurance; that can also make you frustrated and sad. And so it's a vicious circle, with your beliefs leading to problematic ways of coping. Does that make sense to you?

PATIENT: Yes, that's what I seem to be doing.

The therapist is ready to introduce the emotional schema model after illustrating the connections described above. This model will become the basis for case conceptualization and treatment planning.

THERAPIST: Each of us has beliefs about our emotions. Sometimes when we feel sad, we think it makes sense—for example, we feel sad after someone we care about dies. Our sadness makes sense. We may also believe that our sadness will lessen over time, as we go through a process of letting go. We think our sadness is normal. We may believe that other people will validate that it makes sense that we are sad. All of these are our beliefs about sadness in that situation: It makes sense; it won't last forever; other people would feel the same way; we can get validation. But let's say that you had other beliefs about your emotion. For example, you might believe that your sadness doesn't make sense—that it will go on forever, that other people would not feel the same way, that no one could understand you. And you might fear that your sadness will escalate and overwhelm you, and that you will lose control. So you are confused and afraid of your sadness. These two examples illustrate how beliefs about emotion affect you differently.

PATIENT: I guess I have a lot of negative beliefs about my feelings— especially the idea that they will last forever and go out of control.

THERAPIST: Yes, and these beliefs are called "emotional schemas." What this means is simply that you have your own theory about your sadness, for example. So this then leads to several questions. First, does your theory make you sadder? For example, if you think your sadness will last indefinitely, then you might feel more sad and hopeless. Second, does your theory lead you to ruminate, isolate yourself, remain passive, or seek reassurance over and over? Third, if you had a different theory of your sadness—if you believed that it makes sense, that it is temporary, that it is not going out of control, or that there are things that you could do to aim toward positive emotions—would this new theory make a difference for you?

PATIENT: That sounds like a lot to ask for.

THERAPIST: Let's take a look at this diagram (*presenting the diagram of the emotional schema model, Figure 3.2 in Chapter 3*). Notice that you might have a range of feelings—sadness, anxiety, sexual—and then you may or may not pay attention to them. Let's say that you normalized the emotions: You thought that your feelings made sense, that other people felt the same way, and that you could accept those feelings. You might also share them with a close friend who validates you, and you then move on in your life. Wouldn't that be a great way to think about emotions?

PATIENT: Yes. I wish I could. But that's not the way I am thinking now.

THERAPIST: Well, maybe that could change. Now let's look at the diagram again and see if any of this describes you. In some cases, you might think that your emotions don't make sense, that they will last forever, that they need to be controlled—and perhaps you feel guilty or ashamed. You might think that your emotions are problematic. Does any of this sound like you at times?

PATIENT: A lot of the time. Especially since I have been more depressed.

THERAPIST: And perhaps you might think, "How can I get rid of these emotions?" Now some people drink, binge-eat, or use drugs. Other people isolate themselves and avoid experiences. Does any of this sound like you?

PATIENT: I don't drink that much, but I have been eating more junk food.

THERAPIST: And these problematic ways of coping may just add to your sadness. And then the cycle begins again: "I'm sad," "My sadness doesn't make sense," ruminating, isolating, more sadness, more hopelessness. And so it goes.

PATIENT: This sounds like me. But it also sounds depressing.

THERAPIST: Yes, I can see that it sounds depressing. But what if you had different beliefs about your emotions and different ways of coping? What then?

PATIENT: I guess I might feel better. But how can you do this?

THERAPIST: That's what this therapy can help you with.

The therapist and patient may examine how the patient may have difficulty noticing, labeling, and differentiating various emotions. For example, the patient may simply notice that "I felt upset," whereas further exploration reveals that the patient felt frustrated, angry, anxious, sad, confused, and envious. (Patients with alexithymia have more difficulty recognizing and labeling emotions, as well as linking emotions to specific memories.) Rather than normalizing, expressing, learning from, and validating these emotions, the patient may engage in experiential avoidance. This is further related to negative assessments of emotion, such as the belief that these feelings will last indefinitely, are unique to the self, cannot be controlled, and do not make sense. These interpretations further drive the cycle of avoidance, externalization, suppression, and rumination.

In this first phase of emotional schema therapy, the patient learns how the process of noticing, labeling, differentiating, evaluating, and using emotions constructively or problematically contributes to the problems for which he or she is seeking help. In addition, in this phase of therapy, the therapist and patient explore earlier memories of emotional socialization that link dismissive or disorganized styles of parenting with specific beliefs about emotion, which I examine shortly.

Schematic illustrations linking beliefs to emotion regulation help the patient understand how assessment is used in understanding the emotional schemas and strategies that underpin psychopathology. Moreover, the therapist can use such an illustration to assist the patient in differentiating emotions and levels of emotions (primary and secondary emotions), identifying implicit models of the content and function of emotions, determining the causes of emotions, and identifying processes of emotion regulation in self and others. As noted above, the representation of the emotional schema model provided in Chapter 3 (see Figure 3.2) is useful for patients early in therapy.

## LINKING EMOTIONAL SCHEMAS
## TO PROBLEMATIC COPING STRATEGIES

As illustrated in the transcripts above, beliefs about the duration or comprehensibility of an emotion may result in problematic coping strategies, such as avoidance, rumination, and excessive reassurance seeking. The therapist can identify which emotional schema beliefs the patient has endorsed on the LESS II or in the interview, and then examine the consequences of these beliefs. For example, a patient who believes that "My emotions will go out of control" (as the woman in the exchange below does) will activate strategies to suppress or lessen emotional intensity, and, when these strategies fail, may become more determined to suppress the emotion.

THERAPIST: I noticed on the [LESS II] questionnaire that you indicated that you believe that your emotions can go out of control. When you have this thought about your emotions, what do you do next?

PATIENT: I feel anxious. I'm afraid.

THERAPIST: That makes sense. But I wonder if there are ways that you try to get control, or things that you say or do to make yourself feel less anxious.

PATIENT: Sometimes I'll eat junk food. It makes me feel calmer initially. I can just stuff myself with food.

THERAPIST: OK, so when you think your emotions will go out of control, you binge-eat at times. I can see that. Anything else that you might do?

PATIENT: I worry about what's going to happen to me: "Will I go crazy? Will this last forever?" There are times when I thought I couldn't stand the feeling, and thought maybe I would be better off dead. But I wouldn't do anything. It's just something that I thought at times.

THERAPIST: I can understand that it might be very hard. So you worry and then think it's hopeless, and it sounds like you have to pull yourself back from that feeling.

PATIENT: I might call my friend Gillian because, you see, she can calm me down. She can help me feel that it will be OK.

THERAPIST: So Gillian is someone who is very important to you. It's like you are thinking, "The way to get my emotions in check is to get someone else to help me." You think, "Gillian can calm me down." It's like you are thinking, "Someone else can take control of my emotion and help me."

In this case, the patient can see that beliefs about emotion result in problematic coping strategies, and that in some cases she delegates control over her emotions to another person. In each case, there is a lack of self-efficacy; she feels overwhelmed with part of herself and feels the need to escape from herself. This continual battle with herself makes her feel more anxious and depressed, and the cycle begins anew.

One patient who has been introduced in Chapter 4, a widow in her late 50s, would leave work at the end of the day and walk home while drinking whiskey out of a bottle in a bag. By the time she got to her apartment, she was intoxicated. As described in Chapter 4, the therapist asked her, "What would it be like if you got to your apartment and had nothing to drink? What if you were not high?" She indicated that she feared that she would be overcome with loneliness and sadness because her apartment was empty. Her husband had died 2 years ago and she missed him. The therapist then continued: "And what if you did feel lonely and sad, what would happen next?" She indicated that she had not thought this through, but she believed that her sadness and loneliness would just get worse: "It would be unbearable—there would be no end to it." The therapist reflected that she seemed to think she needed to avoid those feelings of sadness and loneliness, and that drinking was the only way to keep her from having her emotions overwhelm her. If she did not believe that her sadness and loneliness would escalate and overwhelm her, there would be no need to drink. We will return again to this patient in a later chapter, but her experience indicates how beliefs about emotion can result in problematic ways of coping.

## IDENTIFYING HOW EMOTIONAL SCHEMAS WERE LEARNED IN THE FAMILY

Emotional schemas are often experienced as automatic responses that an individual does not generally reflect on. For example, until a patient is asked about the belief that an emotion will last indefinitely, the patient may have been going through years with this belief without considering that it might not be accurate. As indicated earlier, gaining distance from a belief is the first step in modifying it. One way to gain distance is to understand how beliefs were taught in the family. If they were learned, then it is possible to unlearn them. Children learn that their emotions make sense through "emotion talk" in the family. That is, when emotion words are used, a parent reflects, labels, and expands on the emotion the child is describing, and the parent assists the child in examining ways to cope. As described in Chapter 3, this "emotion coaching" has been found to be an important component in the development of self-control in children (Eisenberg & Spinrad, 2004; Gottman et al., 1996; Hanish et al., 2004; Michalik et al., 2007; Rotenberg & Eisenberg, 1997; Sallquist et al., 2009). Gottman and colleagues (1996) have also identified several problematic strategies of emotional socialization, also described in Chapter 3: dysregulated, dismissive, and disapproving styles. The dismissive strategy denies the significance of the child's emotions ("Oh, it's nothing. Don't bother yourself. Why are you making such a big deal of this?"); the disapproving style involves criticism and overcontrol of the child's feelings ("Stop acting like such a baby! Why can't you grow up?"); and in the dysregulated style, parents are overwhelmed by their own emotions and reject the child's emotions ("Can't you see I'm having my own problems? I can't deal with your father's drinking and your craziness. Leave me alone!").

Such experiences of being ignored, criticized, humiliated, dismissed, or minimized when upset can have a lasting effect on individuals' beliefs about their emotions and how others will respond. For example, when patients were upset as children, did their parents comfort the children; encourage them to express their emotions; help them understand that their emotions made sense; and assist them in learning ways to solve problems, provide rewarding alternatives, or negotiate conflict? Or did the parents tell the children that they had no reason to feel upset, that they were spoiled, that they were acting like babies? In some cases, like the patient with the wife-identified "anger problem" in Chapter 4, the patient may say, "My father would tell me everything would be OK. He tried to support me." However, on closer examination this reassurance can also be viewed as dismissive of emotion, communicating this to the child: "Your emotions are out of proportion to what is going on. There is no need to talk any further about your feelings, and you should just get over it." The question is whether the parents made time and emotional space to hear the child's feelings. In the following case, this woman had a dismissive father and an overwhelmed mother:

> THERAPIST: When you were upset as a child, which parent did you feel was hard to go to?
>
> PATIENT: Well, my father was always busy with work, and when he came home he was tired and didn't really want to say much. So I learned that it didn't make much sense to talk with him.
>
> THERAPIST: Do you recall any response that he had to your feelings?
>
> PATIENT: Oh, he would say, "Don't worry. You'll get over it."
>
> THERAPIST: How did that make you feel when he said that?
>
> PATIENT: Like he had no time for me. Like my emotions were annoying to him.
>
> THERAPIST: How about your mother?
>
> PATIENT: She was depressed and anxious a lot, and things weren't so good between her and my dad. So she would often talk about her own difficulties. She was sad and lonely and felt that my father was too busy with work.
>
> THERAPIST: So it sounds like the focus was on her feelings, and there wasn't much time for yours?
>
> PATIENT: Yeah. I guess so. She would say, "I'm having a hard enough time myself. Your father is never home. I have to take care of you and your sister. What's bothering you now?"

THERAPIST: So she was overwhelmed with her feelings, and your feelings were going to be a burden to her. How did that make you feel?

PATIENT: Sad . . . and guilty. Yes, guilty that I was making life hard for her.

What emotional schemas were learned here? This patient learned that she did not have a right to her feelings, that she was to blame, that her emotions were a burden to others, that others would not validate her feelings or encourage her to express her feelings, and that her emotions were bad. She did not learn how to label her feelings, differentiate them, make sense of them, or regulate them. The message was this: "Get over your emotion and don't burden people."

The therapist can inquire further about messages about emotions that were learned in the patient's family. Were there certain emotions that were not OK? For example, was it not OK to be angry, anxious, or sad? Was the message that the child's emotions did not make sense, that the child was overreacting, that other people wouldn't feel this way? Or did the parents validate emotions, encourage expression, normalize emotions, and comfort the child? Was the child labeled "out of control," "selfish," "crazy," or "stupid"? Did the parents "overinterpret" the emotions (e.g., "You are really trying to manipulate me with your crying. You won't get away with it")?

Some children are placed in the position of being are asked to take care of their parents' emotions—a form of "reverse parenting." For example, one patient described her mother as continually anxious and worried about her own anxiety. The father was angry, distant, and unpredictable. The mother turned to the child—when she was 8—as a source of comfort. "I remember my mother saying she was worried about pains in her chest, and could I get her some aspirin? She would say, 'Maybe you should stay home and not visit your friend.' I felt like I had to take care of her." As an adult, this patient continually wondered whether her emotions made sense, whether the therapist would understand, and whether her emotions were going to go on forever. The reverse parenting that she experienced in taking care of her mother's emotions led her to feel that no one would protect her or take care of her. As a result of this lack of emotional parenting, she married an overly controlling man who doted on her but encouraged her to believe that she was incapable of taking care of herself. When she became more successful at work, he belittled her, saying that she was selfish. She had moved from a home where her mother controlled her with guilt and fear, to a home where her husband controlled her with the message that she was weak and incompetent.

What emotional schemas were learned in this case? The reverse-parenting child learned that she could not express her feelings, that she would not be validated, that her emotions would be a burden to others, that she needed to take care of others, that she needed to defer to what others wanted and take care of their needs, that her emotions did not make sense, and that no one shared her feelings. Her mother seldom engaged in soothing of emotions, so she did not learn how to self-regulate her feelings or how to improve things for herself. She sought out a parental figure in a partner to compensate for what was missing when she was a child. She expected her husband to take care of her emotions.

Recognizing how emotional schemas are learned helps a patient gain distance from them, since the patient can understand that his or her beliefs about emotion are largely due to problematic parenting. The goal, however, is not to get stuck in blaming the parents for the adult's difficulties with emotion, but rather to help the patient understand that beliefs about emotion can vary, depending on the learning environment. Furthermore, understanding the experience of emotional socialization assists the patient in making sense of emotion and feeling less guilty about not having learned more adaptive beliefs and emotion regulation strategies. The therapist can say, "You can't blame yourself for something your parents never taught you."

THERAPIST: So you can see how you learned certain beliefs about emotion when you were a kid. It's not your fault that your parents were not helpful. You might even wonder how they developed such negative beliefs about emotion. Maybe their parents were critical and dismissive about emotion. Is that possible?

PATIENT: Yes, my mother's mother was highly critical. She was what you call a "narcissist." Everything was about her. She thought that my father wasn't good enough for my mother. And even today, my mother seems to be afraid of her. I can tell.

THERAPIST: Well, your parents were limited in helping you understand and deal with your emotions. Maybe their limitations go back to their childhood. But the good news is that you can learn new ways of thinking about your emotions and dealing with them.

PATIENT: That would be good. (*Pause*) It's about time, I guess.

THERAPIST: Yes, it is about time. But wouldn't it be great if you could learn that your emotions make sense, that other people might have the same feelings, and that your emotions will not go on forever and overwhelm you? Wouldn't it be great if you could learn to accept some emotions as experiences that you are having for the moment, while realizing that you can produce other positive emotions in yourself and live a life that has room for all of the emotions—the positive and negative?

PATIENT: That would be wonderful. But I don't even know how that is possible.

THERAPIST: Well, we can find out. That's something that we can work on together, if you want to. That's something that we can try to do.

The therapist can explore further which emotions were not acceptable in the family. An extreme example of such emotions can be seen in the case of a 24-year-old former semipro football player who suffered from a conversion disorder. He was unable to work and lived at home with his mother, with whom he experienced a great deal of frustration, since she regularly criticized him. He complained that he had difficulty sitting up and would lie on the floor in the therapist's office. He claimed that he had "dirty anger" and that he wanted to eliminate any angry thoughts and feelings. He indicated that his religious faith (he claimed to be "born-again") prohibited angry feelings, although he could not specify what teaching in his faith explicitly prohibited feelings. The medical examination indicated that there was nothing physically wrong with him that could account for his need to lie on the floor. "I feel more comfortable lying here," he said. The therapist asked him about anger in his family:

THERAPIST: When you were growing up, what was it like when you got angry?

PATIENT: We were told that anger was a sin, that you should never get angry with anyone in the family. That you were bad.

THERAPIST: So you were made to feel guilty about being angry? You were told you were bad?

The therapist noticed, over the course of several sessions, that when the patient was questioned about his mother, he started to feel angry about her critical treatment of him; as his anger increased, he sat up on the floor and appeared physically stronger. When the therapist commented on this observation, he retreated to lying on the floor and said that his anger was bad. This is a dramatic example of how messages instilling guilt about anger in a child can result in severe psychopathology.

Another patient who appeared alexithymic had difficulty identifying his emotions. He had been out of work and had been looking for a job for over 7 months. He showed little expression on his face when he spoke about emotional issues. He also commented that he didn't know how he really felt about his girlfriend. When asked whether he had ever been in love, he commented, "Maybe—in retrospect. I don't know." The therapist asked him whether he had ever talked to his parents when he was a kid about his feelings.

PATIENT: They don't want to hear about your feelings. They are entirely concerned about achieving things—getting into the right schools, being a success. No, to talk about feeling would be a waste of time.

THERAPIST: How about now?

PATIENT: If I told them how I feel, if I told them that this was a hard time for me, they would use it against me. It's a sign of weakness.

Thus, in this patient's family, emotions were off limits; they were not consistent with the values of achievement and status; and emotions conferred interpersonal vulnerability.

## CLARIFYING HOW CHANGING EMOTIONAL SCHEMAS CAN AFFECT PSYCHOPATHOLOGY

In building the motivation to change, the therapist can now use some of the information about the patient's beliefs about emotions and maladaptive coping to illustrate that changing beliefs can help address the patient's presenting concerns. Patients who have been relying on passivity, avoidance, substance misuse, rumination, bingeing, and other unhelpful coping strategies can begin to examine how changing their beliefs about emotion can make these strategies unnecessary. For example, in the example of the widow who returned intoxicated to her apartment, if she could come to recognize that her sadness pointed to her higher values of love and dedication (something to feel proud about), that her sadness and loneliness could be viewed as temporary reminders of someone she loved, and that these feelings could come and go without overwhelming her, she might have less need for alcohol as a means of avoiding or suppressing her feelings.

The therapist can inquire about specific emotion regulation strategies during the initial interview and can augment this with the use of questionnaires. A measure that targets a variety of general emotion regulation strategies has been developed by Aldao and Nolen-Hoeksema (2012a). The Emotion Regulation Strategies Questionnaire (ERSQ) is shown in Figure 5.1. This simple questionnaire provides a quick evaluation of whether patients use problem solving, cognitive restructuring, acceptance, suppression, distraction, or self-criticism; hide feelings from others; worry or ruminate; seek reassurance; or "do something else" (take a breath, drink, eat, etc.). In addition to the ERSQ, which may be used at intake (see Chapter 4), the therapist can inquire about other behaviors that patients use, expanding on the category of "do something else." For example, does the patient dissociate, get "lost" in the Internet, peruse pornography, self-mutilate, engage in compulsive behaviors (e.g., compulsive cleaning), contact people

| YOU TRIED to | Not at all | A little | Somewhat | A lot |
|---|---|---|---|---|
| come up with ideas to change the situation or fix the problem | O | O | O | O |
| think of the situation differently in order to change how you felt | O | O | O | O |
| allow or accept your feelings | O | O | O | O |
| "push down" your feelings or put them out of your mind | O | O | O | O |
| do something to take your mind off things | O | O | O | O |
| criticize yourself for your feelings | O | O | O | O |
| hide your feelings from others | O | O | O | O |
| worry or ruminate about the situation | O | O | O | O |
| talk to others | O | O | O | O |
| do something else (took a deep breath, drank alcohol, ate to feel better) | O | O | O | O |

**FIGURE 5.1.** Emotion Regulation Strategies Questionnaire (ERSQ). From Aldao and Nolen-Hoeksema (2012a). Copyright 2012 by Elsevier. Reprinted by permission.

in ways that are inappropriate, cry, throw temper tantrums, or engage in other problematic behaviors? Of particular importance to depression is the use of passivity and avoidance as coping strategies. For example, when the patient feels "down," does he or she lie in bed for long periods of time, avoid interacting with people, not respond to communication from other people, sleep for long periods of time, ruminate, and withdraw in general? Patients may not see these as "coping strategies" or "things that they do"— but, ironically, doing "nothing" may be the most common coping strategy.

The therapist can identify the typical strategies and then link them to beliefs about emotion. For example, consider a woman who lies in bed for most of Saturday, complaining of having no energy and no motivation, and describing herself as feeling sad. Depressed patients often complain of "no energy" and "no motivation," and then "logically" conclude that they "can't do anything." Her belief about her energy or motivation is that it is finite and depleted, and that doing something would deplete her even more. She wants to conserve whatever energy she has. She also believes that interacting with people would make her more sad and frustrated.

The patient is using passivity and avoidance as coping strategies. The therapist can ask her about her sadness and energy, and inquire what would happen if she actually got out of bed, left her apartment, did some exercise, and saw some friends:

PATIENT: I would be exhausted. I just can't do it.

THERAPIST: What if you had a different belief about your motivation? For example, what if you believed that your motivation to do something would increase once you started to do it? For example, what if you believed that your motivation to exercise would increase once you started to exercise?

PATIENT: I would get out of bed and exercise, I guess.

THERAPIST: Then, if you imagined yourself exercising, getting out and doing something, how do you predict you would feel?

PATIENT: I might feel better. But I don't have the energy.

THERAPIST: What is the worst thing that could happen if you exercised and had little energy?

PATIENT: I would feel more tired, I guess.

THERAPIST: What is the best thing that could happen if you exercised, but started with little energy?

PATIENT: I might have more energy.

THERAPIST: That might be a way to jump-start you out of your depression. You might experiment with doing something active when your emotions tell you to stay passive and avoid.

The therapist can indicate that it is possible to act without motivation.

Many patients believe that they have to be "ready" to change or motivated to change. They think, "I need to want to do it," as if the desire must always precede the action. The therapist can say, "What if you saw me walking back and forth in front of this building, looking down the street as if I am waiting for a bus to show up? You would ask me, 'What are you doing?' and I would reply, 'I am waiting for my motivation to show up so I can go to work.' What would you think then?" This example is quite helpful to patients who avoid doing uncomfortable things because they do not feel motivated or ready. They think that they have to have the energy, the desire, or the motivation. One way to respond to this belief is to say, "Don't you do things every day that you are not really motivated to do, simply because you have to do these things—like go to work?"

Since rumination is a common maladaptive emotion regulation strategy, the therapist can link this to problematic emotional schemas, such as difficulty accepting emotion or difficulty accepting "conflicting" feelings. For example, a young man ruminated extensively after a breakup with his girlfriend: "I can't make sense of this. I don't understand what went wrong." He had a high intolerance for the uncertainty of the situation, but also realized that he could not accept the breakup and he could not "reconcile" his mixed feelings about her—that he still loved her, but also was angry and disillusioned with her. Thus he activated rumination as a strategy to gain closure, make sense, and avoid similar problems in the future. The therapist pointed out that what was driving his rumination was his belief that he could not accept the sadness that he felt, could not accept his mixed feelings, and could not accept the fact that he might have missed some signs about the relationship. Rumination, then, became a strategy of avoiding acceptance. This was helpful to him in motivating him to look at the role of rumination as a strategy that had failed.

## USING CASE CONCEPTUALIZATION TO DEVELOP A TREATMENT PLAN

Case conceptualization, which has been discussed in Chapter 4, and treatment planning are linked together in emotional schema therapy. During the initial stage of therapy, the therapist and patient are collecting information about the patient's beliefs about emotion; typical maladaptive coping strategies; the origin of some of these beliefs about emotion; and the impact of these beliefs and strategies on depression, anxiety, anger, interpersonal relationships, motivation, and work. This is an ongoing process throughout therapy, as new insights are gained about the impact of emotional schemas and how they are currently maintained. A general outline of a case conceptualization is provided in Chapter 4, and a model for case conceptualization is provided in Figure 4.3.

Consider the following example of a patient whose emotional schemas affected her interpersonal functioning and self-care. Veronica was a married woman with a long history of marital conflict. She feared sexual intimacy with her husband, who had betrayed her on several occasions and who had indicated from the beginning of the marriage that he didn't think he wanted to be married. Her beliefs about her emotions (sadness, anger, confusion, anxiety) were that her emotions did not make sense; that she had to get rid of these feelings immediately, or they would go out of control; that she did not have a right to these feelings, since she was not a "good wife"; that no one would understand her; that she could not express these emotions, or she would never stop crying; and that others would not feel the same way. Veronica indicated that her mother, a pediatrician, never had time for her feelings and would tell her, "You shouldn't complain about anything. Do you realize the kind of problems that the children I see have?" She was taught that her feelings were a burden to her mother, that she was selfish and childish, and that her mother felt disgusted with her "neediness." As a child she often felt lonely, and during early adolescence she developed both anorexia and bulimia nervosa. She believed that her mother paid little attention to her eating disorders and claimed, "You are only trying to get attention from me." She described several years in college when she abused drugs and had numerous sexual partners with whom there was little emotional intimacy. She thought that sexual intimacy would give her emotional closeness, but it seldom gave her any real emotional satisfaction. It further confirmed her belief that she was there to satisfy the emotional needs of others and that no one really knew her. At present, she was still married and living with her husband—but she was also carrying on an extramarital affair with a married man, with whom she saw no future. She would ruminate about her situation, but was afraid of making a change, since "this is the best that I can get." She was well thought of at her job, but was reluctant to push for advancement, thinking that she was undeserving of it. She had learned that she had no right to her emotions, and therefore she felt entitled to little else in life.

After several sessions of therapy and evaluation, the therapist developed a case conceptualization with Veronica, and a diagram of this is shown in Figure 5.2. The diagram illustrates how she learned about her emotions while growing up; which maladaptive strategies she had used as a child

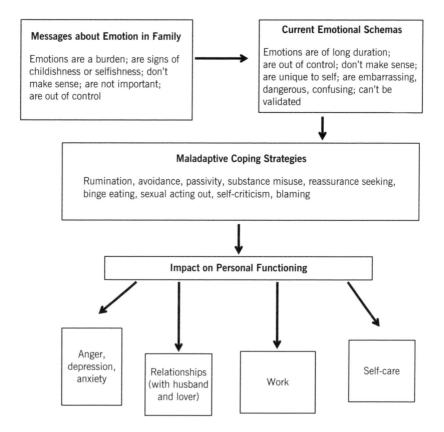

**FIGURE 5.2.** Diagram of Veronica's case conceptualization.

(isolating herself, suppressing her feelings, binge-eating, restricting food, perfectionism about weight and appearance); and how her beliefs about emotion and her belief that she was undeserving of love led first to her sexual acting out and substance misuse in college, and then to her feeling that she was trapped in a loveless marriage and an impossible extramarital affair. The goals of therapy, then, would be for her to examine these beliefs about emotions, modify her beliefs about deserving love and attention, find more adaptive strategies to handle the issues of her marriage, develop a "bill of rights" and a list of needs, use problem solving to move forward, learn to accept herself as a fallible human being who did not need to be perfect, and develop strategies to cope with powerful emotions when they occurred.

The treatment plan is developed directly out of the case conceptualization. Beginning with assessment and with socializing the patient to therapy, the plan progresses through identifying and modifying emotional schemas, eliminating problematic strategies of coping with emotion, developing more adaptive emotional schemas and coping strategies, identifying values and virtues to direct behavior and choices, and using positive psychology to build a more emotionally full life. As emphasized throughout this book, the ultimate goal is not necessarily to feel better; it is to have a more complete life.

## SUMMARY

Socialization of the patient to the emotional schema model is an ongoing process, sometimes continuing throughout all phases of therapy. The case conceptualization is often the first time the patient has understood that his or her beliefs about their emotions were determined by problematic socialization experiences, which then set the patient on a course of unhelpful strategies to get needs met or to cope with emotions. These patterns have continued through relationships, work, self-care, and other areas of life, and they may have led to a sense of hopelessness about having a more meaningful life. Indeed, the case conceptualization may be one of the most validating experiences that the patient may have: It may indicate that someone else understands, that the patient's emotions do make sense, that he or she can talk about emotions without decompensating, and that there is a plan to change.

In the chapters of Part III (Chapters 6–9), I focus on a select group of emotional schema dimensions: validation, duration, control, guilt, acceptance, simplistic view of emotion (intolerance of ambivalence), and values. Other dimensions, such as comprehensibility, numbness, rationality, consensus, rumination, expression, and blame, are discussed throughout the book in descriptions of various problems that patients present.

# PART III

## SPECIFIC INTERVENTIONS FOR EMOTIONAL SCHEMAS

# CHAPTER 6

# The Centrality of Validation

We must learn to weep for the plague, not just cure it.
—MIGUEL DE UNAMUNO

The concept of shared emotion and suffering is part of what the Spanish philosopher and novelist Miguel de Unamuno (1921/1954) described in a book titled *Tragic Sense of Life*. Contrasting the approach of rationality and pragmatism with the experience of shared suffering—and the inevitability of suffering in life—de Unamuno told a story of a young man (representing rationality and pragmatism) confronting an old man (representing the tragic vision). The old man is sitting by the side of the road, weeping. The young man says, "Old man. Why do you weep?" The old man replies, "My son has died. I weep over the death of my son." The young man, in his rationality, responds, "But weeping avails nothing. Your son is dead." And the old man replies, "I weep precisely because weeping avails nothing. We must learn how to weep for the plague, not just cure it." de Unamuno believed that life is not simply about problem solving, not simply about utility, and not simply about rationalizing away the inevitable suffering of human beings. For de Unamuno, the "tragic sense" is a world view acknowledging that terrible things happen, that they can be shared and witnessed, that catharsis is part of being a witness to the difficulties each of us will experience, and that there is nobility in the feelings of strangers. Tragedy, according to de Unamuno, is not pessimism, and it is not morose. It is a recognition that we weep because things matter, and that we like to know we are not alone.

Validation is the recognition that while it is hard enough to suffer, it is worse to suffer alone. In emotional schema therapy, the therapist recognizes the essential nature of validation: In the therapeutic relationship (and in all other meaningful relationships), solving problems may first begin with sharing the problems, and with recognizing that the person who suffers also needs to feel heard, understood, and ultimately cared for. Validation is the means by which the therapist will help develop the patient's sense of emotional safety. That is, the patient can believe, "My vulnerability is safe here. I can trust this person with my feelings. This person wants to know me, to take care of me, even to protect me." Validation is a fundamental component of all attachment. People who are vulnerable want their problems solved, but they also seek safety and understanding.

This is what de Unamuno meant by weeping for the plague, not just curing it. Certainly no one will expect that a therapist will literally weep for a patient, or that the therapist will suffer the same feelings that the patient is sharing. But if the patient is talking about his feelings, weeping, and openly letting emotions out, then the therapist needs to create a sense that what is said is being truly heard—that the emotions have registered with the therapist, that there is some mirroring, some reflection, some connection. The patient will want to believe that the therapist has some idea about what it is like to feel what is being felt, and that those feelings are respected. Too quick or facile "disputation" of the content of what is being said may communicate, "We need to move away from your feelings as quickly as we can." But giving the patient time and space to express the emotions, even to sort through what is being felt—in other words, to give the patient opportunities to "let the emotions happen"—communicates that "Your feelings matter. Your experience is important. I have time for you. I am here for you." No one wants to be rushed through a painful expression. One wants to be heard—and cared for. To share one's suffering is to trust the other person.

This chapter examines what validation is—and what it is not. It reviews some common misconceptions that patients and therapists have about validation, and ways in which they can get stuck in seeking validation to the exclusion of change. Just as therapy may involve both acceptance of what is given and the possibility of change, validation involves both recognition and respect for the feelings and meanings of the present moment, and the exploration of new ways of coping, interpreting, and feeling. It is this dialectic—an apparent contradiction for some—that can lead to impasses in the process of change.

## WHAT DO WE MEAN BY "VALIDATION"?

"Validation" (finding the truth in what we feel and think) is the fulcrum between "empathy" (recognizing the feeling that another person has) and "compassion" (feeling *with* and *for* another person, caring about the suffering of that person, and extending kindness toward that person) (Leahy, 2001, 2005c, 2011b). Many years ago, Carl Rogers (1951) described the qualities of "unconditional positive regard"—a therapist's ability to reflect the understanding and acceptance of a patient's feelings, so as to create an emotionally safe environment for change. In the emotional schema model, validation includes unconditional positive regard, but it goes further: It encompasses a consideration of what invalidation means to an individual, the individual's standards for validation, and the consequences of being invalidated.

When I empathize with you, I am able to identify the feeling that you are having—for example, "It sounds like you are feeling sad and lonely." When I validate you, I not only identify your feeling, but I also communicate that I understand the reasons why you are feeling the way you feel: "I can see that you are sad and lonely, and I can understand that it makes sense, given the loss of the relationship and how much it means to you to connect with people you care about."

Finding the "truth" in other persons' feelings—even if this truth involves "distorted" thoughts or "biased" sets of rules, or even if the other persons' suffering has resulted from their own pride or jealousy—allows us as listeners to bear witness to the fact that the other persons' suffering means something to us. Validation is about meaning, and no one ever wants to feel that he or she is the only person who can understand that meaning. Meanings are to be shared and understood by others; meanings are the basis of conversation. This is why people struggle to make their meanings clear. It is why they say, "Do you know what I mean?" In validation, we listeners are the witnesses who see the speakers' "truth," and we are affected by their suffering. For the persons who are sharing their suffering, it is not enough for us simply to understand the content of what is being said; it is not enough to paraphrase or to repeat back verbatim what the speakers have told us. The speakers may want something more: They may want to know that we understand "what it is like to be going through this." Validation is not simply a recording of "facts" (i.e., "This is what happened"). It includes some sense that a listener understands what an experience was like, what it felt like, and what it meant. It conveys that the listener can imagine what it would be like for him or her to have this experience, to stand in the shoes of the speaker. It is a temporary joining of minds, relinquishing the barrier between self and other.

A speaker can express emotions directly (talk about feelings, cry, complain, describe, rejoice)—but if this expression falls on deaf ears, if the expression is not heard, reflected, understood, cared for, or experienced in some way by the listener, and given shared meaning, then the expression has not led to the connection that validation gives. Validation does not merely involve the *recording* of an expression ("I see that you are upset"). Validation is *responsive* to what is heard: It hears the feeling and the meaning; it respects the moment that the person is in. Validation is part of the attachment system. That is, it shares elements with the process of a caregiver's picking up an infant as the infant cries. It shows connection; it demonstrates care. Validation gives the speaker the sense that "You have heard me. You understand how I feel. You care." Validation creates a safe emotional environment—one where the speaker's suffering (or joy) is respected, the meaning is grasped, and the speaker no longer feels alone.

## ATTACHMENT THEORY AND VALIDATION

Bowlby (1969, 1973) and Ainsworth, Blehar, Waters, and Wall (1978) proposed that infants are innately predisposed to form and maintain attachment to a single figure, and that interruptions in the attachment bond will activate behavioral systems that seek completion until attachment is secured. Bowlby's ethological model of attachment stressed the evolutionary implications of attachment in establishing proximity to adults who could protect infants, feed them, and socialize them in appropriate behaviors, thereby assuring their survival. Attachment theorists further elaborated this model to emphasize the importance for an infant or child of establishing a sense of *security* in attachment—not simply proximity (Sroufe & Waters, 1977). This security entails the predictability of the caregiver's responsiveness to the child.

Bowlby proposed that security (or insecurity) in attachment is established through the development of an "internal working model," or cognitive representation, of a reliable (or unreliable) attachment figure. Specifically, an internal working model for a securely attached infant includes confidence that the caregiver will respond to cries of distress, will be responsive in soothing the infant through reciprocal interactions, and will be predictable in providing positive (rather than punitive) interactions. Greater responsiveness of the caregiver to the infant's expressed needs sets the foundation for a more secure representation of functioning in the world (Feeney & Thrush, 2010; Mikulincer et al., 2001). To know that the parental figure responds with care to one's suffering is to begin to believe that the world is predictable and safe. The assumption guiding attachment theory is that this internal working model—established in early childhood—will affect subsequent attachment experiences with other individuals in the person's life. It is this responsiveness, as described by Bowlby and others, that marks the early foundation of validation schemas.

Ainsworth and her colleagues and successors have differentiated four attachment styles: "secure," "anxious," "avoidant," and "disorganized" (Ainsworth et al., 1978; De Wolff & van IJzendoorn, 1997). Other classification systems that have been employed differentiate three types: "secure," "avoidant," and "ambivalent" (Troy & Sroufe, 1987; Urban,

Carlson, Egeland, & Sroufe, 1991). Research on attachment styles suggests that early childhood attachment is predictive of social functioning in middle childhood and early adulthood—specifically, peer relationships, depression, aggression, dependency, and social competence (Ainsworth et al., 1978; Arend, Gove, & Sroufe, 1979; Cassidy, 1995; De Wolff & van IJzendoorn, 1997; Elicker, Englund, & Sroufe, 1992; Englund, Kuo, Puig, & Collins, 2012; Kerns, 1994; Urban et al., 1991). Adults who classify themselves as "secure" describe their early experience with their caregivers as one of responsiveness to emotions (Hazan & Shaver, 1987). Although attachment experiences may have long-term implications, it is also possible that there may be genetic differences in attachment styles related to inherited personality traits (Donnellan, Burt, Levendosky, & Klump, 2008). The importance of attachment experience and responsiveness is a central component of mentalization theory as advanced by Fonagy, Bateman, and others (e.g., Bateman & Fonagy, 2004; Fonagy, 1989).

The ability to represent the mental states of self and others is a reciprocal process of reflection and learning, according to mentalization theory, and is an important component of self-regulation. These early attachment dynamics are viewed by mentalization theorists as central to the emergence of borderline personality disorder and other forms of psychopathology.

It is argued here that validation in meaningful relationships is reflective of attachment issues. First, during the process of forming and maintaining attachment during early childhood, the rudiments of validation include a caregiver's responsiveness to a child's distress, which reinforces the child's mental representations that "My feelings make sense to others" and "Others hear me." If the child has a working model that "My attachment figure is unreliable, rejecting, or indifferent," then problematic schemas will develop about validation and invalidation. For example, the working model "My feelings don't matter to others" will lead to a continued sense that "People will invalidate me," "People will be dismissive of me," and "My feelings are experienced alone and without the support of others."

Second, responsive soothing of the child's feelings by the caregiver encourages the child to believe, "My distressed feelings can be soothed." Initially, this soothing occurs through the caregiver's attention and reassurance, but it is later internalized by the child in self-calming and optimistic self-statements. Such statements eventually become an internal working model, in Bowlby's sense—an internal representation that "My feelings make sense and can be calmed." However, if the internal working model is that "My feelings will not be soothed," then negative emotional schemas may be created and activated, such as "My feelings will go on indefinitely," "My feelings are out of control," or "My feelings are dangerous."

Third, the child's communication of feelings to the caregiver becomes an opportunity not only for expressing feelings, but for the caregiver to link emotional states to external events that "cause" the feelings (e.g., "You're upset because your brother hit you"). This attempt by the caregiver to comprehend the cause of the child's feelings, and to share this with the child, can also assist the child in differentiating these feelings ("It sounds like you are angry and hurt") and in constructing a theory of mind that can be applied to both self and others. Indeed, without an adequate theory of mind, the child will be impaired in showing empathy, validation, and compassion toward others—and will be unable to soothe the feelings of other people. Moreover, without an adequate theory of his or her own mind and emotions, the individual will be impaired in recognizing, differentiating, and controlling these emotions.

Patients in therapy enter the therapeutic relationship with different adult attachment styles—secure, anxious, avoidant, or disorganized, in the typology of Ainsworth and her followers. The anxious attachment style, characterized by clinging behaviors and need for reassurance, may result from and cause fears that validation will not be obtained. Individuals with an anxious attachment style may have idiosyncratic beliefs about validation (e.g., "You have to feel what I feel to understand me"), and may fear that the therapist will become critical or withdrawn. Nevertheless, these anxious individuals still will seek validation and eventual attachment to the therapist. In contrast, the avoidant attachment style will be reflected in wariness and distance; patients with this style will avoid closer contact and openness in the therapeutic relationship—as they do in other relationships. These individuals may avoid disappointment by hoping for less and avoid rejection by sharing less. Patients with a disorganized attachment style may have difficulty identifying needs—or may escalate the expression of these needs, for fear that they will not be heard, and therefore the needs will never be met. Conflicts in earlier attachment experiences may result in vacillation between seeking validation (often through escalation of demands, complaining, or emotional expression) and wariness of validation (since the attachment figure is seen as unpredictable).

## META-EMOTION AND VALIDATION

As mentioned in earlier chapters, John Gottman and his colleagues have proposed that parents differ in their beliefs and values about emotional experience and expression, which they describes as "meta-emotion philosophies" (e.g., Gottman et al., 1996). For example, some parents view their children's experience and expression of "unpleasant" emotions—such as anger, sadness, or anxiety—as negative events that must be avoided. Such emotions are to be suppressed or avoided, and only positive emotions or neutral emotions are tolerated. These negative emotional views are communicated through interactions in which a parent will be dismissive of, critical of, or overwhelmed by a child's emotions. For example, a dismissive parent may say, "It's no big deal. You'll get over it"; a critical parent may say, "You're acting like a big baby. Grow up"; and an overwhelmed parent may say, "I have my own problems, so I can't deal with your problems." In any of these three cases, the child's emotions are invalidated, dismissed, and marginalized.

In contrast to these problematic styles of emotional socialization, Gottman and colleagues (1996) have identified an "emotion-coaching" style that entails the ability to recognize even low levels of emotional intensity, to use even "unpleasant" emotions as opportunities for intimacy and support, to assist a child in labeling and differentiating emotions, and to engage in problem solving with the child. The emotion-coaching parent sounds a lot like a parent using Rogers's client-centered approach, with unconditional positive regard, acceptance, and exploration; added to this reflective and empathic listening, however, is the willingness to differentiate and label various emotions, while also suggesting that the child can utilize problem solving to cope with difficulties. Parents who adapt the emotion-coaching style are more likely to have children who will be able to soothe their own emotions. That is, emotion coaching assists in emotional self-regulation.

Furthermore, children of parents using emotion coaching are more effective in interactions with their peers, even when appropriate behavior with peers involves the inhibition of emotional expression. Thus children of parents utilizing emotional coaching are more advanced in "emotional intelligence"—knowing when to express and when to inhibit expression, and knowing how to process and regulate their own emotions (Eisenberg et al., 1998; Eisenberg & Fabes, 1994; Mayer & Salovey, 1997; Michalik et al., 2007). Emotional coaching does not simply reinforce a cathartic style in children; rather, it allows them to identify, differentiate, validate, self-soothe, and problem-solve. It assists in theory of mind regarding emotion. An emotional schema therapist helps a patient identify current and past experiences of invalidation, while helping the patient experience validation in the therapeutic relationship. However, because many (if not most) patients have experienced dismissive, punitive, and contemptuous responses when seeking validation from others, the therapist will help focus the patient on what the experience of invalidation has meant in the past (e.g., "My emotions are a burden") and why attempts at validation in the current therapeutic relationship may appear to fail (e.g., "You are taking their side").

## WHY DOES VALIDATION MATTER?

As indicated in Chapter 3, our research indicated that invalidation was a key predictor of depression (Leahy, Tirch, & Melwani, 2012), and that among the 14 emotional schema dimensions, low validation was the best predictor of marital discord. It was also the key predictor for alcohol and other substance misuse, and was the third best predictor for borderline personality. Validation was related to 12 of the other 13 dimensions of emotional schemas. A multiple-regression analysis indicated that the best predictors of validation among the other dimensions were blame, duration, and incomprehensibility. That is, people who believed that they were validated were less likely to blame others, less likely to believe that their emotions would last indefinitely, and less likely to believe that their emotions were incomprehensible. Validation thus appears to be a central component of emotional schemas, psychopathology, and interpersonal relationships.

My own experience as a therapist reflects the importance of validation—and of its failure. Some years ago, armed with my cognitive therapy techniques, I found myself at an impasse in working with a rather inhibited man who was trying to figure out what to do about his job and his intimate relationships. As I used one technique after another to identify his automatic thoughts, categorize them, examine the costs and benefits, and consider the evidence, I found that he withdrew more and more from our interaction. My initial response, of course, was to think that he was "resistant" and (naively on my part) to push against this "resistance"; inevitably, this led to more withdrawal. I was getting nowhere—but, more importantly, he was getting nowhere. So I asked him, "It seems like you are withdrawing from our discussions. What is going on for you?" He looked at me, somewhat puzzled (since this kind of statement was unlike me), and he observed, "You don't seem to be listening to what I am saying. You are just using your techniques."

He was right. I was making a fetish of techniques.

As we discussed what the experience was like for him, he commented that he felt all alone in the room, as if no one could hear him. We explored how this experience was similar to other experiences he had had. He realized that his mother had been very dominant and critical, and that she considered her viewpoint the only valid viewpoint. He also said that he had a hard time sorting out his feelings and thoughts, that he would feel anxious and get blocked, and that the cognitive therapy techniques reminded him of his mother's criticisms. He also observed that his girlfriend also seemed a little domineering, which made it hard for him to connect with her.

I wish I could tell this man how grateful I am for setting me straight. He changed me as a therapist. I realized—as he made clear for me—that in order for me to be heard, he had to be heard. His feelings, his thoughts, his confusion, and his inhibition were all that mattered in our discussions. I had to learn to hold myself back and give him time and space to find what he was feeling. I had to set aside the agenda, set aside the techniques, enter into his world, and accept his confusion; I needed to recognize that the route from here to there was not always a straight line, and that I was not the one drawing the lines. I followed his lead. He could now speak because I was more willing to listen.

I must confess that this was not the only time I realized that I could be invalidating. Indeed, even when I tried to be validating, it could come across as invalidating. But what I have learned from my interactions with this patient and others is that exploring the invalidation, recognizing it, admitting to it, sharing it, and even acknowledging my own blind spots is validating. And once these patients believed that I would validate them, they could trust me.

## THE PATIENT'S PAST AND CURRENT INVALIDATING ENVIRONMENTS

### Invalidation in Childhood

The emotional schema model recognizes the importance of early experiences of emotional socialization. It shares with the theory behind DBT (Linehan, Bohus, & Lynch, 2007), with mentalization theory (Fonagy, 2002), and with the model underlying compassion-focused therapy (Gilbert, 2009) the recognition of the importance of emotional invalidation, lack of responsiveness, and lack of compassion in the emergence of problematic beliefs about self and others. While these other approaches clearly highlight the importance of invalidating environments, the emotional schema model is particularly focused on the beliefs about emotions and others that are activated as a result of these experiences—that is, on the social-cognitive content of invalidation. For example, once the therapist has identified the patient's problematic negative views of emotions (e.g., "I cannot get validated," "My emotions are shameful," "My emotions are not similar to those of others"), the therapist and patient can reflect on how these beliefs about emotion were learned during childhood. The therapist can ask, "When you were a child, how did your mother [father] respond to you when you were upset?" and "If you were upset, would you turn to your mother or father?" Patients reporting negative emotional schemas often describe invalidating emotional environments. The following are typical responses:

"My father was distant—never there, it seems—and when he was there he was cold, like he had no interest in us."
"My mother was always talking on the phone or going out to see her friends. She made me feel like I was interrupting her."
"I was always worried about my mother, who had so many problems with my father, who was always angry. There was no room for my emotions because I had to calm her down."
"My mother was a pediatrician, and when I would talk about my problems, she made me feel guilty. She would say, 'Don't you realize that your problems don't compare to those of the kids I am helping at work?'"

These invalidating and dismissive comments still seem to be painful for patients to recall.

The therapist can then inquire, "Given what you describe as these invalidating and dismissive comments by your parent, what did this make you think and feel?" The patient with the cold and absent father thought, "No one is interested in my feelings—or in me." The patient with the mother who was always on the phone thought, "People don't care about me unless I make them know that it really is terrible. I have to make myself heard." Veronica, the patient with the dismissive pediatrician mother (see Chapter 5), thought, "I must be selfish and spoiled to have the needs that I have." The range of feelings is also important—from anger, anxiety, shame, guilt, sadness, and helplessness to indifference, resignation, and confusion. Such patients never say they felt better.

In addition to the experience of dismissive, invalidating, and critical interactions, the therapist can inquire about what the patient did to be heard or to get his or her emotions validated. Some patients with dismissive parents (who were too busy for their emotions) describe how they would try to get heard by complaining of physical symptoms, creating emergencies, throwing tantrums, or getting into trouble. One patient, who seemed to intensify her emotions on a regular basis, described how she tried to be "the good girl"—dressing in the "right way," being well mannered, and trying to please her mother. When that would not work, she would create emergencies—acting as if she was extremely upset, crying, or complaining loudly. Another patient described withdrawing into dolls, fantasy, and reading books where "things were safe." Another patient channeled his efforts into being a good student and getting recognition from his teachers. Finally, a patient who was ignored by his father and bullied by his peers described how he took on an unemotional philosophical stance, almost sounding like a junior Stoic practicing indifference. In therapy, he would appear rational and cordial, but not particularly emotional, while describing how his wife complained that he was out of touch with her emotionally.

## Compensations for Invalidating Environments

Compensations for invalidating environments (either the childhood environments described above, or the current environments described below) fall into several categories: (1) seeking alternative sources of validation, such as another parent, a relative, or a friend; (2) attempting to please and impress the invalidating parent in order to be accepted; (3) escalating the expression of emotion; (4) somatizing in order to get reassurance; (5) retreating into fantasy; (6) engaging in excessive sexual acting out in order to feel cared for and wanted; (7) intellectualizing and denying emotional needs; (8) misusing alcohol or drugs in order to self-soothe; and (9) reversing attachment roles by caring for others, especially the invalidating parent (reverse parenting). Each of these "adaptations" has implications for psychopathology, such as dependency, emotional dysregulation, over-dramatic displays of emotion, health anxiety, repressive emotional style, alexithymia, substance use disorders, and self-defeating relationships.

Let us consider these various compensations for invalidation. First, the individual may seek out other sources of validation. Some children may recognize early that their parents are not good at validating, but that a grandparent or friend may be helpful. They shift their attachment interests to these other people. It can be helpful for the patient to identify the people during childhood (or currently) who have been (or are) sought out for emotional support. Having alternative sources of validation can help the patient realize that the invalidation was distinctive to a parent and cannot be generalized to all others. In addition, identifying validating and compassionate figures in the patient's life can be helpful in invoking a compassionate representation—a process discussed later. However, "validating" figures in the patient's life can also be problematic figures. For example, a woman described how her father had angry outbursts and her mother was self-absorbed with her own health anxiety. As a young woman, she turned to and eventually married a man who was very supportive, "protective," and physically affectionate. She believed that she could get her attachment needs met through him. However, he also became alcoholic, controlling, possessive, and demanding, leading her to feel trapped in her desperate attachment to "the only person who understood me." Not all "validating" figures are helpful choices.

Second, the child may work hard at trying to please the parent in order to get validated. For example, one woman described how her somewhat narcissistic, self-preoccupied mother was dismissive and contemptuous of her emotional needs. Recognizing that her mother would not validate her, she attempted to impress her mother with dressing in "pretty girl" outfits, getting good grades in school, and trying to fit into the social set that her mother valued. Rather than getting validated for her emotions or her own individual identity, she realized that she could only get validated for reflecting her mother's narcissistic ideals. As an adult, she became vulnerable to pleasing exploitative, narcissistic people, including her first husband and other family members. The therapist can help the patient identify such compensations for invalidation by asking the patient, "If you believed that you could not get validated for the way you felt, did you try to get approval for other qualities or other behaviors? How did this work out?" Moreover, the therapist can inquire whether today there are similar ways that the patient seeks validation.

A third common response to invalidation for many children (and adults) is to escalate the intensity of expression. Temper tantrums, yelling, making threats, stealing, disobedience, and other problematic behaviors are often responses to the belief "I am not being heard." For example, a young man described his childhood as a fruitless attempt to get validation—or any attention—from his father, who was preoccupied with his business pursuits. As a result of this failure to be recognized, the boy would throw temper tantrums, "partly to punish my father and partly to get any attention." The therapist asked him, "What was the most positive memory you have of your father growing up?" He replied, "I remember when I was about 5 years old and I went into my parents' bedroom, and my father had me on his lap in bed, and he was bouncing me up and down." As an adult, he shifted his attempt for validation to fulfilling his father's dreams about work by becoming an academic, only to learn once again that his father only had limited capacity to recognize and appreciate the individuality of his son. Similar to many people who fail to obtain validation from parents, he viewed the deficiency as residing in himself (not attractive, not interesting, not worthwhile) rather than in the other person. He had come to believe that he lacked the validity for validation; he was not good enough.

Escalation of validation seeking is a common problem for patients who are often described as "emotionally dysregulated." Screaming or yelling is often a response to the belief, "You don't hear me." Unfortunately, people who escalate their yelling are generally dismissed as either "irrational" or not even "worth being heard," further reinforcing their belief that they cannot be validated. The therapist can ask the patient who escalates the intensity of validation seeking:

> "I get a sense that you don't think that people hear you or care about how you feel. Is it possible that you have felt this way many times in the past—for example, as a child? Have you felt this way in other relationships? Do you sometimes feel this way with me as well?"

Or:

> "Perhaps you yell because you believe that this is the only way to be heard, the only way to be taken seriously. When you yell, do people validate you or do they turn away? Do some people yell back? Have you lost friends because of this? If we could find a more effective way for being heard, would that be something that you might want to do?"

Another problematic style of intensifying validation is repeatedly attempting to connect with people who have shown indifference. For example, one young woman repeatedly text-messaged friends whom she had alienated, leading them to feel that she was stalking them. Other individuals may e-mail or text angry and profane messages. These problematic styles of validation seeking lead to further rejection, further depression, further isolation—and, ironically, escalation of the same behavior to seek validation.

Fourth, some individuals focus on somatic complaints, either real or imagined. Frequent childhood absence from school, vague physical complaints, or "undiagnosed" ailments may reflect indirect attempts to seek attachment and emotional soothing. For example, one elderly man with a long history of hypochondriasis described how his wife was dismissive of any emotional expression: "She has always been cold, a bit formal, even cold toward the children. She has no interest in the grandchildren." Initially, he would seek out emotional support from his wife for his vague physical complaints and health worries, but she was dismissive and often contemptuous. He described that he often felt that visiting doctors for examinations was a way in which he socialized: "It's like they invite me in to lunch. They care about me. It's a way for me to get that tender loving care that I don't get at home." Seeking attention for physical complaints may often lead to some support and validation, but it is likely to result in partners' and friends' discounting any medical concerns as "one more false alarm." Moreover, rumination and preoccupation about physical problems will only add to the anxiety and depression that the patient experiences. It is helpful to validate the need for attention and "tender loving care," while suggesting that preoccupation with physical concerns will only add further problems. The need for attention can be obviated by encouraging self-validation and self-compassion as discussed later.

Fifth, some patients replace validation from others with fantasies about an ideal or exciting world. This, of course, is less threatening, since one is not likely to be rejected in a fantasy world. One patient described how she invented an imaginary alter ego when she was a girl, to replace the need to receive validation from her critical and abusive mother. This alter ego—an imagined audience for her—became a repository for comfort. She could also talk to her dolls, since she felt that she had a special connection with them. As a teenager, she replaced these audiences with her cat. The therapist asked, "When you were a teenager, did you think there was anyone that you could talk to, share your feelings with?" The patient replied, "Definitely my cat. I would come home and talk to her and feel like she understood me. I think I'll get better when I get a cat." A man with avoidant personality disorder described how he felt he could get lost in books of fiction, especially adventure books: "I feel I can take on a different personality in these books, imagining myself as part of the adventure. I feel respected and valued in these fantasies." He described how he could daydream for hours about escaping. His relationship with his wife was one of parallel partnership—never having sex, seldom talking about anything important, just going through the motions of acting as if they were a happy couple—while he had an affair with another woman.

Sexual acting out is a sixth means by which some people seek out a replacement for validation. A man who described his wife as dismissive and manipulative would regularly go to prostitutes for massages and sex.

He claimed that they understood his needs and didn't give him a hard time. When he was not visiting prostitutes, he would see his "girlfriend," whom he "helped out financially" by paying for her rent. He claimed that she was someone he could talk to without being rejected. Another man, who was ostensibly religious, would hire a prostitute for conversation rather than sex; he would arrange to have dinner delivered to a hotel room, where he would talk to her and try to impress her with his intelligence. A woman whose parents drank heavily and were dismissive of her feelings indicated that she would seek out anonymous sexual encounters with men, to feel wanted and to feel attracted. She knew that these relationships were dead-end relationships, but "It's easier this way; I won't get hurt."

A seventh type of compensation for invalidation is intellectualizing and denying emotional needs. These individuals believe that their emotions will never be accepted, understood, or cared for by others; as a consequence, they adapt a self-denying, overly rational position regarding emotions. For example, a woman whose alcoholic husband was unwilling to have sex because of his erectile dysfunction began cognitive therapy by claiming that she must be too needy: "After all, we have been married for almost 25 years, and people our age usually don't have sex. Maybe I am too needy." This self-denying intellectualization prevented her from legitimizing her frustration and kept her stuck in a self-defeating relationship. As she later validated her needs for sex and affection, she began to assert herself, which finally led to significant changes in her husband's drinking and improvement in their intimate relationship. A man described earlier who complained about the lack of support from his parents for his difficulty in finding a job withdrew into an overly rational strategy: "I know that I must be irrational to think that I need understanding and support. I should be able to get by without that." When asked what he thought about sharing his emotions or feeling emotions, he replied, "Emotions are a waste of time. They get you nowhere." He added, "When people see that you are emotional, they take advantage of you." This retreat into an antiemotional, overly rational position is not uncommon and may be one reason why some of these individuals seek out cognitive-behavioral therapy. One patient was surprised that I was even talking about emotions and validation: "I thought this was a rational approach. I didn't think that we would be wasting our time with emotions."

The antiemotional, overly rational response to a history of invalidation can be a difficult barrier to therapy, since patients may try to use cognitive therapy against any emotional experience. For example, patients may say, "I know I don't need that; I just *prefer* something," as if humans do not have desires and needs that are universal. "I know it shouldn't bother me that my husband isn't interested in sex. I am being too emotional, too needy." The emotional schema therapist can reframe the goals of therapy as "knowing what you need and getting your needs met," and can point out that "emotions may tell us about what we need, what is missing, what to ask for." Therapy is not an exercise in rearranging the true and false statements in a logical "truth table." It is the process of patients' discovering the truth about who they are, what they need, and where to get those needs met. By overemphasizing rationality, a patient risks ignoring the needs to which emotions give a voice. The therapist can say, "You can't get your needs met if you don't allow yourself to feel their absence."

The eighth response to invalidation is reliance on drugs, alcohol, or food to self-soothe. Our research on emotional schemas indicated that the best predictors of a history of alcohol dependence in a linear regression were validation, control, and blame (Leahy, 2010b). Thus individuals who believed that their emotions were not validated or were out of control, or who blamed others, were more likely to report a history of alcohol dependence. In the current context of compensation for invalidation, some individuals will rely on substance misuse or binge eating to self-soothe, since they believe that they are unable to gain acceptance from others. Research on risk factors for adolescent substance abuse indicates that family, social, and school connectedness (reverse-scored) are predictors of abuse (Sale, Sambrano, Springer, & Turner, 2003). Indeed, the importance of validation and social connectedness in the treatment of alcohol and drug misuse may be one of the reasons why many of these patients can benefit from group therapy or Twelve-Step programs, which emphasize sharing experiences, reducing a sense of isolation, and validating the difficulties involved. Affiliative behavior increases oxytocin levels, and increasing oxytocin levels decreases vulnerability to alcohol or drug misuse (McGregor & Bowen, 2012). Individuals who self-soothe with alcohol, drugs, or binge eating may be satisfying emotional needs not met through validation by activating oxytocin levels.

Finally, a ninth response to invalidation is compulsive caring for others, especially, reverse parenting. Bowlby (1969, 1973) proposed many years ago that disruptions in early attachment may lead to compulsive caretaking of others. Individuals with insecure attachments may adapt by directing their attachment behavior to taking care of other people—including reverse parenting (children's taking care of parents) and compulsive caregiving for other people (spouse/partner, children, strangers, or even animals). This redirected affiliative behavior may provide the soothing effects of social connectedness that are missing from lack of validation, but may also serve the function of assuring the dependence of others on the self—and thereby "assuring" that others will not leave. Moreover, focusing on the needs of others may obscure the ability to focus on one's own needs. A woman who experienced years of invalidation from her father, and later from her husband, focused excessively on attempting to soothe every negative mood that her daughter with borderline personality disorder expressed. She believed that to be a good mother meant that she had to take care of all of the needs that her daughter experienced, and that it was catastrophic if her daughter was unhappy. The emotional schema approach was to shift her away from a dichotomous view of her daughter's needs and her needs, and to help her balance her self-care with reasonable attention to her daughter while establishing workable boundaries. She acknowledged that she felt that she was selfish when she established boundaries or worked on her own needs, and that this was the message that her mother had conveyed when she was a girl asking for support from her mother.

## The Current Invalidating Environment

The current invalidating environment is also relevant, since it may reinforce negative views of emotion. As indicated in a study described in Chapter 3, partners in marital or cohabiting relationships described the negative responses of their partners toward their emotions. These perceived negative responses of partners accounted for almost 50% of the variance in relationship satisfaction and were also highly predictive of depression. The therapist can use the RESS (see Chapter 4, Figure 4.2) to inquire about the current emotional interactions that the patient is experiencing: "When you are upset, how does your partner respond to you? Does your partner make you feel guilty about your emotions? Does your partner help you understand that others would feel the same way?" and other questions related to the specific dimensions of emotional schemas. For example, the hypochondriacal older man described earlier said that his wife would tell him he would never change, he was being foolish, he should "get over it," and he was "bizarre" for feeling the way he did. Another patient described her husband as verbally abusive and contemptuous of her emotions: He would say, "You are just being a big baby. You have nothing to complain about." Another patient initially said that her husband was supportive and encouraging, but on closer inquiry she observed that he would say, "Don't worry, it's no big thing; you will get over it." Until examining this, she did not realize that she actually felt he was being dismissive and somewhat condescending, even if his intentions were positive.

The therapist can inquire about the nature of social support: "When you are feeling down, to whom do you turn for support? How do they respond? How do you feel about their response? What is missing? What would you like them to say?" In addition, the therapist can inquire about significant individuals in the patient's life who do not validate him or her: "Is there anyone that is part of your life that you would be reluctant to seek validation and support from? How have they responded? How did that make you feel?" Sometimes patients may seek support from individuals who are continually critical, dismissive and punitive—and, unfortunately, often these can include their spouses or partners. Initially, the therapist can suggest that the patients may choose to refrain from seeking validation from critical people, and either seek validation from those who are supportive or validate themselves. However, the therapist can also suggest that couple work—focused on the emotional schemas and responses of the other partner—may help in developing a more validating environment. For example, a patient complained that her husband was aloof, overly intellectualized, and dismissive. In couple therapy, he indicated that he wanted to be supportive of his wife, but he thought that listening to her complaints only reinforced her complaining. His emotional schema was that talking about feelings was a waste of time. The therapist was able to get the husband and wife to role-play active listening and validation; to the surprise of the husband, he discovered that he very much valued having his feelings validated. This led to more motivation and willingness on his part to use active listening and validation with his wife.

## Coming to Terms with the Past Invalidating Environment

Once past and present invalidations have been discussed and clarified, the therapist can ask the patient what he or she wished the parents had said or done when the patient was upset. Veronica, the patient with the cold pediatrician mother, commented, "I wish my mother would have sat down with me and talked to me about how I felt. I just felt all alone. When I was a teenager I developed an eating disorder, but my mother still didn't seem to have time for me." The therapist asked, "What do you wish she could have said or done?" Veronica replied, "It would have really made me feel better if she'd just said, 'Your feelings matter to me. I've been too busy at work. Let's talk about how you feel and what is going on. I'm sorry I haven't been paying as much attention to you. You matter to me.'" Another patient said, "I wish that my father would have just given me a hug and told me how special I was." Several patients say, "I wish that my mother [father] had said, 'I am sorry.'"

Some patients with invalidating experiences say that as a result of these, they had a hard time making sense of their emotions, expressing them, and accepting them. The lack of validation led them to believe that their emotions were a burden to others and/or a waste of time, that their emotions were not the same as those of others, that they were selfish for having these feelings, and that they could only be heard if they escalated their emotions. Others learned that it was better to suppress emotions (perhaps by concentrating on superficial appearance or school achievement), or to "just get over it." One woman said, "It was easier to look pretty than to get someone to care about my feelings."

Some patients complain that their parents often "interpreted" their emotions for them: "They would tell me how I really felt." Perhaps as a result of the influence of psychoanalytic thinking, some parents believed that their children's reports of their feelings were only a cover for deeper feelings and intentions, which were often pathologized by the parents. Veronica (the pediatrician's daughter) said, "When I was upset because my mother didn't have enough time for me, she would say, 'You just want to be the center of everything. Since you don't get your way all the time, you want to punish me.'" This made Veronica feel angry, guilty, and confused, and led her to believe that she really did not even know her own feelings. Another patient observed that her mother would try to make her feel guilty if she wanted to visit her friends: "You really don't care about me. You don't care if I get sick and die. Sure, go off and see your friends and leave me alone here. You really don't care about me." Some patients describe how their parents would interpret their crying as manipulation: "You're not going to make me feel guilty with your crying. Stop trying to manipulate me. The more you cry, the more I will ignore you." Parental feedback or interpretations of "how you really feel" often lead patients to a sense that they cannot trust their own perceptions of their own feelings and have to rely on others to interpret these feelings. Indeed, some such patients come to develop considerable dependence on reassurance from others about decisions, feelings, and perceptions. For example, a patient whose mother would interpret his feelings and tell him what he really felt became obsessively indecisive: "What do you think I should do?"

Invalidating environments touch on every dimension of emotional schemas. For example, parents (and partners) give messages about duration ("You will go on forever with your crying"), lack of consensus ("Other kids don't act this way"), guilt/shame ("You are just being spoiled"), lack of acceptance ("You are just going to have to change the way you feel," "I can't put up with this"), control ("You don't have any control over your feelings. You have to snap out of it now!"), and incomprehensibility ("You don't make any sense. I have no idea what you are talking about"). These messages about emotion become internalized, and the children come to view their own emotions in the manner that their parents instructed them. One man described his mother, busy on the phone while dismissing him when he tried to get attention, made him believe that his feelings did not matter. In therapy, he replayed this angry response at being dismissed by misperceiving the therapist's intentions: "You are just like everyone else. You don't listen to me." He described how he continually complained at work about the workload and what he perceived to be unfair compensation, not realizing that he was undermining himself at work. His attempts at getting people to take his feelings seriously included repeated complaints, name calling, angry outbursts, and passive–aggressive pouting.

I have found it useful to ask a patient to fill out the LESS II the way the patient thinks each parent (or the spouse/partner) might fill it out: For example, "If your mother were filling this out in terms of how she thinks about your emotions, what do you think she would say?" This often leads to immediate insight into the parent's (or partner's) negative emotional schemas—revealing that the other person believed the patient's emotions did not make sense, the patient did not have a right to his or her feelings, the patient's feelings were going on forever, or the patient should have other feelings. The patient can then fill it out the way he or she wishes the other person had thought about the patient's emotions. For example, one patient said, "I wish my mother had encouraged me to talk about my feelings and tell me she understood why I felt the way I felt. I wish she had told me that other kids feel this way." When the patient realizes that he or she has internalized the other person's problematic theory of emotion, greater insight and distance from this belief system can be achieved. "It's not me—she just didn't know how to be a mother," one patient observed.

## THE FIVE STEPS IN VALIDATION

What does ideal validation sound like? I would suggest that it includes four steps: rephrasing, empathizing, finding the truth, and exploring. Rephrasing what the other has said entails the listener's repeating back to the speaker what the listener has heard, without inferring or interpreting: For example, "So what you are saying is that your boss isn't really treating you fairly, and you believe that you are doing a good job and should get paid more than you are being paid." Rephrasing also asks for feedback, in order to determine whether the listener really got the correct message—that is, "Did I hear you correctly?"

Empathizing involves identifying the emotions that the speaker is communicating—not inferring them, but mirroring back what the emotions explicitly are: "It sounds like you are feeling frustrated and angry about the situation." The ideal validator does not infer other emotions (e.g., "You must be feeling sad, too"), since this is not a reflection of what is being heard. Therapist listeners should keep in mind that some individuals who have experienced invalidating parents or partners are often told by others what they "really" feel—which is invalidating. Staying with the information that the speaker gives is important. Again, too, the listener should ask for feedback: "Did I understand correctly what your feelings are or did I miss something?"

Next, validation entails finding the truth in the right to have those feelings, given the events and the speaker's interpretation of them: "I can see that it would make you angry and frustrated, since you think that you are putting in so much time and effort, and you don't see your pay reflecting that. So you are angry because it seems so unfair to you." Again, the listener should not go beyond what the speaker is saying. Interpretations or inferences, such as "Yes, this sounds like your mother to you, which is why you are so angry," should be avoided. These gratuitous interpretations can sound dismissive and condescending, suggesting to the speaker, "You don't have a valid feeling here because you are overreacting due to your bad experience with your mother." These interpretations can be explored later, after validation has occurred, but if given too early they invalidate and alienate the speaker.

Finally, the listener can explore other thoughts, feelings, and memories that the speaker might have, in order to open up the experience for the speaker: "Are there other thoughts and feelings that you have about this?" or "Can you tell me more about the experience that you had?" These exploratory "opening" and "inviting" questions set the stage for the speaker to share his or her experience with a listener who is conveying a nonjudgmental, nondirective role in listening and accepting what is being heard.

In validation, the speaker does not attempt to change the listener or to instruct the listener on better ways of coping. That can come later—*or not at all*. Some therapists may intervene too early, without helping their patients feel heard, accepted, and understood. For example, if the therapist in the situation above were to begin interpreting the anger—"You are not angry at your boss; you are angry at your mother"—the patient would experience this as another critical or dismissive response on the part of a prospective listener. Indeed, the listener would sound like the patient's mother. Or, if the therapist jumps in too quickly with "rational disputation"—"What is the evidence for and against the idea that you are being treated unfairly?" or "Is it possible that you are personalizing and mind-reading?"—the patient may believe that the therapist is dominating, criticizing, and controlling. This belief is very likely to alienate the patient further.

The goal with validation in therapy is to establish a *safe emotional environment* for the patient to trust the therapist with his or her vulnerability. The patient who has described earlier experiences of invalidation, or whose partner is critical and invalidating, or whose responses on the LESS II indicate negative views of emotion—especially the belief that the patient cannot express emotions or is not validated—is a good candidate for more direct emphasis on validation. Moreover, validation is not limited to the first sessions or to the process of getting to know the patient; it is part of the ongoing process of establishing and maintaining trust.

## MICROSKILLS

"Microskills" are essential aspects of validation, but are not sufficient for validation. These general therapeutic behaviors include attending, questioning, focusing, confrontation, reflection, and other skills that facilitate active listening and an improved therapeutic alliance (Ridley, Mollen, & Kelly, 2011a, 2011b). Proper pacing, reflective listening, attending to nonverbal behavior, open-ended questioning, and empathic reflection and summarizing are all helpful in setting the stage for effective validation. The validating listener communicates verbally and nonverbally a warm, accepting, nonjudgmental style. As indicated above, microskills are often part of the validating response. The therapist can communicate this trustworthy and warm response by pacing the interaction to avoid rushing the patient through discussion; allowing silence and pauses so that the patient can gather his or her thoughts and feelings; using a voice that is soft, warm, and with appropriate intonation of emphasis on words that matter to the patient ("It sounds like you really didn't feel *respected*"); and maintaining appropriate body posture (open, relaxed), eye contact (direct but not fixed gaze), and facial expression (mirroring the emotions that the patient may have—e.g., if the patient is expressing fear, the therapist's face expresses concern and understanding).

In addition to the microskills described above, the skilled therapist can practice a "therapeutic Sherlock Holmes" approach in observing the patient. Often a patient's emotional experiences and manner in relating to others are observable in how the patient "appears" in therapy. The observing therapist can notice the manner in which the patient is dressed and groomed (overly meticulous, slovenly, anhedonic, provocative); the intonation of the patient's voice; the expression on the patient's face; any tendency by the patient to look down or away; and hesitations in speech, body posture, inappropriate laughter, long sighs, and other cues. For example, a man who is dressed in a meticulous manner may also be overly concerned with how he appears to others, concerned that his appearance must be perfect in order for him to be accepted. A sexually provocative patient may believe that through relating in a sexual manner, other vulnerabilities can be hidden and the self can be accepted as a sexual object, or the self can gain control by seducing, controlling, or harassing others. Downward casting of the eyes may suggest that the patient feels embarrassed (or at least uncomfortable) in talking about certain topics. The intonation of the patient's voice may suggest that a topic is being either glossed over or emphasized. In any case, the therapist cannot know what is going on with the patient emotionally unless he or she inquires.

THERAPIST: I noticed that your voice became quieter when you began talking about your mother and how she seemed not to care. Why was your voice quieter?

PATIENT: I guess I was feeling guilty. I was feeling like, you know, I shouldn't be criticizing her.

THERAPIST: So it sounded like you almost put yourself on "mute" when you began recognizing how your mother was distant from you. Did you feel like you were on "mute" when you tried to get her attention?

PATIENT: I guess I never thought of it that way—but, yes, that seems like what it was like.

THERAPIST: And did you think that I might be like your mother and not hear you, not care?

PATIENT: I wasn't really thinking when I was speaking. I was beginning to space out. Maybe I felt that it is hard to be here and talk about these things.

THERAPIST: So if you space out when you are talking about difficult memories and difficult feelings, you can escape for a moment. And especially if you think that no one can hear the pain that you are feeling.

## USE OF THE THERAPIST'S OWN EMOTION TO VALIDATE

The emotional schema therapist recognizes that his or her own emotions are a source of information about the experience for the patient. This can take two forms: "What am I feeling as I listen to this?" or "If I were this person, what would I feel?" I recognize that I have a range of feelings in listening to my own patients describe the difficulties that they have experienced. These feelings include sadness, concern, anger, and the desire to protect or defend the patients. Of course, these may reflect my idiosyncratic responses, but they also tell me what the patients may have been missing from others. For example, a woman disclosed in therapy that she had been raped at her high school prom. When she told her parents, they blamed her for getting drunk and hanging out with the "wrong crowd." She felt ashamed, abandoned, and betrayed, and believed that no one would defend her or protect her. She ironically turned to the rapist as a protector, since he was tough and confident, and she became his girlfriend for a while. Her choices in male partners after that were men she realized she could not rely on; this enabled her to discount any need to trust or rely on them, and she was continually unfaithful to each man she partnered with. Since she had not felt defended and protected by her parents, she would always keep part of herself separate, choosing men with whom she knew she could only have dead-end relationships. As her therapist, I felt a wish to protect her and anger toward the rapist and the parents, while recognizing that this was exactly what was missing in the patient's experience with her parents. Being blamed for her own victimization led her to wonder whether she deserved to be treated badly and whether her only value was as a sex object. I asked her what feelings she wished her parents had communicated to her, and she replied, "I wish that they could have seen it wasn't my fault. I wish that they could have defended me rather than blamed me." I asked her how that might have affected the way she felt about relationships—whether she might have kept herself from commitments because she could not trust someone to be completely there for her. She realized that she could not trust herself to trust a man, since they might leave her, betray her, or find fault with her. Once in a relationship, she would look for problems—slight flaws, disappointments, or imperfections that would give her permission to see another man on the side. She realized, she said, that she always knew she could get out of a relationship because there was always another man who would find her attractive. She continually hedged her bets. Although she claimed that her goal was a permanent marital relationship, the more important goal was to keep herself from getting too attached to one person.

Indeed, her sense of shame over the earlier victimization was reflected in the fact that it took her months to tell me about the rape. She had to establish that I was on her side, that I was not judgmental, and that I could be trusted. She observed that she had felt she was to blame—partly because her mother had told her that she had been dressed provocatively and that she had been drunk: "What do you expect?" Putting myself in her shoes, I realized that the shaming and guilt induction that her parents (especially her mother) directed at her would have made me feel marginalized and distrustful. So feeling distrustful about vulnerability was a natural consequence for her. It made sense not to trust me because I could have been like everyone else she had formerly trusted.

Some therapists like to believe that therapy is simply about rational responses, the "right" behaviors, or solving problems. This is sometimes true of less experienced therapists who have formed an allegiance to a school of therapy and have become "true believers." But the life stories that patients tell us are not so easily fixed and not so easily put in perspective. Theories, diagnostic categories, and techniques are not the same thing as understanding another individual. Indeed, I would argue that we never really *completely* understand another person; we can never really know what it is like for that person. Our validation and our understanding are always incomplete, always a possible disappointment for the other. Knowing our imperfections as listeners may be the first step in validating the difficulty that our patients have in feeling understood, since all that we as listeners can really do is try. Creating a safe emotional environment for a patient is not the same thing as fixing a problem. Certainly fixing a problem is important—maybe even essential. But the therapeutic relationship is more about a patient's being cared for, valued, accepted, and even nurtured. It is about attachment needs, especially for those who have been invalidated or abused. When our patients cry out, it is important that they are heard.

## RESPECT FOR SUFFERING AND THE CURRENT MOMENT

People seek out therapy because, on some level, they are suffering or have suffered. The experiences they have had and their difficulties in coping with these have led to sadness, anxiety, anger, helplessness, and hopelessness. Respecting the feelings that reflect suffering communicates that sometimes suffering makes sense; sometimes it is inevitable; sometimes the current moment feels just awful. This does not mean that a therapist cannot help a patient cope more effectively and, with some effort, put an end to suffering. But it suggests that at the present time, "You are hurting and I understand how hard it is." *Before you can fix the pain, the therapist must hear the sound of pain.* The therapist can say something like this:

> "I can see that you are suffering with this breakup. You are telling me how much she meant to you, how you were planning your whole life together, and how this breakup is just devastating. Your pain tells me that things matter to you, that you have depth in your feelings, and that it is hard to go through this. It is hard because losing a relationship with someone you love is hard. Taking a moment to recognize that you are suffering right now is the honest thing to do. It tells you where you are at this moment."

In the comments above, the therapist is communicating respect for the current moment—the moment of suffering. Like the wise author of Ecclesiastes 3:1–4, the therapist and patient may together become witnesses to the recognition that life brings a wide range of experiences, and each has its time to be experienced: "To every thing there is a season, and a time to every purpose under heaven: a time to be born, and a time to die; a time to plant, and a time to pluck up that which is planted; a time to kill, and a time to heal; a time to break down, and a time to build up; a time to weep, and a time to laugh; a time to mourn, and a time to dance." Respecting the moment conveys the idea that there is a moment for every emotion and every experience, but that moments come and go, and that these experiences and emotions change likewise. This idea of respect for the moment and for the fluidity of moments is a key feature of emotional schema therapy, since emotions do not have indefinite duration unless a person gets stuck in them.

THERAPIST: And, knowing that you are suffering, you can say to yourself, "At this moment I am very unhappy. I am suffering. Right now, this is how I feel. That is the feeling I am having right at this present moment." Yes, recognizing that you feel this way at this moment, respect it; hear the feeling; acknowledge that you are the person with the feeling. And that moments change, but each moment has its validity, each moment is part of your life.

PATIENT: It's so hard, so hard.

THERAPIST: Yes, I hear how hard it is for you right now. We can talk about your feelings and what this means to you, and we can try some techniques and try to do some things. But right at this moment it hurts, and so some of the things I say may not be as helpful to you right now. Perhaps later, but right now you are where you are.

This validation of the current moment—"You are where you are"—communicates acceptance of the patient's feelings in the present moment, while implying that there may be ways to change those feelings. Paradoxically, when the therapist shares with the patient a respect and acceptance for these painful feelings, the patient may be more trusting of the therapist's suggestions for change. Saying, "It may not help so much right now," gives the patient two possibilities: Either it helps now (which can move the patient toward change), or it does not help right now (which is what the therapist is actually suggesting). But if it does not help right now, the patient can conclude that the therapist recognizes the temporary difficulties in change and holds open the hope that things might change. In contrast, imagine what would happen if the therapist said, "If you thought this way, everything would change for you." This kind of affirmation of change would sound dismissive of the current moment, would minimize the suffering that is the patient's current experience, and would thus be unlikely to produce change—adding to the hopelessness that the patient may feel. Change is an "option" for the emotional schema approach, since it needs to be balanced with respecting and accepting the current moment. For the patient seeking validation, showing acceptance and respect for the current moment may be the first step in pursuing change from that moment.

## WORKING WITH VALIDATION FAILURES

### Inevitable Empathic Failures

Kohut (1971/2009, 1977) recognized that an inevitable part of the therapeutic relationship is that the patient will recognize that the therapist cannot completely empathize or validate what the patient is feeling. Kohut referred to this as an "empathic failure" and suggested that addressing these inevitable failures is an essential part of therapy. Similarly, I have described how many patients will believe that the therapist does not understand or even care enough about the patients' difficulties—partly because some patients may have idiosyncratic beliefs about what constitutes validation, and partly because no two people can completely understand the other, since most experiences are private and many cannot be adequately articulated (Leahy, 2001, in press; Leahy, Tirch, & Napolitano, 2011). For a patient who has a long history of experiencing invalidation, new invalidation experiences with a therapist can contribute to a sense of hopelessness and eventually to premature termination of therapy.

The therapist can say something like this to anticipate the patient's inevitable experiences of not feeling understood:

> "It is very likely that at times I may not completely understand your feelings and experiences in a way that you feel understood. This may be because any two people are limited in connecting completely, or it may be because of shortcomings that I might have in really understanding you. That can be frustrating. But I wonder if we can agree to discuss these misunderstandings when they arise. I wonder if you would be willing to let me know if you feel that I am not really getting where you are coming from."

This anticipation sets the stage for further validation of future frustration in connection between patient and therapist. The therapist communicates that he or she already knows the limitations and knows that this will be frustrating. We might call this "anticipatory validation" because the future occurrence of empathic failures is already recognized, and the stage is set for discussion and mediation of these:

THERAPIST: I think that understanding and respecting your feelings is one of the most important things that I can do for you, but I also wonder what it will be like when I don't do that effectively. I mean, there will be times that I don't really validate what you are feeling—times that I might fail you. Is that possible?

PATIENT: Oh, no, you are doing a good job. You don't need to worry about that.

THERAPIST: I appreciate your faith in me, but I also know that all of us will eventually let people down, and it may be that there are certain feelings, certain sensitivities that I don't tune into. So, if that happens, I wonder what your response will be.

PATIENT: Oh, I understand no one is perfect.

THERAPIST: Yes, you are really understanding, and I appreciate that. But let's look at the past experiences that you have had. Your father seemed to be wrapped up in his work, and your mother was busy dealing with her own problems and you felt that there wasn't much room for your needs. And you told me last week how you felt that your friend Lara doesn't seem to validate you, that she seems to be critical or more interested in herself. And, in what we are doing together here, validation is really key. So I appreciate your being understanding of me, but I wonder if you could tell me when I am validating you and when I am not.

PATIENT: I guess I feel right now that you are validating the experiences that I have had.

THERAPIST: Would you feel hesitant in telling me when I do invalidate you? You recall that you told me that your mother didn't listen to those concerns, so I would wonder if you might think that I would be dismissive too.

PATIENT: I guess you are right. I either hold my feelings in and don't say anything, or I burst out with anger that seems to come out of nowhere. Or I just stop seeing the person.

THERAPIST: Yeah, those are my concerns, too. How do you think I would respond if you told me that I wasn't really understanding you or that I wasn't validating you?

PATIENT: I guess I think, talking with you now, that you would be understanding.

THERAPIST: Of course, we don't know unless we try. OK. Can you think of any time in the last few weeks that I didn't seem to connect with you on something?

PATIENT: (*Pausing*) Well, I know you are trying to connect, but when I told you about my relationship with my boss—and how she seems not to really give me credit—I didn't feel really validated. You seemed to change the topic.

THERAPIST: Oh, yes, I remember that. Yes, you were feeling that you are working really hard and she never acknowledges your hard work. I can imagine that that sort of thing would be upsetting, and I could have really explored that more, and we could have talked about how that felt and what you thought. In fact, when I think of that sort of thing, I can see that this would be upsetting to most people—feeling like our hard work isn't recognized.

PATIENT: Thanks. You get it—I mean, got it.

Empathic failures—inevitable misunderstandings—occur in almost any close relationship. Some individuals become especially distraught when their spouses or partners do not validate them—and one would hope that there would be some validation in an intimate relationship. But, as later discussions of the therapeutic relationship and of, intimate relationships will make clear (see Chapters 12 and 13), dealing with the disappointments of validation is an essential part of balancing a relationship between unrealistic expectations about emotional and relationship perfection and the realities of human frailty.

## Examining the Meaning of Invalidation

As noted earlier, our research shows that the perception that one is validated is correlated with most of the other emotional schema dimensions.

Validation and invalidation have meanings for the patient. The therapist can explore these meanings with the patient by inquiring what it means in the therapeutic relationship or in any relationship when the patient feels invalidated. People have a wide range of interpretations about invalidation:

"You don't care."
"If you don't care, you can't help me."
"I'm just another patient for you. I am not an individual."
"No one cares about me."
"My feelings don't matter."
"My feelings don't make sense."
"You are taking their side. You think I'm to blame."
"You need to understand everything that I am thinking and feeling."
"If you don't understand all of my feelings, you will never help me."
"You are just like my mother [father, wife, husband, friend]."
"I am all alone."
"I don't matter."

The therapist can take such interpretations and examine them by using validation, cost–benefit analysis, evidence for and against, the double-standard technique, giving advice to a friend, and other cognitive therapy techniques. Here is an example:

THERAPIST: I can see that you think that if I don't understand all your feelings, then I can't help you. That must be really upsetting to think that I can't help you, since we are here to work together to try to help you, and understanding how you feel is so important. I can see that is frustrating, annoying, and even a little scary.

PATIENT: Yeah. No one seems to get me.

THERAPIST: That's a difficult place to be, feeling no one gets you. Like feeling alone in the world and that no one cares.

PATIENT: Look, I know you care, but sometimes you don't let me finish.

THERAPIST: Yes, there are a lot of feelings and thoughts that you have, and I know that I may cut you off. I can see that when I do that, it feels like I don't care.

PATIENT: I know you care, but that's how I feel. That's how I see it.

THERAPIST: Here is the dilemma that all of us face in our relationships. It's that we might really care, but we might not be able to understand all of the feelings that the other person has. We might struggle really hard to connect with what seems at the moment the more important feeling that someone has, but we might miss what is really important to the other person. Could that be what is going on with you and me?

PATIENT: Yes, I guess it is. But it still is painful.

THERAPIST: So let's think about this together, OK? Let's imagine that you go through your relationships expecting that others should understand everything that you are feeling. What is the consequence for you of that expectation?

PATIENT: I guess I feel the way I do—pissed off and disappointed.

THERAPIST: Is there any advantage of getting people to understand everything?

PATIENT: Yeah. Maybe I will finally feel understood.

THERAPIST: That would be good, too, but I wonder, is it working for you? Are you feeling understood a lot of the time?

PATIENT: I generally feel people don't get me.

THERAPIST: What if you had a friend that really expected you to understand every feeling and thought that she had? What advice would you give her?

PATIENT: I would tell her, "You will never get what you want."

THERAPIST: What would you tell her to aim for if she can't get everything that she wants?

PATIENT: I don't know. I guess when it comes to feelings, it's important to be understood. But I guess she would have to decide which feelings are the most important ones and which are not, and go with that.

## Self-Validation

A therapist (or other people) cannot be around to validate a patient all the time. Many patients who have experienced invalidating environments often try to suppress their emotions, or they ruminate about what is wrong with them that they have these feelings. For such patients, it can be extremely helpful to stand back and recognize that it makes sense to feel bad when bad things happen. Owning an emotion, respecting the emotion, and allowing themselves the right to have a feeling does not mean that they are self-indulgent, insane, or out of control, or that the emotion will last forever. Self-soothing, compassionate messages to the self are helpful antidotes to the invalidating experiences that a patient has had (Gilbert, 2009; Neff, 2009). Compassion-focused therapy techniques can be quite helpful for individuals experiencing distressing emotions (Gilbert, 2009). A patient who feel lonely and sad can imagine the face and voice of a compassionate and loving person, imagine this person expressing loving kindness, and imagine how that kindness is soothing and calming the self. Self-validating can also include self-statements about how a patient's emotions "make sense," how others would feel the same way, and how the patient "understands that I understand myself." Statements that patients can affirm—for example, "I am only a human being. I am feeling lonely at the present moment, and that is part of being human"—can help calm the patients, giving them a sense that their compassionate self-reflection is always with them and that they are always capable of supporting themselves. The message is that a patient does not have to get rid of an emotion at the present moment, as long as the patient feels understood, cared for, and supported by the self.

Yet some individuals may continue to believe that validating themselves—or expressing compassion toward themselves—is not merited and even increases the risk of their becoming conceited, dismissive of others, and thus rejected by others. For example, a woman with a long history of binge eating, weight problems, and chronic depression viewed self-validation as "New Age nonsense." She feared that if she engaged in it, she would become soft, self-pitying, and another "loser." She would continually discount any progress that she would make ("Why should I be a cheerleader if it's what I am supposed to do?" she would say in a sarcastic voice). The therapist examined her use of a double standard: "Why are you kinder toward others than toward yourself?" She realized that she wanted to think of herself as a tolerant and loving person, but that she believed she did not deserve to give love to herself.

> THERAPIST: So you don't think it's right to reward or praise yourself because you don't deserve this kindness? Why do others deserve kindness?
>
> PATIENT: Well, everyone does. Except me.
>
> THERAPIST: Why not you?
>
> PATIENT: I don't know; that's just the way I am. I should have done better. There really is no reason that I am depressed.
>
> THERAPIST: Well, think about your reasoning on this: "I am depressed. I don't deserve my kindness. That makes me more depressed. Then I don't deserve any kindness." It sounds like you are punishing yourself for being depressed, which keeps you depressed.
>
> PATIENT: I know. It sounds illogical. But I guess I am afraid if I start blowing my own horn, I will sound conceited.
>
> THERAPIST: Maybe you can blow the horn so that you are the only one who hears it.

Self-validation can take the form of self-directed messages that are compassionate, kind, and supportive:

"I'm trying, so I really need to give myself credit. Life is hard, and I am working on making things better. I want to love myself, support myself, be kind to myself. Painful feelings are part of life for all of us, including me. There are a lot of good things that I can experience. I need to be a friend to myself."

The therapist and patient can then set up an "experiment" to see whether giving the self these validating and compassionate statements leads to arrogance and difficulties with other people. In addition, the therapist can do a "feared fantasy" role play, in which the therapist plays the role of a voice saying that being kind to the self is going to lead to terrible outcomes.

THERAPIST: (*As negative voice*) You know when you say kind things to yourself, you are really misleading yourself. I mean, the little things that you do don't really matter.

PATIENT: (*As rational responder*) Every positive step I take can matter—including being supportive to myself. If I keep being rewarding to myself, I might feel better.

THERAPIST: But you don't deserve to feel better. People who are depressed deserve to feel bad.

PATIENT: That's absurd. Depression is an illness for a lot of people, and everyone deserves a chance.

THERAPIST: Yeah, everyone except you. If you start saying positive things about yourself, you will become conceited and arrogant and alienate everyone.

PATIENT: That's crazy. I can quietly—silently—say supportive things to myself, and that will probably make me less depressed. And if I am less depressed, I probably will be more fun to be around.

## SUMMARY

This chapter has reviewed the need for validation as a basic need for understanding and connectedness. This need arises from the original child–caregiver attachment system, which seeks completion or fulfillment throughout the lifespan. Validation is related to—and can produce improvement in—a wide range of other emotional schemas, such as helping the individual make sense of emotion, recognizing that others have similar emotions, allowing for expression, reducing rumination, and helping the individual realize that the experience of emotion need not last indefinitely and will not go out of control. Some individuals have problematic beliefs about validation, expecting total and complete agreement and mirroring; these beliefs inevitably lead to empathic failures. The emotional schema therapist can anticipate such failures as potential roadblocks by raising the issue, exploring the meaning of the invalidation when it occurs, and developing a mutual acceptance of the possibility of disappointment. Finally, self-invalidation and the resistance to directing compassion toward the self can be addressed by using the double-standard technique and other cognitive techniques, engaging in "feared fantasy" role plays, and setting up behavioral experiments to determine what the real outcomes of self-validation are.

# CHAPTER 7

# Comprehensibility, Duration, Control, Guilt/Shame, and Acceptance

> Be grateful for whatever comes,
> because each has been sent
> as a guide from beyond.
> —JALAL AL-DIN RUMI[1]

After the patient has been assessed and the therapist has described the emotional schema model, each session will focus on understanding the specific emotions that are troubling the individual and the ways in which specific beliefs about emotions and strategies of emotion regulation maintain or exacerbate problematic coping. Similar to a cognitive therapy model that identifies cognitive biases, the emotional schema model encourages the patient to consider the implications of specific beliefs about emotion and to determine how different beliefs and strategies can be more adaptive. In this chapter, I provide guidelines for identifying and modifying five specific dimensions of emotional schemas: beliefs about emotions' comprehensibility, duration, and control; the extent to which emotions induce guilt and shame; and the degree to which emotions are accepted.

Various cognitive therapy techniques (e.g., advantages and disadvantages of a belief, evidence for and against the belief, collecting data, the double-standard technique), as well as behavioral experiments and

---

[1] From Rumi (1997). Copyright 1997 by Coleman Barks and Michael Green. Reprinted by permission of Coleman Barks.

experiential exercises both in and between sessions, are utilized to address these five dimensions. The emotional schema therapist utilizes imagery induction and rescripting (Hackmann, 2005; Smucker & Dancu, 1999), detached mindfulness (Roemer & Orsillo, 2009; Segal, Williams, & Teasdale, 2002), techniques to enhance psychological flexibility (Hayes et al., 2012), clarification of values (linking painful emotions to higher values) (Wilson & Murrell, 2004), positive psychology techniques (Seligman, 2002), DBT techniques (Linehan, 1993, 2015), and compassion-focused therapy techniques (Gilbert, 2009). Using these techniques to help modify these five types of problematic beliefs about emotions will increase patients' ability to tolerate and utilize emotional experience, and will help them interrupt the links between emotional schemas and problematic coping strategies (Leahy, Tirch, & Napolitano, 2011). Thus a wide range of techniques can be used to address beliefs about comprehensibility, duration, control, guilt/shame, and acceptance of emotion within the more encompassing and integrative emotional schema model.

## COMPREHENSIBILITY

Emotions may appear to "come out of nowhere" for some people: They may say, "I don't know why I feel the way I do." The consequences of the belief that "My emotions don't make sense" are that these persons feel confused, helpless, and hopeless. If emotions appear to be incomprehensible, the individuals may fear their emotions, believe that they are losing control or going insane, or conclude that they have no control over what they do not understand. In addition, individuals who believe that their emotions do not make sense may ruminate: "I can't figure out why I feel this way," or "What is wrong with me?" Making sense of emotions is a key element of emotional schema therapy.

Some patients are alexithymic; that is, they have difficulty in labeling and differentiating emotions, and in recalling events associated with various emotions (Lundh, Johnsson, Sundqvist, & Olsson, 2002; Paivio & McCulloch, 2004). These individuals often have difficulty comprehending why they have a negative feeling. These patients may report vague or diffuse complaints ("I feel down," "Something is wrong") and have difficulty finding words for emotions, recalling events associated with different emotions, or linking emotions to their thoughts. The emotional schema therapist may assist such patients in noticing the onset and experience of various emotions, linking them to events and thoughts, and making sense of them in the context in which they occur.

First, traditional cognitive therapy provides a strong rationale for linking emotions to specific automatic thoughts, assumptions, or core beliefs. For example, a patient's emotions of shame and sadness make sense if these emotions are linked to automatic thoughts such as "People think I am a loser," or "I need the approval of everyone to feel good about myself." Further, cognitive therapy can link core beliefs such as "I am inadequate," or "I am unlovable," to emotions such as sadness and shame. Second, the therapist may also suggest that depression or anxiety may have a biological component—especially if there is evidence of early onset or familial history of psychopathology. Thus biologically based psychopathology may account for both an emotion (e.g., sadness) and the cognitive biases associated with the emotion. Third, a behavioral model can be useful in making sense of emotion. If sadness is associated with passivity, isolation, and experiential avoidance, then the patient can examine whether the sadness increases or decreases in connection with these processes. Moreover, by experimenting with behavioral activation, the patient can determine whether the sadness can be modified simply by taking action and confronting feared or uncomfortable situations. Indeed, behavioral activation can address other dimensions of emotional schemas, such as durability, control, and the belief that one is helpless over an emotion.

Fourth, some patients claim that they do not understand why they feel or think a particular way, since they recognize on a "rational" level that "I have nothing to feel bad about." That is, these individuals believe that their automatic thoughts (e.g., "I am a failure") have no rational basis, and therefore there is no "reason" to feel bad. The therapist can indicate to such patients that depression or anxiety may arise for a variety of reasons, that emotions can cause negative thoughts or be consequences of these thoughts, and that the believability or credibility of thoughts may change over time. Thoughts that are associated with negative emotions do not have to be true in order to maintain these emotions; they just have to be credible. Patients may claim, "But I don't really believe these thoughts. I know that they are irrational." The therapist may suggest that the degree of belief may change with situations that the patient encounters. For example, a man who experiences a breakup may claim, "I know I will be able to find someone else"—but when he recalls the ex-partner, he is flooded with thoughts that elicit depression: "I can't be happy without her," or "I screwed it up." These thoughts may be context-specific, suggesting that rationality takes a back seat to emotional evocation in a specific context. Furthermore, emotions may arise from biological imbalances that are not clearly related to the situation or to automatic thoughts; that is, emotions may arise "spontaneously" as a result of a biological diathesis. For example, a woman in her 30s who was being evaluated could not understand the reason for her extreme mood variations. The therapist suggested that she might have a bipolar disorder, and that this was largely a biological predisposition with a high heritability. Although initially skeptical of this diagnosis, she was able to confirm it with the help of her psychiatrist and with her husband's description of her history. Thus "making sense" of wide variations in mood through appropriate diagnosis not only can confer more comprehensibility, but also can suggest a course of treatment—in this woman's case, a combination of cognitive-behavioral therapy and medication.

In order to address the issue of comprehensibility, the therapist can ask the following questions: "Do the emotions make sense to you? Which emotions are most difficult to understand? Which are less difficult to understand?" For example, some patients may have little difficulty identifying their angry feelings, but more difficulty identifying sad feelings. They may more easily recognize that "I am angry because someone offended me," than understand that "I am sad because I think I will always feel sad." A married woman could not understand why she was sad, since "I have a good marriage, a good home. We are financially secure." Her depression probably had a biological component, but she had also given up her professional identity as a lawyer in order to be a full-time mother. She did not realize that this was a loss of some identity and sense of competence; she thought, "I should be happier." Underestimating the impact of major life events often leaves patients with a sense that their current emotions are incomprehensible. The therapist can explore possible reasons—biological vulnerability, childhood experiences, recent sources of stress, loss, or conflict, or memories that might account for an emotion. The following questions can be raised:

> "What could be some good reasons why you are sad [anxious angry, etc.]?"
> "What are you thinking (what images do you have) when you are sad [etc.]?"
> "What situations trigger these feelings?"
> "What does this emotion remind you of?"
> "Are there any difficulties that might account for your feeling this way?"
> "Can you recall the earliest memories that are associated with these emotions?"

As discussed below in the section on duration of emotion, understanding why one feels a certain way can be facilitated by identifying the situations that trigger the emotion and the thoughts that accompany the feelings. For example, the mother who had set aside her career as a lawyer recognized that she felt sad when her husband left in the morning and when she heard about former colleagues from her office. The husband's leaving in the morning triggered her thoughts devaluing her role as a mother: "I have wasted my entire education. I have nothing to contribute." When she heard about former colleagues, her thoughts were "I gave up a good career. They're going to think I am a loser."

Sometimes patients have a better understanding of their emotions when they consider how other people might respond or feel. The therapist can ask, "If someone else experienced this, what kinds of different feelings could they have?" Realizing that emotions make sense from others' point of view is a key element in normalizing and making sense of these feelings. Individuals are less likely to ruminate, feel guilty, or isolate themselves when they think others might feel the same way as they do. In addition to normalizing emotions, asking about how others might respond can elicit ideas about more adaptive ways of coping. The former lawyer reflected, "I remember that Sally left her firm a few years ago and initially felt great being home, but then she had a lot of doubts. One of the ideas that she had was that she was going to try working part-time in a smaller local firm after her child was 2 years old. I remember that she felt better with that plan."

People have beliefs about what it means that they do not understand their emotions. These are "meta-emotional beliefs" and may lead to problematic ways of coping. (Note the similarity between these meta-emotional beliefs and the model of metacognitive therapy advanced by Wells [2009].) The emotional schema model proposes that there are specific theories about emotion, just as there are theories about the role of thinking as noted in the metacognitive model. Specific questions to address beliefs about the incomprehensibility of emotion include the following: "If you think your feelings don't make sense right now, what does this make you think? Are you afraid that you are going crazy or losing control?" Some patients who believe that their emotions do not make sense begin to think that there is something deeply wrong with them. For example, patients with panic disorder believe that they have some deep vulnerability that has to be watched and controlled, lest they lose all control and go completely insane. Other patients who are emotionally dysregulated believe that there is some deep, dark secret that cannot be uncovered, or that their current emotional dysregulation is a permanent handicap from which they will never escape. Others believe that "unless I have a really good explanation that ties together everything, then my emotions make no sense." As Ingram, Atchley, and Segal (2011) indicate, different levels of "explanation" may account for vulnerability, ranging from the behavioral and cognitive to the neurological and developmental. "Making sense" of an emotion does not mean that there is only one way of understanding it, and in most cases, there is no deep, dark secret that needs to be uncovered. Individuals who believe that there is some such secret will ruminate in a search for the "truth," and will reject other interpretations as not dealing with the "real problem."

However, there are cases in which the current emotional theory does relate to earlier experiences, although these are not necessarily repressed experiences or deep secrets to be uncovered. Patients' understanding of why they feel the way they do can also be facilitated by examining earlier child-hood or adult experiences: "Are there things that happened to you as a kid that might account for why you feel this way?" Developmental origins of current emotions are not always useful; indeed, they may sometimes lead to overpathologizing the current emotional experience, since the patient may come to believe that "all the damage has already been done." Theories of the causation of a vulnerability or an emotion may reflect beliefs about personal qualities as fixed, immutable, and pervasive (e.g., "My mother made me feel like my emotions weren't important, so I guess I will always think my emotions don't matter"). This belief in "emotional determinism" is often reinforced by popularization of psychodynamic or "inner wounded child" models, which some individuals incorrectly interpret as models of permanent emotional disability.

However, for patients who believe that their current emotions do not make sense, this line of inquiry can be helpful. For example, the former lawyer mentioned earlier recalled that her mother's professional career was curtailed by parenthood, and that this was a source of regret for her. Indeed, her mother took a great deal of pride in the academic accomplishments of her daughter—but also took a great deal of pleasure in becoming a grandmother. These "mixed messages" led to a sense of unfulfilled potential, while she herself appeared to vacillate (understandably) between the roles of professional lawyer and loving mother.

Relatedly, recalling images or scenes from childhood can elicit more emotions and thoughts, further illustrating the link between current emotions and past experiences. The current emotion—for example, loneliness—may be "induced" by asking the patient to imagine what it would be like to feel really lonely. The patient may be encouraged to close his or her eyes and repeat gently, "I am so lonely," while observing the images, memories, and other emotions that accompany the feeling of loneliness: "Notice the feelings in your body, the feelings in your chest, the sense of emptiness and loss. Notice the sadness that you have because you are lonely, and notice any other emotions that may come. Now gently observe any image that comes to your mind. Watch it and see it unfold." One patient began to weep as she recalled lying in bed alone while her parents were out, feeling that she was all alone. The therapist asked, "What thoughts come to you in this image?" The patient responded, "They don't really care about me. I don't matter." Her current anxiety and sadness were elicited by her husband's going on business trips. She recalled that she had missed her father most of all when she was a child; he had died suddenly when she was 12, and she was left with a mother who she thought resented her.

Finally, even with the most thorough attempts to link emotions to bio-logical diathesis, early childhood experiences, emotional socialization in the family, automatic thoughts, and personal schemas, some patients still may find that their emotions do not make sense. Such patients appear to believe in "insight perfectionism"; that is, they believe they must understand everything about their emotions (or themselves) in order to function effectively. Their sense that "I can't figure out what is making me feel this way" often leads to a ruminative search for "real meanings" and "complete understanding": "Unless I can really get to the bottom of this, I don't know how I can make any decisions about how to live my life." The apparent rule is that complete insight is a necessary condition for change, just as some patients feel that complete motivation is a necessary condition. The therapist can ask whether it is always necessary to understand why one is feeling the way one is feeling, or whether it is more important to determine which goals, values, or behaviors are productive.

The etiology of an emotion—or an emotional schema—may be less important than how a current emotion is interpreted and "regulated." For example, the patient whose current sadness may seem incomprehensible may conclude, "If I do not understand my emotion, then I am helpless to change it." This belief in the necessity of understanding can be examined by setting up behavioral experiments illustrating that specific activities or situations are associated with more pleasant emotions and that "insight" may not always be necessary for change. Insight may sometimes be an advantage, but it may not be a necessity. Understanding may be less important in certain situations than effectiveness.

## DURATION

Our research (see Chapter 3) indicated that a major predictor of both depression and anxiety was the belief that emotions will last indefinitely (Leahy, Tirch, & Melwani, 2012; Tirch, Leahy, Silberstein, & Melwani, 2012). As also indicated in an earlier chapter, the perception of durability of emotion is a consistent finding in research on "affect forecasting" (Wilson & Gilbert, 2003). Research on beliefs about "discount rates" (i.e., the emphasis on shorter-term gains while discounting cumulative longer-term gains) results in short-term gratification at the cost of longer term gain (Frederick et al., 2002; McClure et al., 2007; Read & Read, 2004). The belief in durability of emotion is a consequence of anchoring predictions to the current emotion ("I feel sad now; I will always feel sad"); focusing on one element to the exclusion of other mitigating factors (e.g., "I don't have a partner now"—nothing else is considered); and underestimating intervening mitigating or compensating factors (e.g., not recognizing that other relationships and valued alternatives might emerge). Furthermore, implicit beliefs about emotion as either fixed (entity theories) or changeable (incremental theories) are related to emotion regulation capabilities (Castella et al., 2013).

Modifying the belief in the duration of emotion is a key factor in increasing affect tolerance. For example, a man with OCD who had fears of contamination believed that if he engaged in exposure and response prevention, his anxiety would last indefinitely and would escalate throughout the day. Similarly, patients with panic disorder may also believe that their anxiety will be interminable. Belief in the durability of thoughts and emotions can likewise be identified as a key element underlying hopelessness and depression: "I will always feel hopeless," or "I will always believe that life is not worth living." Indeed, among the central tenets of mindfulness training is the recognition that thoughts, feelings, sensations—and even "reality"—are in constant transition, coming and going, rising and ebbing. Fluidity and flexibility are in contrast to durability (Hayes et al., 2012; Linehan, 1993, 2015; Roemer & Orsillo, 2009; Segal et al., 2002).

We give priority to addressing beliefs about durability, since these beliefs are so central to other beliefs (e.g., belief about control and acceptance). Knowing that a difficult emotion is temporary makes it easier to tolerate. The need to control a temporary emotion may seem less urgent; the perception of danger and impairment should be decreased; and the underlying beliefs in hopelessness about the emotion should abate. The therapist can raise the issue of durability by asking,

> "I see that you believe that the emotions that you have right now are likely to go on indefinitely. That must be a difficult experience for you, since it is so difficult right now. We often do feel immersed in the way we feel, and it just seems that it will last a very long time. In fact, some emotions may seem to 'engulf the field'—they often capture us and carry us away. Let's take a look at this and see what we can find. Which specific emotions do you think will last indefinitely?"

Since patients often have a variety of emotions—anxiety, anger, sadness, confusion, and even relief—it is valuable to begin differentiating among these emotions to see whether some are less durable than others. The therapist can inquire how a patient can account for why certain emotions are durable while others are not. In particular, the therapist can ask whether feelings of happiness are durable—and, if not, why not. Why would the present negative emotion (e.g., sadness, hopelessness, anger) be the only emotion that is durable? Will the same conditions become permanent, or will anything change? Will the patient always think the same way? Some patients use "emotional reasoning" about the durability of their emotion: "It feels so terrible, I can't imagine that it would go away." This belief that the intensity of an emotion is equal to its durability appears illogical, but many individuals suffering from intense pain reach this conclusion. The therapist can ask, "Are there very intense emotions that you have had in the past?" As the patient enumerates other intense emotional experiences, such as sadness, anger, anxiety, and jealousy, the therapist can ask how long the emotion with the greatest intensity lasted. Since every one of these emotions will have abated at some point, the patient can begin to consider that the current intense emotions also might change.

As with many beliefs, the patient's motivation to change needs to be addressed. The therapist can do this through cost–benefit analysis: "What are the costs and benefits of believing that your emotion will last indefinitely?" Some patients fear getting their hopes up about change, and therefore will defend the permanence of a negative feeling. If so, the therapist can ask, "What would change for you if you came to believe that these emotions will change—become less intense, less bothersome?" There are consequences to the belief in durability, since this belief adds to a sense of helplessness/hopelessness and results in basing future predictions on the present emotional state. Beliefs in durability also often lead to dysfunctional coping, such as avoidance, isolation, inactivity, rumination, worry, binge eating, and substance misuse. To assess such coping, the therapist can inquire what the patient does "next" when the thought that the emotion will last indefinitely occurs:

> "When you think that your negative emotion will last indefinitely, does this lead you to do certain things or avoid certain things? For example, do you just give up, isolate yourself, become passive, or turn inward? Do you dwell on the bad feeling? Do you project into the future how bad it will be and then dwell on that? Do you try to soothe yourself momentarily by overeating, drinking, using drugs, or getting lost in some other activity?"

"If I think that my negative feelings are permanent then I tend to think *what* or do *what*?"

Recognizing the costs of durability beliefs may increase the motivation to change them, although some patients may view such questions as invalidating or as raising false hopes. The therapist may address the issue of validation by observing that the current feelings and beliefs are very powerful and painful, and that validating their existence does not mean that considering alternatives would negate the "reality of the experience" for the patient at the present moment:

> "Imagine if you had terrible physical pain caused by a splinter that was stuck in your foot. The doctor observes how much pain you are in and says that the splinter really is the cause. If the doctor asked if it would be OK for her to pull the splinter out, would you think she was

invalidating? Perhaps if you left the splinter in, the pain would last for hours. Which would be the best course of action?"

Although durability may trigger the desire to avoid or escape the emotion, the therapist can suggest that there are times when "You must go through it to get past it."

The lack of motivation stemming from a belief in durability can also be examined: "Would you be motivated to do things to make things better if you had *doubts* about the durability of your emotion?" Some patients may believe that it makes no sense to take the risk of making changes if their emotions are going to last indefinitely. "Why bother if it is hopeless?" one man said. Belief in the durability of an emotion may thus become a self-fulfilling prophecy. The therapist can point out, "If you believe that your emotions will not change, then it makes sense to do nothing." Moreover, belief in the durability of emotion prevent patients from engaging in exposure to overcome their fears. The man with OCD mentioned earlier believed that if he did exposure to overcome his fears of contamination, then his anxiety would last indefinitely. The long duration (and rising intensity) of his emotion seemed a high price to pay to "test a theory about exposure."

Beliefs about durability and the danger of emotion are central in engaging patients in exposure exercises in the treatment of specific phobia, social anxiety disorder, OCD, PTSD, and any other disorders where activating fear is an essential component in treatment. For example, the patient with fears of contamination was asked how intense his anxiety would be and for how long it would last should he engage in exposure to the "contaminated" objects in his apartment. He commented that his anxiety would escalate to 100%, he would completely deteriorate, he would not be able to function, and his anxiety would ruin the entire week. When asked for evidence for these predictions from his experience of past exposure exercises, he observed that he had not done exposures before, but that he "felt it was true." Exposure exercises can function in a number of ways—sometimes allowing habituation of anxiety, but often allowing the patient to test beliefs about willingness to engage in exposure and beliefs about the duration, tolerability, and danger of anxious arousal. In this case, the disconfirmation of the patient's beliefs about emotional arousal (and about the resulting impairment) helped him to undergo further exposures to other "contaminations."

In order to collect information about durability, the therapist can ask the following:

"Do your most painful emotions increase and decrease during the course of the day or week? What does this tell you about how emotions change? Do your emotions change because you are doing something different, because you are thinking differently, or because you are around other people?"

These beliefs can then be tested by having the patient use an activity schedule (see Leahy, Holland, & McGinn, 2012, or see below) to monitor actions and the emotions associated with them for each hour of the week. By observing that all emotions rise and fall in intensity—and that the intensity varies with situation, time of day, and the thoughts that accompany the emotion—the patient can observe that variation, not durability, is the rule. Further evidence against durability can be obtained by asking about past emotions: "Have you ever had a negative or positive emotion that never went away?" The patient's personal history of the fluidity and transient nature of emotions can help illustrate that even very painful emotions from the past have changed.

Another factor underlying affect forecasting is that people tend to ignore intervening events that might mitigate a current emotion. Predictions about future emotions that are anchored solely to a current emotion do not take into consideration new relationships, rewarding experiences, opportunities, or simply the decay of memory about a past event. The therapist can ask, "Think back about those painful emotions that went away in the past. What happened that led these emotions to decrease in intensity for you?" Tracing the history of the decay of an emotion is helpful, since it may illustrate that "You have had these beliefs about durability in the past—for very painful experiences—but even those emotions changed." By refocusing on events and experiences that modified difficult emotions, the patient can come to realize that all painful emotions eventually decrease because new sources of reward, meaning, and experience emerge. A woman who believed that her current feelings of desperation, loneliness, and hopelessness would last indefinitely recalled that she had had the same emotions after a previous breakup. On reflection, she realized that she had idealized her former partner, and that the prior breakup (although difficult) had created opportunities for new relationships.

To further examine possible reasons why emotions will not be durable, the therapist may inquire about all of the events that might occur in the next week, month, year, and 5-year period. How will the patient feel about these? Many patients with durability beliefs are myopic about affect forecasting, predicting that their current emotion has been plaguing them for days and will continue indefinitely. Often such patients will focus on one source of reward as the reason why they will continue with the current emotion: "I lost my job, so I really don't have any sense of what to do," or "Without my partner, I have no life." Alternative sources of rewards and meanings—both related and unrelated to the current loss—may then be examined. The therapist can inquire, "What are some sources of pleasure, meaning, challenge, growth, or reward that might come your way in the next week [month, year, 5 years]?" For example, a man who lost his job realized that he had many other sources of rewards independent of his current job. These included his child, his wife, his friends, his extended family, exercise, hobbies, reading, and other activities. In addition, he considered the possibility that a new job closer to home might have certain benefits over the lost job, which had required considerable daily commuting.

Figures 7.1 through 7.3 provide guidance for the therapist and patient in examining the patient's beliefs about the duration of emotions. (Note that these figures are provided for guidance purposes only and are not intended to be reproducible.) Figure 7.1 is a set of questions for testing the patient's duration beliefs. Figure 7.2 is a schedule the patient can use to chart the daily fluctuation of emotions in connection with his or her activities. Figure 7.3 enables the patient and therapist to draw conclusions from the activity schedule about emotions and activities.

## CONTROL

Our research shows that the perception of an emotion as out of control is a key factor in anxiety and is associated with a wide range of psychopathology (Leahy, Tirch, & Melwani, 2012). Indeed, the idea of "emotion regulation" implies that uncontrolled emotions can have significant negative effects on adaptive functioning. Some patients believe that they need to get rid of a negative feeling immediately and completely. This sense of urgency and need for complete elimination set almost impossible standards for emotion regulation. These standards then lead to a sense of futility (e.g., "I am still anxious!"), further exacerbating anxiety and helplessness. Or patients must immediately figure out what is wrong.

The sense of time urgency is linked to beliefs about control, escalation, comprehensibility, and even intolerance of uncertainty (a simplistic view of emotion). Such patients may believe that if they don't get control immediately, then their emotions will unravel, escalate to intolerable levels, and completely impair them. Or, if they do not figure things out immediately and understand exactly what is going on, they will never be able to cope with their emotions. Time urgency is similar to the concept of "looming vulnerability" that Riskind and colleagues have delineated in a number of studies, indicating that anxiety may also be the result of the belief that a threat is fast approaching and that the ability to cope or avoid is disappearing (Riskind, 1997; Riskind & Kleiman, 2012; Riskind, Tzur, Williams, Mann, & Shahar, 2007).

The first question to ask of the patient is which emotion is out of control. Again, we find that some patients have "no problem" with one emotion's (e.g., anger's) being out of control, but they fear that other emotions

**Instructions:** Please write out your answers to the questions in the spaces provided. If you changed some of your beliefs about emotion, would it affect anything in your life? Would you feel more hopeful, less helpless, less anxious? What could be some more adaptive ways of viewing your emotions?

Which specific emotions do you think will last indefinitely?

_____

_____

_____

What are the costs and benefits of believing that your emotion will last indefinitely? What would change for you if you came to believe that these emotions will change—become less intense, less bothersome?

_____

_____

_____

Have you ever had a negative or positive emotion that never went away?

_____

_____

_____

Think back about those painful emotions that went away in the past. What happened that led these emotions to decrease in intensity for you?

_____

_____

_____

Does your most painful emotion increase and decrease during the course of the day or week? What does this tell you about how emotions change? Do your emotions change because you are doing something different, because you are thinking differently, or because you are around other people?

_____

_____

_____

**FIGURE 7.1.** Questions for testing beliefs about how long emotions last. (Do not reproduce.)

**Instructions:** In the spaces provided, please write down briefly what you do and how you feel each waking hour of each day. For example, if you have breakfast between 7:00 A.M. and 8:00 A.M. and you feel sad and lonely, write "Breakfast, sad, lonely." If you are working between 10:00 A.M. and 11:00 A.M. and you feel challenged and interested, write "Working, challenged, interested." See if there is a pattern to your emotions that is related to what you are doing, the time of day, and the people you are with.

| | Mon | Tues | Wed | Thurs | Fri | Sat | Sun |
|---|---|---|---|---|---|---|---|
| 6:00 A.M. | | | | | | | |
| 7:00 | | | | | | | |
| 8:00 | | | | | | | |
| 9:00 | | | | | | | |
| 10:00 | | | | | | | |
| 11:00 | | | | | | | |
| Noon | | | | | | | |
| 1:00 P.M. | | | | | | | |
| 2:00 | | | | | | | |
| 3:00 | | | | | | | |

| | | | | | | | |
|---|---|---|---|---|---|---|---|
| 4:00 | | | | | | | |
| 5:00 | | | | | | | |
| 6:00 | | | | | | | |
| 7:00 | | | | | | | |
| 8:00 | | | | | | | |
| 9:00 | | | | | | | |
| 10:00 | | | | | | | |
| 11:00 | | | | | | | |
| Midnight | | | | | | | |
| 1:00 A.M. | | | | | | | |
| 2:00–5:00 | | | | | | | |

**FIGURE 7.2.** Keeping track of activities and emotions. (Do not reproduce.)

When is your negative emotion the most intense?

_____

_____

_____

When do you feel better?

_____

_____

_____

What would happen if you did more of the activities associated with feeling better?

_____

_____

_____

Can you assign these activities to yourself?

_____

_____

_____

What if you decreased the negative activities?

_____

_____

_____

How can you do that?

_____

_____

_____

You thought that your negative emotions didn't change. What does your activity schedule tell you?

_____

_____

_____

What conclusions can you draw from this exercise?

_____

_____

_____

**FIGURE 7.3.** Conclusions about emotions and activities.

(e.g., anxiety, sadness) can go out of control. In such a case, the therapist can ask why it is OK for certain emotions to go out of control, whereas other emotions cannot be tolerated. Narrowing the focus on the emotions that are out of control allows the patient to examine why it is so bad if some emotions are out of control while others are not. Second, the therapist can inquire whether the patient actually experiences the emotion as out of control, or only *fears* that it might go out of control. For example, most patients with panic disorder do not report that their anxiety is out of control; rather, they fear that the anxiety, once activated, will escalate out of control. This perception of a "chain reaction" or "nuclear reaction" leads some patients to focus on the smallest sign of emotional arousal and jump to conclusions about further escalation. Thus unwanted sensations or thoughts become "signals" that avoidance or safety behaviors "need to be activated" to prevent a catastrophe.

Third, the therapist can inquire what the signs are that an emotion is going out of control. For some patients, the very experience of a lower-intensity emotion signifies that the emotion will intensify and result in loss of control. For instance, increased heart rate, physical tension, more rapid breathing, and feeling anxious or annoyed become signs that total loss of control is imminent. Related to this is the hyperfocus on arousal, which simply increases arousal and results in further perception of being out of control. The therapist can ask the patient to test the idea that an emotion will go out of control by intentionally intensifying the emotion or sensations—for example, through running in place, spinning, staring into a light bulb, recalling unhappy events, or even repeating feared thoughts. Encouraging the patient to stay with this exercise for enough time to allow for habituation can dispel beliefs that emotions and sensations need to be eliminated immediately.

Fourth, the therapist can ask, "What do you think would happen if you couldn't get rid of that feeling entirely?" Patients with panic disorder may claim that they will lose control, start screaming, and make fools of themselves. Sad and anxious patients with borderline personality disorder may say that they will become so depressed and anxious that they will need to cut themselves to reduce the tension. Patients with OCD who are asked to engage in exposure to their fears may claim that their anxiety will escalate to catastrophic levels and that they will go insane. The question in each case is this: "What will the impairment be if you lose control?" The therapist may ask, "Are you afraid that having a strong feeling is a sign of something worse? Going crazy? Losing complete control?"

Fifth, rather than focusing on total control, the therapist can ask what the advantages would be if the patient viewed emotions along a moderating continuum. For instance, anxious arousal on a 10-point scale might be observed to rise to 9, drop to 6, rise to 7, drop to 3, and drop to 1. Observing that emotions may fluctuate in intensity, and indeed decay with time, can suggest that emotions are self-regulating—very much like a thermostat. Rather than viewing the onset of an emotion as a predictor of unraveling, the patient may learn to observe that this onset begins a process of rising and falling. Taking an observing and describing role toward the emotion can be helpful:

> "Imagine that you are watching the waves coming in and out on the beach. You are sitting up on the boardwalk away from the water, but you can see the waves rising and falling. Now imagine that the waves are higher for a few moments, and you see them crashing down onto the sand. The water pulls back, and another wave comes crashing in. With time, you begin to notice that the waves are less intense—more calmly coming ashore, more calmly going out to the water. Now you are observing that the water is more still—just gentle waves coming in, lapping the beach, and gently going out. Now think of your emotions as waves that come and go, rise and fall, intense, now calmer, now gentle. But you stand on the boardwalk and observe and feel the breeze from the ocean on this warm summer day."

Images of emotion as a fluid can also be helpful if the patient can imagine him- or herself as a large and ever-expanding container that has more and more room to contain an emotion, rather than as needing to put up a wall to keep the fluid emotion out. The ebb and flow of the emotion can also confer the sense of temporary and changing experience, rather than a sense of fixed durability.

Sixth, the therapist can use analogies of other sources of arousal that rise and fall—for example, hunger, or arousal due to caffeine:

> "You seem to think that your emotion is going to rise to uncontrollable and catastrophic levels. But let's take a look at some other sources of arousal. Let's imagine that you just had two cups of really strong coffee. You now have a caffeine buzz. You are tense; your heart is pounding; you are tense, maybe a bit irritable. What do you think will happen if you just wait it out to see if the buzz decreases over the next hour or so? You might say to yourself, 'I guess I had too much coffee, so I will be a bit buzzed for a while. Oh, well.' Allowing yourself to accept arousal and just wait it out may be less anxiety-provoking than demanding that you have to get rid of arousal immediately. The sense of urgency about an emotion adds to the arousal, which adds to the sense of urgency, thereby causing increased anxiety."

Seventh, some patients believe that they have to control an emotion because it is a "bad" emotion. Examples of emotions that are labeled as "bad" include anxiety, sadness, loneliness, anger, and sexual feelings.

Seldom do people claim that they have to get rid of a "good" emotion, such as happiness, satisfaction, hope, appreciation, or gratitude. The therapist can suggest that an emotion is neither good nor bad, but simply *is*:

> "All of our emotions are there because they have been adaptive to our ancestors and to ourselves. For example, anxiety may be helpful in suggesting that there may be something wrong or that something bad might happen. It's an alarm. Sadness may tell us that there is something missing that we value. It reports on what has happened. The emotions themselves are neither good nor bad; they are experiences that we have. They are activities in our brains. Imagine if you could observe your brain activity and see that your anxiety is a current going from one cell to another, passing along a chemical between cells. It is an event in your brain. You can see it. Imagine that you observe the event as it lights up and then it dims down. It comes and goes. It's neither good nor bad. It simply is."

The therapist can suggest that making choices about possible actions would constitute a moral or ethical issue—not the thoughts, images, or emotions that exist independent of action. Indeed, one can feel *temptation* or the desire to do something that is considered unethical, but the decision not to take action is what constitutes a moral or ethical choice:

> "We may not have a choice as to our thoughts, sensations, or emotions, but we do have a choice as to our actions. Imagine that you claimed that you had been totally faithful to your partner for the past year, but we discover that you were on a deserted island. Would we think that you had made a moral choice? In contrast, imagine that there were numerous beautiful and sexy people who showed an interest in you, but you chose not to pursue them. Would that be a moral choice, or would you be immoral simply because you had a desire and felt tempted?"

Eighth, some patients believe that a feeling will immediately become an action. Such a belief is a variation of thought–action fusion. Since an emotion or a thought precedes an action, it may seem natural to jump to the conclusion that the emotion or thought *results* in the action (e.g., "I got anxious, so I ran," or "I got angry, so I yelled at him"). But most emotions and thoughts do not lead to actions; they are simply experienced as internal events. The therapist can inquire, "Isn't there a difference between controlling your actions and controlling your feelings? What is the difference?" Or: "Aren't there lots of feelings that you have that never lead to an action? Do you always eat whenever you have a feeling of hunger? Do you always attack someone when you feel angry? Do you always run away whenever you feel anxious?" The patient with emotion–action fusion fears that the onset of an emotion will automatically lead to an unwanted action, and thus believes that the emotion needs to be totally controlled. The therapist can ask the patient to keep track of a negative emotion (its occurrence and intensity), monitor the activities or situations, and then list the specific behaviors that the patient engages in. This can be illustrated in the session:

> "I understand that you often think that if you feel anxious, you will go out of control. Let's take the last time that you were on a plane. You have told me that you fear that you will get anxious, jump out of your seat, and bang on the exit. OK. Now the last time you were on a plane you felt anxious, you told me, but did you jump out of your seat and bang on the exit door? Why not?"

Thoughts and emotions are internal events, whereas behavior is an external event that is chosen. In this example, the patient realizes that anxious thoughts and feelings are present, but chooses to stay seated. Monitoring the occurrence of anxiety throughout the day and week, along with the specific behavior, can illustrate that an emotion does not control behavior; *the patient controls behavior.* Even if an emotion cannot be controlled, the patient can control what he or she says or does.

Ninth, many patients who believe that they do not have control over their emotions use problematic coping strategies, such as binge eating, substance misuse, rumination, and avoidance. This sense of being out of control is magnified by these coping strategies, since they represent "out-of-control" behavior: "I feel out of control, and then I do more out-of-control things." The therapist can suggest that the occurrence of a feeling is not the real problem, but the interpretations and strategies that are employed:

> "What if you thought that your emotions would rise and fall on their own? Would you feel out of control? What if you thought that there are some really helpful and adaptive strategies to use when you feel upset? Would you feel out of control? Perhaps the problem is not your emotions, but the way that you cope with them at times. If you use unhelpful strategies, it may just add to that sense of being out of control and not being effective. Perhaps we can identify some useful strategies that you can use."

The belief in the need for control can also be addressed by encouraging the patient to do absolutely nothing about an emotion when it arises, but simply to observe it with detached mindfulness. This is similar to techniques advocated by Wells (2009) in his metacognitive approach. Sitting and doing nothing can be a daily mindfulness exercise as the patient intentionally practices remaining still, passive, and detached while intentionally surrendering to the observations of the moment. While doing nothing, the individual can also observe the internal voice that tells him, "You should be doing something—controlling things, getting rid of thoughts, or judging your current experience." Later the therapist can explore with the patient whether he or she has difficulty tolerating doing nothing—just observing, being in the moment, or letting time drift by (Roemer & Orsillo, 2009; Wells, 2009). The need to do something evokes emotions and maintains them, since goals continually need completion. In addition, the patient can practice imagining disappearing completely while observing that the world continues without him or her—or imagining standing above everything on a distant and elevated balcony while observing other people going about their lives. By disappearing, or rising above, or observing, the patient can experience the sense of detachment and distance that can provide the peace of losing all goals for the moment (Leahy, 2005d). Since emotions are directed toward goals, relinquishing goals by abandoning oneself—by "disappearing"—leads to relinquishing the emotion.

Figure 7.4 delineates some of the maladaptive and adaptive strategies that can be used in emotion regulation. Maladaptive strategies include avoidance, suppression, worry/rumination, and substance misuse or other forms of acting out (e.g., self-cutting). We have identified a number of

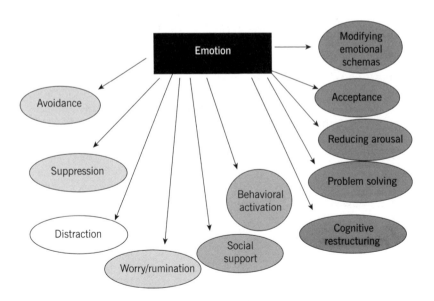

**FIGURE 7.4.** Some examples of adaptive and maladaptive emotion regulation strategies. Maladaptive strategies are at left, lightly shaded; adaptive strategies are at right in darker shading. Based on Leahy, Tirch, and Napolitano (2011).

helpful strategies that can be used to replace the maladaptive strategies (Leahy, Tirch, & Napolitano, 2011). These include cognitive restructuring, acceptance, modification of emotional schemas, problem solving, DBT skills, communication skills, relaxation (and other arousal reduction techniques), behavioral activation, mindfulness, compassion-focused techniques, distraction (to some extent), social support, and emotion-focused therapy techniques. The therapist can suggest that knowing that there are adaptive strategies can reduce the fear of an emotion:

> "If you fell into the water and it was 20 feet deep and you thought that you couldn't swim, how would you feel? Anxious, terrified? But what if you fell in the water and you knew that you were a strong swimmer—that you could stay afloat for hours. How would you feel? If you had techniques and tools that could gradually calm you down and make things better, would you have less fear of losing control?"

## GUILT AND SHAME

Some people feel guilty or ashamed about their thoughts, sensations, behaviors, or emotions. I refer to "guilt" as a belief that one's qualities are inconsistent with an ideal view of the self. For example, a woman who views herself as peaceful and rational may feel guilty over having feelings of anger and the desire for revenge. A husband who loves his wife may feel guilty over his sexual fantasies about other women. Other examples of guilty thoughts about emotion are: "I shouldn't feel sad; I have so much to be thankful for," or "Anger is a bad emotion; it means that I am an angry, terrible person." "Shame" entails beliefs that it would be intolerable for other people to know about one's emotions. Shame is linked to embarrassment and humiliation as well as, a desire to hide from others what one is truly thinking, sensing, or feeling. Patients may feel ashamed that they have sexual feelings, especially "unconventional" desires (however they may define these). Or anxious patients may feel ashamed that they are anxious, and apprehensive that others will notice their anxiety and think that they are weak. Whereas shame involves the desire to hide from others, guilt involves a tendency to criticize the self. In reality, people often feel both ashamed and guilty about their emotions—embarrassed that others might know, and guilty and self-critical that their emotions conflict with their view of themselves. (See also Tangney, Stuewig, & Mashek, 2007, for a detailed discussion about the differences between guilt and shame and their implications.) Figure 7.5 illustrates the process of guilt about an emotion, and Figure 7.6 illustrates that of shame.

It is instructive to learn which emotions a patient feels shame or guilt over. Some people feel ashamed that they have sexual or aggressive

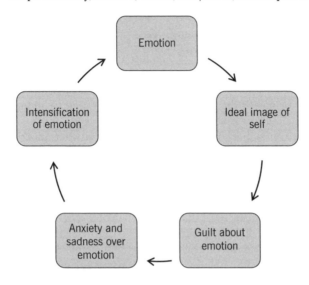

**FIGURE 7.5.** The process of guilt about an emotion.

emotions, but not ashamed that they feel sad or anxious. Others may have the reverse pattern—ashamed of sadness or anxiety, but not ashamed of anger or aggression. The therapist can ask, "Why are certain emotions good and others are bad? How do you know if an emotion is bad?" For example, a man described in earlier chapters had an ideal view of himself as competent and rational; he felt ashamed that he was sad and anxious, but was not ashamed of his anger. His ideal self-image (strength and self-control) led him to view sadness and anxiety as weaknesses. On inquiry as to why he felt ashamed that he was sad and anxious, he indicated that people would view him as weak and take advantage of him. He viewed his

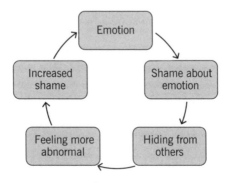

**FIGURE 7.6.** The process of shame about an emotion.

parents as condescending, controlling, and judgmental, and said that they would criticize and humiliate him for his "weakness." However, he believed that his anger was legitimate and was justified by the unfair conditions of his current life. He believed that anger showed his strength, and that he needed to get rid of any emotions that showed weakness. He feared that he might cry in front of others and that they would judge him as "unmanly." As a result, he felt alone with his feelings.

Another man believed that his sexual feelings for women that he would see in cafes or bars indicated that there was something wrong with him and that he might lose control and betray his wife. He believed that he should only have sexual desire for or fantasies about his wife, and that he was not a good husband because of these feelings. He was ambivalent about these desires—sometimes placing himself in situations where he might interact with other women, but then feeling guilty that he had these feelings. He would monitor his fantasies, thereby increasing their intensity and further supporting his guilt. The former lawyer discussed earlier, who left her job to take care of her child, felt guilty about her depression because she believed that she was not entitled to feel down, given that her husband "provided" her with such a high quality of life. Her ideal view of herself was that she should be appreciative and satisfied, and that her depression reflected a selfish and immature quality in her. In addition, she also felt ashamed when speaking with former colleagues or with other women with careers because she believed that they thought less of her.

The therapist can begin to evaluate the patient's guilt and shame about emotions by asking, "Which emotions do you feel guilty about? That is, which ones do you criticize yourself for having? Which emotions are you *not* guilty about? When you feel guilty, what kinds of thoughts go through your head?" As indicated above, patients may have self-critical thoughts about some emotions but not others. Differentiating the evaluations of a variety of emotions can assist the patients in recognizing that it is not emotion per se that they feel guilty about, but only specific emotions. Examples of "thoughts that go through your head when you have an emotion" include "I shouldn't feel this way," "I must be a bad person," "What's wrong with me?," or "I must be weak."

The therapist can ask similar questions about shame: "Are there certain emotions that you feel ashamed about? That is, would you be concerned that others might find out that you have these feelings? What are those emotions? Are there other emotions that you have that you are *not* ashamed about? Why are you ashamed of some emotions but not others? What thoughts go through your head?" Again, as discussed earlier, some patients may feel ashamed about some emotions but not others. They may think that others would think less of them if they knew that they had sexual fantasies or desires or that they were angry. For others, the pattern may be reversed.

As discussed in earlier chapters, many people adhere to a belief in "emotional perfectionism" or "pure mind." That is, they yearn to have only "good" emotions, and only "decent," "rational," and "good" thoughts. Based on an illusion that human nature must be "good" and that they must strive for perfection in their feelings, they feel ashamed and guilty about emotions such as anger, resentment, jealousy, and envy. The emotional schema model embraces the universality of all emotions and views them as constituting the full range of human potential. This includes all of the "imperfect," "undesirable," or "bad" emotions that some believe should be relegated to an ash heap. Rather than viewing human nature as a possibly perfectible condition, the emotional schema therapist recognizes that we humans are capable of almost anything and that these fantasies, sensations, thoughts, and emotions can arise for any of us. The therapist will avoid the role of "guru" who tries to encourage patients to believe that they are capable of perfect emotional peace; positive emotions on demand; or freedom from temptation, desire, resentment, or the urge to get revenge. Rather than relegating or eliminating these emotions, the therapist can suggest:

"Acknowledging the full range of our human emotional nature allows us to be aware and accepting of the thoughts and emotions that we have, so as to view them as a 'given' from which we can stand back and consider valued action. Just because you feel envious does not mean that you are 'an envious person' or 'a bad person,' and it does not mean that you will attempt to destroy those who surpass you. Rather, acknowledging your envy allows you to realize that—like all of us humans—you are capable of these feelings, but that you also make choices as to your actions. Emotions are the 'given' that cannot be wished away, judged away, or suppressed. None of us is so good that we aren't capable of feeling almost anything."

In this way, the therapist can introduce the idea that emotions can be viewed as a "given" or an experience that "simply is." Like hunger, thirst, pain, pleasure, or sensations of various kinds, an emotion can be viewed as an "experience" that one has, rather than a sign of moral degradation, personal weakness, or lack of control.

The therapist can then continue:

"What if you suspended judgment about your emotion and simply viewed it as another experience that you might have? You could say to yourself, 'I am feeling sad right now,' or 'I am feeling jealous at the moment.' Is there any advantage in judging your emotions? Are there any disadvantages in judging your emotions? What would be the costs and benefits of accepting an emotion as an experience that you are having at this moment?"

Some patients believe that they need to judge their emotions in order to notice their feelings and be able to control them: "If I simply accepted my jealousy, I might let my guard down and act out," or "If I simply accepted my sadness right now, I might just give up and become even more depressed." The therapist can illustrate the bind that the patient is in: "You are feeling sad, and then you criticize yourself for your sadness, which makes you feel guilty and then more sad. You are feeling bad about feeling bad." In addition, the therapist can introduce the idea that accepting that one has an emotion, without judging the emotion, does not imply that one does nothing to make life better: "Is it possible to accept that you feel sad, but are still able to choose to do things to make your life better at this time? You can say, 'OK, I feel sad, I accept that; it's the experience for the moment. But there are some rewarding things that I can do to have other feelings.'" Figure 7.7 illustrates the process of accepting an emotion as a "given" and focusing instead on valued goals.

The therapist can examine the patient's rationale for shame or guilt over specific emotions. This rationale can then be examined by using cognitive therapy techniques, such as cost–benefit analysis, evidence for and against, the double-standard technique, and role play. The therapist can ask, "What are the reasons that you think your emotions are not legitimate? Why shouldn't you have the feelings that you have?" The man who felt guilty about his sexual desires for other women said, "A good husband should not want other women. If he does, then it means that there is something wrong with him, and he might go out of control." As noted earlier,

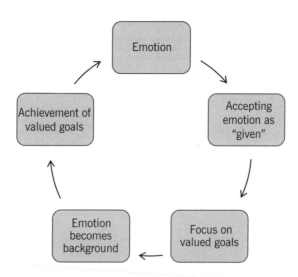

**FIGURE 7.7.** The process by which accepting an emotion as a "given" and focusing instead on valued goals can lead to the achievement of those goals.

his guilt over his fantasies then led him to monitor them, which increased his anxiety, increased his fantasies, and led to failed attempts to suppress his desires. The lawyer who was raising her child believed that a nice home and supportive husband should be enough to fulfill any needs that she had. Indeed, she believed that she should not have a need, or desire, for a professional career. Again, this was linked to her mother's experience of giving up her professional career to raise a family. She believed that she should be satisfied with the arrangement that her mother had, even though, ironically, her mother had not been satisfied with it.

The therapist can also help normalize the patient's emotions: "Is it possible that others could have the same feelings in this situation?" Often patients who feel ashamed of their feelings or emotions do not share them with others, further contributing to their sense that their emotions are not "legitimate." The man who had fantasies about other women equated desire with defectiveness in his marriage.

THERAPIST: You think that your desire for other women means that there is something wrong with your marriage. Do you have desire for your wife?

PATIENT: Yes, I find her very attractive.

THERAPIST: Could it be that your desire for other women simply means that you are alive, you have strong feelings, and that you find women attractive—very much like other heterosexual men do all the time? Maybe you find them attractive because *they are attractive.*

PATIENT: I guess that's possible.

THERAPIST: Imagine if someone said, "The only woman in the world who I find attractive is my wife." What would you think?

PATIENT: I would think he was lying.

A young woman reported feeling guilty and ashamed that she was jealous of her partner's ex-girlfriend, with whom he had recently had dinner: "I don't want to be that girl who is crazy and insecure." She believed that she should be sophisticated and flexible and not have feelings of jealousy, since to her they reflected insecurity. The therapist asked her how her friends might feel about their boyfriends' having dinner with an ex-girlfriend, and the patient actually took an informal poll. Almost every one of them said that they wouldn't like it, although two of them shared her self-critical thought, "I should be able to tolerate it." I examine jealousy in more detail in Chapter 10, but normalizing emotions such as jealousy can help reduce shame and guilt about them.

As indicated earlier, some people equate an emotion or sensation with an action—a variation of thought–action fusion. The therapist can ask such patients, "Can you see that having a feeling (e.g., sexual fantasy) is not the same as acting on it (e.g., being unfaithful)?" The man who felt guilty and anxious about his sexual desires for other women feared that his fantasies would rapidly lead to action, and that this would destroy his marriage and family life. The therapist observed that the patient had sexual fantasies about other women for years and had never acted on them:

> THERAPIST: What do you make of the fact that you have these fantasies but do not act on them?
>
> PATIENT: I must have a lot of self-control.
>
> THERAPIST: OK. Let's think this through. Imagine that you did act on these fantasies and began going to bars and having sex with strangers on a regular basis. Where would that lead?
>
> PATIENT: It would wreck my marriage. And it would not be consistent with the way I see myself.
>
> THERAPIST: You seem to think that you should never have any feelings of temptation. But the only way to make a moral or ethical choice is to have temptations that you choose to resist. In fact, each time you have a fantasy, you might say to yourself, "Yes, I am alive, and it makes sense to have desire, but I can think ahead as to what is in my best interests and choose not to act on my desire."

The patient later reported that by feeling less guilty and anxious about his fantasies, he was able to enjoy himself in public and felt less guilty around his wife. He also recognized that he was making conscious decisions not to act out because he valued his marriage, not because there was something wrong with him or his relationship with his wife.

Distinguishing between an emotion or feeling and an action is an important step in alleviating guilt. Actions are what harm others, not the emotions that one is having. The therapist can ask, "How is anyone harmed by your emotions?" Or the therapist can be more specific:

> "Imagine your emotions are a headache that you are having for about 30 minutes. It is painful and unpleasant. You may even think it will never go away, or you might get catastrophic and think that you have a brain tumor. Should other people be afraid that your headache will cause them harm? Emotions are internal events, brain activities—chemical and electrical events in your brain. It is not an emotion that harms others; it is an action. If there is no behavior, there is no harm."

Alternatively, some patients fail to recognize that their emotions may reflect that there *is* something wrong in their lives or in their relationships. They may focus on their sensations or symptoms, rather than on the interpersonal conflicts that they are facing. It may be less threatening to be concerned about one's own emotions or sensations than about one's relationship with another person. For example, a married woman complained about her fear that she would have a panic attack while driving or traveling. Her ideal view of herself was of someone who was well grounded, strong, independent, and rational. In her initial meetings with the therapist, she claimed that her husband was very understanding and supportive, and that her marriage was almost ideal. The initial approach in therapy with her was the traditional cognitive-behavioral approach: providing her with a conceptualization of panic as false alarms and catastrophic interpretations; panic induction; exposure to situations likely to elicit panic; and decastrophizing her symptoms. Although these interventions were somewhat effective, she still had considerable anticipatory anxiety and worry, and expressed concern that she had difficulty being as independent as she once was. She felt embarrassed about "needing" therapy. Further inquiry indicated that her marital relationship was less than ideal. Her husband was often late returning home, with unexplained absences. She reported that she did not trust him, but that she was hesitant to assert herself because she feared he would leave her. She was encouraged to assert herself more directly with her husband about her concerns over his absence. Through a friend, she learned that her husband had had an affair with another woman. She confronted him with this infidelity and expressed considerable anger toward him. He begged forgiveness. After her direct assertion with him, she reported no further panic attacks and no worry about having panic attacks.

Another young man complained about his fear that he would not be able to maintain an erection with a new partner. He worried that he was "unmanly" and that his anxiety suggested that he was deeply disturbed. His erectile dysfunction had begun during a relationship with a former girlfriend, who would alternate between saying she loved him and then rejecting him and saying she wanted her freedom to pursue other men. The therapist asked him how he felt when she rejected him, and he replied that he had no right to feel angry because she had a lot of psychological problems. He indicated that it was his role to be supportive to her. The therapist suggested that his penis was trying to tell him something: "It is unsafe emotionally to be vulnerable with her." The therapist asked, "What if you looked at feelings and emotions as experiences that tell you that something is bothering you—like a caution sign, a stop sign, or a flashing red light?" His anxiety and emotional ambivalence toward her were similar to a warning sign, "Danger ahead." However, rather than looking ahead to verify the danger, he felt anxious that he had a sign. The therapist suggested, "Maybe your penis is smarter than you are. The sign tells you that something is wrong. It might be useful to obey the sign."

Finally, guilt or shame over an emotion often results in problematic coping strategies. A common strategy is rumination: "What is wrong with me that I feel this way? What could be going on?" The patient believes that the rumination will provide an answer that will "explain" why he or she has an emotion that is "wrong" to have. Other strategies include avoiding triggers for the emotion. For example, the lawyer who was now a mother felt ashamed of her depression and reduced her contact with former colleagues, further adding to her sense of isolation. Other strategies may include binge eating, substance misuse, and hypersomnia. The rationale is that since the emotion is "wrong" or "shameful," then any situations that elicit the emotion should be avoided—or, better still, the emotional experience should be numbed. Some people believe that they should be punished for their emotion: "I don't deserve to be happy. I deserve to be depressed."

## ACCEPTANCE

Many patients who endorse negative emotional schemas believe that they cannot simply accept having an emotion. They often equate acceptance with letting their guard down, losing of control, being defeated or overwhelmed, and inviting further escalation of emotion and significant impairment. Indeed, it is almost as if these individuals believe that the emotion is "attacking" them, beating them down, or taking over, and that the best defense is an offense. In contrast to this refusal to accept—or even fear of acceptance of—emotion, there is considerable evidence that relinquishing the struggle against an emotion can have palliative effects: It often gives people greater flexibility in taking action and willingness to engage in behaviors, *even in the presence of unpleasant emotions* (Hayes et al., 2006, 2012; Linehan et al., 2007). The willingness to accept an emotion (or sensation) while pursuing action toward valued goals is a hallmark of ACT, behavioral activation therapy, and DBT (Hayes et al., 2006, 2012; Linehan et al., 2007; Martell, Dimidjian, & Herman-Dunn, 2010). The emotional schema model draws on each of these approaches to help modify negative beliefs about acceptance of emotion.

The emotional schema model proposes that individuals have specific beliefs about the meanings and consequences of accepting unpleasant emotions. Modifying these beliefs through cognitive, behavioral, and experiential techniques can help develop more adaptive beliefs about acceptance, which can facilitate productive action and decrease the credibility of beliefs that one must eliminate unwanted emotions immediately. The goal is to achieve belief in this paradox: By temporarily relinquishing control, one will feel less out of control. When one gives up the goal of the impossible (controlling everything), one can live in the world of the possible (what is).

First, the therapist can inquire as to the patient's beliefs about the implications of accepting an emotion: "What will happen if you allow yourself to accept an emotion? Will you act on it [feeling–action fusion]? Do you fear that if you accept an emotion, it won't go away?" Some patients believe that if they accept an emotion, it will escalate in intensity and overwhelm them. One patient described his beliefs about anxiety: "If I simply accept the anxiety, I think it will get worse and worse, and I will have a panic attack." The therapist asked, "Then what will happen?" He replied, "Well, if I am on the plane, I see myself losing control, getting up, screaming, and trying to open the door." Many patients with intense anxiety believe that their emotions will quickly turn into action ("thought–action fusion") and that they must catch the emotion and eliminate it before it unravels. Standard cognitive-behavioral techniques, such as exposure to interoceptive stimuli, can help dissuade such patients from the belief that accepting—or even allowing—an unchecked emotion will lead to dangerous escalation (Barlow, 2002). For example, the patient who feared having a panic attack on the plane was able to tolerate intense arousal in session that was induced by practicing hyperventilation. Similar in-session exposure techniques can also be used, such as inducing dizziness in session (though spinning in a chair or staring at a mirror) while practicing acceptance of the emotion. This can disconfirm the belief that the patient must do everything possible to eliminate arousal in order to have it abate. Indeed, the goal in this kind of exposure exercise is to do nothing, but allow the sensations to come and go.

As mentioned in the section on control, the patient can also test the belief that "I need to do something about the emotion" by practicing "mindful detachment"—that is, simply standing back and observing that he or she is having an emotion, while intending to do nothing about it (Wells, 2009). Again, mindful detachment is a metacognitive technique. Other metacognitive techniques include viewing an emotion or thought as a telemarketing phone call that one does not respond to, as a train coming in and out of a station, or as a cloud that passes in the sky (Wells, 2009). Other, more "traditional" mindfulness techniques, such as body scan meditation, mindfulness of the breath, and mindfulness of the surrounding environment, can enhance this observing rather than controlling relationship to an emotion (Roemer & Orsillo, 2002, 2009). The emotional schema therapist's question afterward is this: "What has happened with the emotion when you decided to take the perspective of an observer?"

Second, some patients believe that negative emotions are important to motivate them to change. This "negative motivational theory" is a common source of refusal to engage in self-reward following productive action. For example, a woman who would engage in some positive behaviors between sessions believed that it was important to feel bad when she did not engage in positive behaviors, in order to motivate her to do better. Her negative motivational theory also led her to believe that feeling good after positive behavior was simplistic, shallow, and undeserved: "I should be doing positive things, and I shouldn't need to be a cheerleader for them." This patient had a dog and was quite fond of it. The therapist asked, "If you want to train your dog to do something, do you reward or ignore her positive behavior?" The patient commented, "Do you want me to be my own dog?" The therapist replied, "Yes. You might treat yourself better." The therapist then suggested that she experiment with rewarding (through self-praise) any positive behavior she engaged in, keep track of it, and simply say to herself when she did not follow through, "I can try harder next time." When this patient returned for her next session, she commented that she did get more done and she did feel somewhat better. The therapist jokingly commented, "It sounds like you were a good dog." Using humor can often take the sting out of the intense emotions that the patient fears.

Third, attempts to inhibit negative feelings can have problematic consequences, including thought rebound, greater intensity of negative beliefs about suppressed thoughts, and greater stress (Gross, 2002; Gross & John, 1997; Wegner, 1994; Wegner, Schneider, Carter, & White, 1987; Wegner & Zanakos, 1994; Wenzlaff & Wegner, 2000). Indeed, emotional avoidance is a key factor in generalized anxiety disorder, since the cognitive focus on worry temporarily inhibits emotional arousal, thus reinforcing worry as a strategy; the arousal only returns later, however (Borkovec et al., 1993; Borkovec, Ray, & Stoeber, 1998; Mennin, Heimberg, Turk, & Fresco, 2002, 2005). Moreover, attempts to suppress an emotion, rather than accept it as a temporary experience, contribute to a wide variety of problematic coping strategies, such as substance misuse, binge eating, self-cutting, and other self-destructive behaviors. The therapist can ask, "What are the negative consequences of inhibiting a feeling through excessive use of attention and energy? What problematic behaviors do you use in order to get rid of an emotion? If you didn't feel the need to get rid of an emotion—if you could accept it for the time being—what would change for the better?"

Fourth, some patients believe that they cannot accept an emotion, since "it is a bad emotion, and I would be bad if I accepted it." As noted earlier in regard to guilt and shame, such "emotional perfectionism" or "pure mind" underlies a considerable amount of refusal to allow oneself to have an emotion (or a fantasy). Indeed, identifying the self with an emotion or fantasy discounts all the complexity that one experiences. For example, a married woman described herself as worried that she had fantasies about other men, concluding that if she allowed herself to have these fantasies, it was equivalent to cheating on her husband. She described herself as having both positive feelings about the fantasies, and guilt and fear over them. As she attempted to suppress these fantasies, they seemed to become more intense and more intrusive. The therapist suggested that accepting fantasies does not imply that one will act on them or that one even wants them:

> "*The mind has a mind of its own*—it's active, free, sometimes chaotic, sometimes bringing up things you don't like, sometimes bringing up

things you like. You can't order your mind around. You can listen to it and then decide what you will do. You have had these fantasies for over a year, and you haven't acted. Perhaps there is a difference between having an emotion and choosing to engage in an action. What if you simply acknowledged to yourself that you have desires and fantasies, and that it is OK to let them happen and then pass on, and that nothing will happen as a result?"

Similarly, a male patient described his urges to check his pocket for his keys, even though he no longer engaged in behavioral checking. He believed that he should be completely free of these urges to check, and indicated that if he could not eliminate the urges, he would eventually decompensate into the behavioral patterns of OCD that he had experienced for many years before he came into behavioral therapy and relinquished the behavioral checking. The therapist suggested that he had a form of emotional perfectionism that he called "pure mind": "You believe that your mind should be completely free of any urges, thoughts, fantasies or emotions that are not part of your belief in a pure, rational, totally in-control mind." The therapist noted that the brain comprises millions of electrochemical events, almost all of which are outside of conscious awareness. Accordingly, the therapist suggested that the patient replace the belief in pure mind with a more realistic belief in "noisy mind":

"Listen to the traffic of New York City that is right outside this office. You have lived in New York for several years now, and you have accepted the noise. In fact, since I have known you, you have not complained about the noise, although both of us hear it. We accept it as the price to pay for living in this city. Giving up pure mind can allow you to decide which sounds or messages in your mind are worth listening to, and which are just background noise that is always there."

Fifth, the reluctance to accept an emotion may also impair patients' ability to use an emotion to tell themselves about what they need. Emotions can report needs, just as hunger or appetite can tell us that we need nourishment. Even negative emotions, such as anxiety, sadness, fear, loneliness, jealousy, and envy, can tell us about danger, rejection, mistakes, the need for companionship, our desire for commitment, and our desire to do well. Simply eliminating emotions would deprive our lives of meaning, intensity, passion, and information about what might be going wrong. For example, a woman who had been married for 28 years described her relationship with her husband as lacking affection, sexuality, and emotional intimacy. Depressed and angry, she commented, "Maybe I am too needy. Maybe I am expecting too much from marriage. After all, when you have been married this long you can't expect these things." Indeed, she had chosen cognitive therapy because she believed that she could avoid talking about her emotions and could develop a "rational" approach to accepting not having any needs. The therapist suggested that her emotions might provide valuable information about what was missing—and what she did need. He asked, "If you deny that something bothers you, how can you fix the problem?" By accepting that these emotions were "legitimate" and "informative," she could work on facing the unresolved issues in her marriage. As she accepted her emotions as painful reminders that important elements were missing in her marriage, she was able to confront her husband, and eventually to move the relationship toward greater intimacy on all levels. Both partners in the marriage were practicing mutual avoidance prior to this, living parallel lives, seldom touching. Accepting the pain of the emotions—and learning to express them directly in the marriage—allowed them to connect on an emotional level. Acceptance does not mean ignoring or minimizing. It can mean using an emotion.

## SUMMARY

This chapter has reviewed the importance of beliefs in emotions as incomprehensible, having indefinite duration, out of control, guilt-inducing or shameful, and unacceptable. Each of these dimensions of emotional schemas is relevant to the fear of emotional experience, avoidance, rumination, self-criticism, and other problematic strategies of coping. Using a variety of cognitive and behavioral techniques drawn from a wide range of approaches (e.g., cognitive therapy, behavioral activation, ACT, DBT, compassion-focused therapy, emotion-focused therapy) can help patients develop a more helpful understanding of their emotional experience, recognize that emotions can be temporary and tolerable experiences, use emotions to recognize needs that may be unfulfilled, and relate to emotions in a more accepting and productive manner.

# CHAPTER 8

# Coping with Ambivalence

I hate and I love.
How do I know it's true?
My pain tells me so.
—CATULLUS, ca. 60 B.C.E.

## DEFINING AMBIVALENCE AND INTOLERANCE OF IT

"Ambivalence" is generally defined as mixed feelings about choosing an alternative; that is, an individual who is faced with a choice feels pulled in apparently opposing directions. Ambivalence also includes having mixed feelings about aspects of the self and of other people, and it reflects beliefs about the nature of choice. Thus individuals who have difficulty tolerating ambivalence may believe that they cannot make a choice if they have mixed feelings, that they must collect more information in order to make a choice, that their uncertainty is both undesirable and intolerable, and that they should wait to make any decision until ambivalence is resolved. On reflection, almost everyone experiences ambivalence on a regular basis, but individuals with emotional schemas related to ambivalence have difficulty tolerating mixed feelings.

Models of choice behavior suggest that individuals consider alternatives by weighing and comparing the costs and benefits of each one. The assumption in choice theory is that choosing any alternative will involve making tradeoffs, and that "rational choices" are made with the recognition that there is no alternative without a cost. For instance, choosing a restaurant for dinner involves various tradeoffs (price, location, cuisine, quality, ambiance). Indecision also has its costs—primarily, the "opportunity cost" of passing up alternatives. For example, if I choose to put all my money in a mattress rather than making any decision about investing it, I pay the opportunity cost of lost interest on a bank account or lost profits in stocks. Individuals who are intolerant of ambivalence are often indecisive, since they believe that they need to make a decision that has no potential disadvantages. Since this is usually impossible, these individuals will often wait a long time to decide, avoid behavior that would follow from a decision, seek reassurance from others, and search for additional information either to bolster a decision or to defeat it.

Moreover, choices are made in terms of overall goals or values. To return to the restaurant example, my choice between fish or chicken is made with the overall (superordinate) goal of satisfying my hunger. Indeed, I may turn out to be indifferent about the relative desirability of chicken or fish, since both may equally satisfy my hunger. Decision makers fall along a continuum, with those at one extreme looking to get the best possible outcome ("maximizers"), while those at the other extreme are simply looking to satisfy a modest criterion or goal ("satisficers") (Simon, 1956). Maximizers reject alternatives that do not provide the maximum benefits with the lowest costs, often remaining indecisive while ignoring opportunity costs. For example, an extreme maximizer in a restaurant may go through pairwise comparisons for an hour and then not have time to eat dinner. Maximizers operate with an assumption that there is a perfect decision to be made, and that they can collect all the information and consider all the permutations. "Satisficers" (the word is Scottish and was first used by Simon) are willing to sacrifice to settle, recognizing that there are limits on time and alternatives, and that they can move forward in an imperfect world with imperfect choices (Simon, 1956, 1957, 1979). Satisficers are more satisfied with their choices (which seems true by definition), whereas maximizers are more likely to regret their choices. This distinction in decision theory is one of the central components of "bounded rationality"—that is, the recognition that there are limits to "rational choice" wherever there are limits to information and time (in other words, always). We do not have an infinite amount of time to make our choices, and we can almost never know all the information. Satisficers are willing to decide with uncertainty and under time constraints (Kahneman & Tversky, 1984; Kahneman et al., 2006). In contrast to maximizers' overvaluation of more information, decision makers in the "real world" often rely on rules of thumb, or "heuristics," to reach decisions rapidly. Indeed, these heuristics are often more accurate than the search for additional (and often irrelevant) information (Gigerenzer & Selten, 2001).

Individuals who have difficulty with ambivalence often act as if there are no realistic, pragmatic considerations in making a choice. Their emphasis is on making a perfect decision without significant tradeoffs, rather than a practical decision in real time. An individual who is intolerant of ambivalence is driven by perfectionistic, dichotomous thinking. For example, a man who was in a relationship with a woman recognized that he was not completely happy with some aspects of her behavior. This led to the following string of automatic thoughts: "There is something about her that I don't completely like," "If I am not completely happy with everything, then it won't work out," "Other people are completely satisfied with their relationships," "If it doesn't work out with her, I will never have anyone," and "I will end up alone." This man idealized what he believed others had in their lives, while discounting the excellent qualities of his current relationship. In addition, many individuals who are intolerant of ambivalence run a significant risk of regret and rumination, since postdecision thinking involves measuring a choice against a "perfect" alternative. Unlike individuals who resolve their ambivalence after a choice by bolstering the choice ("dissonance reduction"), ambivalent individuals refocus on rejected alternatives or possible future alternatives as far more desirable than the choice that was made. Thus individuals who are intolerant of ambivalence delay decisions, ruminate about possible alternatives, demand reassurance, avoid situations where decisions need to be made, regret decisions that are made, discount the positives of the chosen alternative, and ruminate about rejected alternatives.

Intolerance of ambivalence has similarities with intolerance of uncertainty (Dugas, Buhr, & Ladouceur, 2004; Sookman & Pinard, 2002). In both cases, an individual wants either a perfect alternative or perfect predictability. In both cases, the individual is inclined to worry or ruminate about the absence of perfection or certainty, believing that this repetitive negative focus will yield the crucial information that will allow a decision. In both cases, the individual is regret-oriented—both anticipating regret and, once a decision has been made, experiencing regret. Similar to the "Zeigarnik effect," which characterizes difficulty in letting go of an incomplete task, intolerance of ambivalence and intolerance of uncertainty both involve seeking complete closure rather than the incompleteness almost all choices entail.

Intolerance of ambivalence is also associated with a wide variety of cognitive distortions, including dichotomous thinking (as mentioned above), labeling ("This is an unacceptable alternative/a bad choice"), discounting positives ("Yes, there is that positive, but there is also that negative"), negative filtering (focusing primarily on the negative aspects of the alternative under consideration), fortunetelling (predicting that the ambivalent choice will lead to a bad outcome), catastrophizing (anticipating the bad outcome as unbearable), emotional reasoning ("Because I am ambivalent, it must be a bad choice"), and "should" statements ("I should be completely happy with the choice," "I should not be ambivalent").

Intolerance of ambivalence is particularly associated with negative filtering, which, as just noted, involves a confirmation bias focused on anything less than perfect in the alternative under consideration. For example, the man described above would often focus on any negative qualities his partner had or any negative moods he experienced. He then interpreted these observations and experiences as evidence that he would be stuck with the wrong choice. When he experienced boredom, he interpreted this as evidence that there must be something terribly wrong with the relationship: "People who have good relationships do not get bored." Adding to the power of this negative filtering is the belief that there is an idealized world where others may be experiencing consistent bliss, or that the choices one could make will lead to everlasting happiness. This idealization is part of the larger problem of "emotional perfectionism" described in earlier chapters, which suggests that somehow one should feel good or happy all the time, and that this is a goal worth striving for.

## MODIFYING INTOLERANCE OF AMBIVALENCE

### Addressing a Simplistic View of Emotions

The ability to differentiate a wide range of emotions in self and others is a consequence of increasing cognitive development (Saarni, 1999, 2007). In the psychoanalytic literature, ego development is characterized by increasing awareness of potentially conflicting qualities of the self; with the emergence of "ego identity," where a central quality is identified while incorporating differentiated emotions or personal qualities (Loevinger, 1976). Thus a younger child might view others (and self) in dichotomous trait terms (e.g., "He is nasty"), while a more differentiated adult is able to recognize variability of personal qualities across time and situations (e.g., "Sometimes he's nasty, but at other times he can be nice"). Research on the person perception of individuals with borderline personality disorder indicates a tendency to use dichotomous statements (Arntz & Haaf, 2012; Veen & Arntz, 2000). The problem with dichotomous thinking is that it leads to stable trait attributions about self and others, without allowing for the recognition of situational or temporal variability and flexibility. If I think of myself as a sad person, then my life narrative will be one of selective memory, attention, and emphasis on information confirming this belief—a form of confirmation bias. If I think of myself as capable of a wide variety of emotions and behaviors, then I can imagine myself being far more flexible—which is a much more adaptive view of myself. Therefore, addressing a simplistic view of emotion—which is one of the 14 dimensions of emotional schemas discussed in earlier chapters and assessed with the LESS II—is among the first tasks in increasing tolerance for ambivalence in emotional schema therapy.

Dispelling the myth of dichotomous thinking about one's personality or emotions is a key element in increasing acceptance, reducing rumination, and enhancing flexibility. Unlike the Jack Nicholson character in the movie *Anger Management*, who continually barbs the timid Adam Sandler character with "But how do you *really feel*?", the emotional schema therapist embraces and encourages the acceptance of mixed feelings and ambivalence. Some patients believe that they should "figure out how I really feel" by questioning the legitimacy of the emotions or by "digging deeper" for the "underlying emotion." The idea that there is some basic emotion, true feeling, or underlying secret only precipitates a string of ruminative thinking in a search for the "answer." The true "answer" lies in accepting the complexity and the contradictions.

For example, the man described earlier was trying to figure out his "real feelings" about his girlfriend.

> PATIENT: I think she's attractive, she's really nice to me—really nurturing at times—but she can say some things that really bother me.
>
> THERAPIST: What does she say that bothers you?
>
> PATIENT: Well, she's not as interested in politics as I would like her to be.
>
> THERAPIST: OK. So there is something about her that you are not fond of. Why does it bother you that you don't feel completely positive about her—about everything?
>
> PATIENT: Well, maybe she's not the right one for me.

This is a typical train of thought for people who are attempting to make important decisions but unable to accept ambivalence. Again, it reflects perfectionism and "pure mind." In this case, the individual was seeking "existential perfectionism": "Shouldn't I be sure before I decide?" In this particular case of "emotional perfectionism," the man's doubts about his girlfriend led to excessive focus on the negative, rumination, discounting the positive, hesitancy about his commitment, and distancing from the girlfriend. His underlying beliefs were "I should only feel one way," "I should be sure about what I feel," "I can't be in love if I have mixed feelings," and "I can't make a decision to commit if I am ambivalent." Such idealization of univalent emotion often results in the inability to deepen intimate relationships.

A further aspect of the intolerance of ambivalence is the belief that one will be stuck with regret if the "wrong decision" is made. The search for a perfect alternative is an attempt to avoid this regret. I recall years ago talking with someone who had a problematic relationship. I asked him if he had any regrets. He attempted to sound completely rational and replied, "No. Every decision I made was my decision, so I take responsibility for those decisions." This struck me as rather unrealistic, if not naive. How could one learn from mistakes, how could one be true to one's feelings, if there was no room for regret? Indeed, regrets often tell us that we could do a better job of making decisions. And even if regrets are unrealistic, having them does not mean that one must be completely immersed in and permanently "stuck with" the regrets. One can momentarily acknowledge, "I regret I am on the Second Avenue bus in the morning stuck in traffic," and soon get off the bus. Finally, regrets may simply be part of any difficult decision, as Søren Kierkegaard (1843/1992) observed: "I see it all perfectly; there are two possible situations—one can either do this or that. My honest opinion and my friendly advice is this: do it or do not do it—you will regret both."

## Examining the Costs and Benefits of Tolerating Ambivalence

As with most emotional schemas and strategies, a key element in changing schemas related to fear of ambivalence is to examine the motivation to modify the schemas. With no pun intended, most individuals who are intolerant of ambivalence have mixed motives: there are costs to this intolerance, and there is the perception that there are benefits. The therapist can ask, "What are the costs and benefits of not tolerating ambivalence?" Many patients are readily able to acknowledge the costs: dissatisfaction with their lives, rumination, worry about the future, and inability to enjoy the current moment. The therapist can help focus these individuals on the possibility that tolerating ambivalence, rather than eliminating it, might result in a more adaptive way of living. For example, tolerating ambivalence can lead to acceptance of reality as it is, ability to appreciate what one has, reduced rumination, less regret, and greater ability to make decisions.

The therapist can address the consequences of seeking simplicity or definitive feeling: "When you keep questioning how you *really feel* [or have difficulty accepting mixed feelings], what are the consequences for you? What are the advantages of not accepting mixed feelings? What are the disadvantages?" The disadvantages may be the inability to make a decision, rumination, avoidance (of situations that evoke mixed feelings), self-doubt, self-criticism ("What's wrong with me that I don't know?"), excessive reassurance seeking, and negative filtering.

Some people believe that an advantage of not accepting mixed feelings is that they will not make a decision that they will regret. Others believe that there must be some basic feeling that they should identify, so that they can "know for sure." As noted earlier, this search for "how I really feel" is a classic characteristic of those who cannot tolerate uncertainty—"I need to know for sure" (Dugas, Freeston, & Ladouceur, 1997; Ladouceur, Gosselin, & Dugas, 2000). Uncertainty may be equated with a bad outcome ("I will end up making the wrong decision" or "I will be misled"), lack of responsibility ("I should know how I really feel"), or lack of control ("If I don't know how I really feel, then how will I be able to control how things turn out?"). These beliefs can be addressed directly. The therapist can ask,

"Is it possible that you can know for sure that you have specific feelings that are different? For example, can you know for sure that you feel angry at one moment, sad at another moment, happy at another moment? Knowing how you feel does not have to mean that you always feel the same way toward yourself or someone else. In fact, is it possible to say, 'I know for sure that I have mixed feelings'?"

Another way of addressing uncertainty is to question whether there is certainty about anything that is complex: "Do you have mixed feelings about your job?" or "Have you seen a movie that you liked but that there were parts that you did not like?" Mixed feelings can be reframed as complexity, honesty, awareness, and richness of experience, and as also suggesting that there are no perfect alternatives in an imperfect world where people and events are always in flux. Indeed, acknowledging ambivalence can normalize that difficulties, challenges, and disappointments are inevitable in life—and acceptable.

Some patients believe that having a variety of feelings means that they are "contradictory": For example, "There are some things about him that I like and some things I don't like. I don't know why I have these contradictory feelings." The assumption is that all feelings should be univalent—that is, either entirely positive or entirely negative. Labeling feelings as contradictory may trigger beliefs in the necessity of linear thinking and beliefs about either–or exclusion ("It can't be 'A' and 'not A'"). This binary belief system may lead to a rejection of a range of feelings as logically self-contradictory and therefore wrong. An alternative is to replace "contradictory" with a "range of feelings"—or, better still, a "richness of feelings." The therapist can say:

"Imagine a painting that is a beautiful image of a field of flowers. There are red, pink, yellow, purple, and white ones, and green grass, and a blue sky in the distance. Are these colors contradictory? What would the painting be like if it were in black and white? If you were able to see all the colors and appreciate each one as something distinct and vibrant and real, would this be a problem for you? Or imagine that you are eating at a buffet. You taste one dish, and it has a bit of salt; another dish is spicy; another dish is sweet. Would you say that there should be only one way that food tastes?"

Emperor Joseph II reputedly said to Mozart about one of his operas, "Too many notes," to which Mozart allegedly replied, "Exactly as many as are necessary, Your Majesty." This story can be used as well.

In addition, the therapist can address the issue of complexity and richness as a source of perceptiveness and awareness: "Perhaps you are quite complex and sophisticated in your perceptions, so that you can recognize the range and richness of experience. You are aware of many feelings, and this may simply reflect your greater capacity for seeing things clearly." One way of differentiating emotions is to recognize that there are different emotional responses to different stimuli at different times:

> "Is it possible that you might feel sad when you are thinking really negative thoughts, and that you are feeling happy when you are doing things that are rewarding? If your feelings change depending on what you are thinking, they may simply reflect that different thoughts and experiences lead to different feelings."

## Linking Intolerance of Ambivalence to Problematic Coping Strategies

Many individuals with intolerance of ambivalence activate problematic strategies to cope with their mixed feelings. An obvious strategy is indecision—which often involves waiting for more information that might tip the balance. The indecisive, ambivalent individual may fail to move a relationship forward or fail to make a decision about an important purchase, thereby foregoing the possibility of enjoying a more fulfilling relationship or enjoying the alternative. As suggested earlier, one way of addressing this is to point out that as the individual stays indecisive, he or she suffers the opportunity cost of the unaccepted alternatives. Another problematic coping strategy is rumination: "I need to keep thinking about this until I finally feel just right about it." Other ambivalent individuals may cope by seeking reassurance from others, repeatedly asking for advice about what the right feeling or decision should be. In some cases, an ambivalent person may "test" another individual to find out whether the other really cares or if the person actually has an undesired quality. Finally, some individuals feel guilty about their ambivalence and engage in self-criticism. They view ambivalence as a personal failure, believing that they should be completely certain in the midst of complexity and apparent contradictions.

## Recognizing Current Acceptance of Ambivalence

In many cases, an individual is focusing on one area of ambivalence while ignoring the many areas of life where he or she already comfortably accepts ambivalence. For example, a woman was concerned about her ambivalent feelings about her partner; she interpreted this ambivalence as a "bad sign" and believed that she should feel "completely 100%" about him. This indicated a view of ambivalence as an undesirable and unacceptable emotional state. However, when the therapist inquired about other areas of her life where she might feel ambivalent, she acknowledged several:

PATIENT: Yes, I do have mixed feelings toward each of my friends. There are some things I like about them, some things I don't like. Come to think of it, I have mixed feelings about my work, too, but I guess I accept it. And I have mixed feelings about living in New York City. It's expensive and noisy; sometimes people are rude. But there are a lot of things about New York that I like, so—in balance—I can accept it.

THERAPIST: If ambivalence is by nature so bad, then why do you accept it with your friends, your job, and where you live?

PATIENT: Well, I guess I need friends, I need a job, and I need to live somewhere. I don't have a choice.

THERAPIST: If you want to have an intimate relationship with someone, then it may be that ambivalence comes with the territory. Is it possible to really know someone well and not have some ambivalence?

## Normalizing Ambivalence in the Lives of Others

Even if the patient recognizes that he or she already accepts ambivalence in many areas of life, the patient may have an idealized view of the lives of others. One such patient was the man with ambivalent feelings about his partner:

PATIENT: I guess I idealize other people. I think that my sister has a perfect relationship with her husband, and that my friends have perfect lives. But then if I think about it, I can see that my sister also has some difficulties and that things aren't perfect. She has to struggle sometimes.

THERAPIST: Do your friends ever express doubts about their relationships or their jobs?

PATIENT: Of course they do. In fact, just the other night I was talking with my friend Dan, and he was telling me that he was having some problems with his marriage. And we talked about it, and he realized that on balance there are a lot of good things, too.

The therapist can suggest:

"Accepting tradeoffs in relationships, work, where you live, and what you do may be a universal part of the human condition. It may allow us to live our lives in a real world. In a real world, there is uncertainty, frustration, disappointment, and challenge, and this may be balanced against rewarding and meaningful experiences in committed relationships and in work. Could it be that a more helpful way to look at this is whether it makes sense to accept some tradeoffs in order to enjoy some of the benefits? Is this what other people that you know are doing?"

## Examining Cognitive Distortions Underlying Intolerance of Ambivalence

As indicated earlier, intolerance of uncertainty is often characterized by a wide range of cognitive distortions. Each one of these may be addressed by using standard cognitive therapy techniques. For example, dichotomous thinking—"It's either right or not right," "It's either all positive or negative"—can be examined by considering the evidence of other decisions:

> "Are there other decisions that are not black and white—where there are pros and cons for each alternative?"
> "If you buy a car after considering other cars, haven't you indicated that there are positives about other cars that you might not have with the car you've decided on?"
> "How could there be a choice without a cost?"
> "Doesn't the car cost something?"

In a case of labeling ("This is an unacceptable alternative/a bad choice"), the therapist can examine the meaning of the label, "choice":

> "Doesn't 'choice' suggest that there is another choice with appealing qualities?"
> "When you make a choice, aren't you measuring the tradeoffs of alternatives, so that you could make an argument in favor of either one?"
> "Isn't it possible that there are not good and bad choices, but rather alternatives with tradeoffs, both with uncertainty, and with the added uncertainty that you never know how things will work out?"

Discounting positives can be addressed by examining the costs and benefits of discounting positives of the chosen alternative:

> "If all you do is point to the imperfection, aren't you ignoring important information about the positives?"
> "What are the positives? What would be the advantage of appreciating these positives?"

Negative filtering can also be examined with cognitive therapy techniques:

"If you only focus on the negatives, aren't you ignoring the important positives?"

"Is there any alternative that won't have some negatives?"

"What if you weighed the positives and negatives and included both? Is there another alternative with a significantly better tradeoff of positives and negatives?"

The therapist can help the patient address fortunetelling—that is, predicting that a choice will lead to a bad outcome—through similar questioning:

"We often may predict that we will have certain feelings in the future, but we often are wrong. Have you been wrong about your predictions in the past?"

"Would it be acceptable if you had both positive and negative feelings about your choice in the future, or would you only accept positive feelings?"

"Do you know anyone who feels completely positive about their choices and never has a negative feeling?"

Some people believe that a "wrong choice" would be catastrophic. The therapist can inquire:

"Exactly what will be unbearable if you make this choice?"

"What is the evidence that it will be terrible?"

"Are there positives that might offset any negatives?"

"Are you unable to tolerate frustration?"

"If it *were* so terrible—and we don't know if that will be true—could you reverse your decision?"

Other individuals approach ambivalence with emotional reasoning: "Because I am ambivalent, it must be a bad choice." This is another sign of emotional perfectionism ("I must feel completely good whenever I make a decision, and only good things should follow"). The therapist may inquire:

"Isn't the nature of ambivalence both positive and negative feelings?"

"Could it be that you are reasoning only from your emotion, and not acknowledging that making a choice almost necessarily involves both positive and negative feelings?"

"Have you had a negative feeling about a choice before but realized later that the choice led to some positive outcomes?"

"If you simply looked at the tradeoffs of both alternatives, without using your emotion, would you be able to convince another person of either alternative?"

"Could it be that your emotions might change over time, once you make a choice?"

Many individuals endorse a range of "should" statements: "I should be completely happy with the choice" and "I should not be ambivalent." These beliefs can be examined:

"What are the costs and benefits of believing that you should never be ambivalent when making a choice?"

"What is the evidence that this is a practical and realistic approach to life?"

"If everyone else is ambivalent some of the time, then why should you be different from other people?"

"If ambivalence is defined as recognizing the pros and cons of a choice, should you be making choices without recognizing the pros and cons?"

Finally, many people believe that a bad choice will condemn them permanently to an intolerable outcome. The therapist can examine this belief:

"Let's imagine you make a choice in buying an apartment, and after you move in you realize there are a lot of problems with the apartment—leaks, an unfriendly neighbor, some costly repairs. Even if you had made a poor choice given the information at the time, does it necessarily follow that there are no benefits to be experienced in the new apartment?"

"Can't you make the best of a bad choice?"

"Imagine a football play. The quarterback calls for a particular play, and then notices that the defensive lineman is charging toward him much faster than he anticipated. This was a poor call for the play. But perhaps the quarterback can quickly rush back and throw a pass for a touchdown. Sometimes bad choices have good outcomes."

## Deconstructing Trait Concepts

An assumption underlying the belief that one should not have mixed feelings is that the person who is the object of perception is composed of stable and predictable traits. For example, the belief that one should have only one feeling is based on the assumption that the other person's behavior is consistent across time and situations. However, research on personality suggests that there is considerable variability in a person's behavior, depending on the situation, the behavior being assessed, and the perception of the actor—and that although person variables may provide some predictability, much depends on situational factors (Epstein & O'Brien, 1985; Fleeson & Noftle, 2009; Funder & Colvin, 1991). For instance, persons who might be labeled as "aggressive" by some observers may not be aggressive in most situations; their aggression may be verbal, not physical; and their aggression may be determined by their interpretation of a specific provocation at a specific time.

In addition, perception of traits in others suffers from the "actor–observer bias": Individuals engaged in an action tend to attribute their behavior to specific circumstances, whereas observers of others' behavior tend to attribute that behavior to a dispositional trait (Ross & Nisbett, 1991). For example, you might attribute my arguing a point to the "fact" that I am "aggressive," whereas I might attribute my argument to the "fact" that I am simply trying to make a point. The actor–observer bias may be due to perceptual focus (I am focused on the situation, and you, as observer, are focused on me); access by the actor to information about his or her own variability of behavior (I know that I am generally not argumentative); and differential access to the thoughts that may determine an action (I know what I was thinking when I argued my point, whereas you simply observe my argument).

In addition to the belief in traits, there is a corresponding belief in the malleability of behavior (Dweck, 2000, 2006). According to Dweck, some individuals have a fixed belief that ability is due to innate or inherited traits ("entity beliefs"). Others have a view of ability as incremental or capable of growth ("incremental beliefs"). These concepts are related to differences in motivation and the willingness to persevere. For example, a person with an incremental belief about ability is more willing to try harder and to view learning as an incremental process. These differences are also relevant to beliefs about personality traits—that is, can certain personal qualities change or grow, or are they fixed and immutable? Concepts of traits as fixed and immutable are similar to the "overgeneralized" thinking that is characteristic of depressive vulnerability (Teasdale, 1999). Finally, individuals who believe that willpower is not a fixed or limited quality are less likely to be "depleted" by exercising willpower; that is, they are more likely to persist (Job, Dweck, & Walton, 2010).

## Beliefs in Traits

The first step in deconstructing thinking about traits is to examine the extent to which the individual believes in stable, internally determined personality traits. The therapist can ask:

> "Some people believe that other people have fixed traits—that is, that they have stable qualities, regardless of the situation. If you believe in

fixed traits, then you might be describing yourself and other people in terms like 'aggressive,' 'kind,' 'honest,' 'generous,' 'difficult,' or other general terms. Do you find yourself using ideas like this? Do you describe yourself that way? Other people? What are some examples?"

Some patients may readily recognize that they are using such trait concepts frequently, whereas others may need to self-monitor to see whether they are using these labels. A man who idealized his partner acknowledged that he often thought of her as smart, kind, in control, funny, and interesting. He then went on to say that he believed these traits always characterized her. On further reflection, however, he realized there was a great deal of variability in her behavior, much of it dependent on specific situations to which she was responding.

Next, the therapist can ask: "What are the costs and benefits of thinking of yourself or other people in terms of these fixed and unchangeable traits?" The individual just mentioned described the costs of labeling others in this way as follows: He idealized them or devalued them; in comparison to his ideals of others, he fell short; he then felt self-conscious, and he thought others were judging him on the basis of his traits. He had to think twice about the benefits of trait conceptions, but he eventually described these as follows: He might be able to see people realistically; he could predict what they were like; and he could avoid people he did not like.

The therapist can then use Dweck's distinction between entity and incremental beliefs about ability or personality to inquire whether the patient believes that personality traits—such as "aggressive" or "interesting"—are qualities that can improve with practice and with learning. For instance, if an individual believes that his or her own qualities of being "interesting" are fixed, then there is little motivation or hope for any change.

Finally, some individuals treat their ambivalence as if it is a stable trait: "I will always feel ambivalent." This belief in the consistency or durability of an emotion can also be examined:

"If you believe your ambivalence is a fixed emotion that you will feel consistently, then you are likely to hesitate about decisions. Are there times of the day that you do not feel ambivalent? What other emotions do you have during the course of the day? When you are not concentrating on your ambivalence, would you be able to enjoy anything about this choice? Does ambivalence come and go?"

## Traits versus Variability

As noted earlier, beliefs in fixed negative traits are often supported by selective filtering of negative information—that is, confirmation bias. For instance, a man who believed that he was boring would selectively focus on any information confirming that belief. Modifying beliefs about ambivalence often entails modifying such a confirmation bias:

> "If you believe you [or others] have a specific trait, then it may be possible that you are selectively focused on any examples of that behavior. For example, if you think you are boring, you might selectively interpret your behavior as boring, engage in mind reading that others think you are boring, personalize gaps in a conversation as due to your being boring, and hold yourself to a higher standard of how interesting you need to be. Does any of this sound familiar?"

The "boring" man indicated that he thought he had to be interesting all the time, and would often pressure people with his stories and try to monopolize the conversation. If there were a lull, he interpreted this as evidence that he was boring and that people could see right through him. The therapist asked him, "What would count as an example of saying something interesting?" The patient hesitated and then commented, "Well, I know I say some interesting things at times. People seem interested; they ask questions; they laugh." The therapist then inquired, "Are there examples of when other people can seem sometimes boring, sometimes interesting?" The patient was asked to collect examples of behavior in other people, in order to expand his perceptions of his own and others' qualities.

A therapist can then suggest that behavior varies across time and situations, rather than being entirely due to internal, fixed qualities, and that people differ in terms of their perception of a trait (such as "boring"):

> "Is it possible that sometimes you or another person may say something that is boring at a particular time in a particular situation, but that in another situation you or they say something interesting?"
>
> "Is it possible that what someone else finds boring, another person might find interesting?"
>
> "Is it possible that there is no such *thing* as a boring statement, but that people differ in terms of what they find interesting?"
>
> "Is it likely that your feelings change, depending on the interaction and depending on your interpretation of that situation?"
>
> "If things vary so much, then doesn't it make sense that you would have mixed feelings?"

A therapist can also help a patient identify which perceptions or feelings he or she has that are "troubling." The patient can be asked,

"Are there certain situations that tend to make you feel or think this way? Could you keep track of that feeling or thought, rate it from 0 to 100 in how strong it is, and see if there is any pattern? Do you think that your feelings or thoughts will vary? Why would they vary? If they vary, doesn't this make sense that you would have mixed feelings?"

Again, some people believe they have "contradictory" feelings: "How can I like and dislike the same person? Isn't this contradicting myself?" An assumption about "contradiction" is that feelings need to be logically consistent—"either A or not A." The therapist can suggest that feelings are not the same as logical statements ("It is raining or it is not raining"), but represent emotions that come and go, depending on the focus, interpretation, or other emotions at the moment. For example, I can consider my friend Tom, and feel positively about his kindness and humor, but be a little annoyed that he is late to dinner. These are not contradictory, since I am not asserting that "Tom is late and not late" at the same moment. These feelings are responses to different aspects of Tom. Moreover, when I observe a behavior—"Tom is late"—I may interpret the behavior in terms of a personal intention ("He doesn't respect me"), but I may not know what the reasons are for his lateness (e.g., there was more traffic than usual, he got out of work late, he was unable to call me because his phone was not working, he had an argument with his wife, or he has difficulty with time no matter who is waiting for him). Tom's behavior varies across situations and over time, and—most importantly—I may not have access to information about what has motivated him.

## Reframing Ambivalence as the Richness of Information

As much of this chapter has suggested, the belief that one should not feel ambivalent about self, others, or situations is based on the assumption that all information about a stimulus should be "univalent." That is, it should all point in one direction (e.g., either positive or negative), or it should only confirm or disconfirm an immutable trait (e.g., "He is either aggressive or not aggressive"). This dichotomous view of reality assumes that information is organized in a binary fashion. In contrast, the therapist may inquire whether having complicated or mixed feelings about something or someone simply reflects that the more a patient knows about that person or thing, the better the patient can understand the person's or thing's complexity.

"Consider another example, which might sound a bit trivial but can help me make a point. Imagine that you arrive in a city for the first time. During the first day, you notice that there is a diner that is close by. You go there. As days and weeks and months go by, you eat in different restaurants with different ethnic foods and of different quality. You now have far more information about the restaurants in the city than you had the first day or week. There is considerable variability. If someone asks you, 'Is the food good there?' you might respond, 'It depends what kind of food you like and where you go.' You now recognize the considerable richness of information—the range of restaurants and tastes that people have." Or the therapist might suggest the following, "Imagine a painting that was in black and white and imagine another painting with a range of 100 different colors and shades. Which has more richness of information?"

The therapist can then continue: "Is there an advantage of reframing your ambivalence as simply your awareness of the richness and complexity of people and situations? If things are complex, then why would it surprise you that you would have different feelings, especially at different times? Maybe you are just smart and aware of more information." Or the therapist can say: "Think about someone you know really well—your mother or father or your brother or sister. Do you have a range of feelings about them at different times? What are those feelings?" Recognizing that ambivalence may be a reflection of the complexity and richness of information—and that being "smarter and wiser" may be accompanied by less univalent feeling—may help dispel the view that there is "something wrong" with ambivalence.

## Reframing Ambivalence as Challenges and Opportunities

The search for "How do I *really* feel?" often leads to additional rumination and self-doubt. An alternative to searching for the "one true feeling" is to think about relationships (or situations) in terms of the challenges that they provide—especially the opportunities they open up for growth and curiosity. For example, let's suppose I like a lot of qualities about Susan, a coworker, but that there are certain qualities I do not like (e.g., she may be opinionated; her theoretical biases are not my biases). Once I think, "I really like her," I then realize that she has qualities I like less. Rather than try to reduce my mixed feelings to one feeling, I can be challenged to work collaboratively with someone who has some qualities I do not like. This challenge will require me to use acceptance, to be curious about her point of view, to consider the possibility that I can grow in my capacity for tolerance—or even that I can modify some of my theoretical biases to become more inclusive of alternative viewpoints. I can view accepting and developing a curiosity about people for whom I have mixed feelings as an exercise in living in the real world. I can develop a curiosity as to why another person might view things the way that Susan views them. Rather than activate a judgmental perspective ("I can't stand her point of view") or a reductionist decision ("OK, I just don't like her"), I can separate out the qualities I like and do not like, develop a more differentiated view of her, inquire about her point of view, and decide which of her ideas or qualities are ones that are at all relevant to my goals. Replacing judgment with curiosity and acceptance may create possibilities for more adaptive engagement. Ambivalence may be a reflection of "getting to know what reality feels like."

## Making Room

An intolerance of contradictions reflects a belief that one cannot simultaneously hold conflicting views about something: "Either I like it or I don't." An alternative to this univalent perspective is the recognition that one has enough "space" to contain contradictions. As Walt Whitman (1855/1959) observed in his magnificent poem "Song of Myself," "Do I contradict myself?/Very well then I contradict myself,/(I am large, I contain multitudes.)" Whitman observed that he could love the beautiful and the ugly, the young and the old, the rich and the poor. The technique of "making room" allows the acceptance of whatever comes and whatever one feels. A 13th-century Persian poet, Jalal Al-Dinn Rumi, similarly captured this capacity for acceptance of a wide range of experience in his poem "The Guest House":[1]

> This being human is a guest house.
> Every morning a new arrival.
> A joy, a depression, a meanness,
> some momentary awareness comes
> as an unexpected visitor.
> Welcome and entertain them all!
> Even if they are a crowd of sorrows,
> who violently sweep your house
> empty of its furniture,
> still, treat each guest honorably.
> He may be clearing you out
> for some new delight.
> The dark thought, the shame, the malice.
> meet them at the door laughing and invite them in.
> Be grateful for whatever comes.
> because each has been sent
> as a guide from beyond.

---

[1] From Rumi (1997). Copyright 1997 by Coleman Barks and Michael Green. Reprinted by permission of Coleman Barks.

Consider the following exchange with the man who was ambivalent about his partner:

THERAPIST: I can see you have mixed feelings toward her—there are some things that she says that you do not like and some qualities about her physical appearance that are not completely what you would want.

PATIENT: Yes, this makes it difficult for me, since I like her, but I can see that there are some things I do not like.

THERAPIST: What if you were to think of yourself as having the capacity to contain a large number of feelings, as if you are making room for qualities you like and do not like? What if you were to think of yourself as a very large container, where feelings are like different liquids that flow in and out and there is plenty of room for all of it?

PATIENT: This would help me a great deal. I wouldn't worry so much.

THERAPIST: Perhaps accepting someone or loving someone is like a large container that is never completely full, that always has room.

The advantage of making room for emotions is that individuals need no longer feel the need to reduce emotions to a single emotion; like Walt Whitman, they can recognize that they can be filled with multitudes. Rather than struggle against mixed feelings, they can invite them all in and make room. Many patients indicate that they feel relieved with this approach because they can recognize that mixed feelings are not a sign of something bad, but rather a reflection of goodness and expansiveness.

## Overcoming Resistance to Accepting Ambivalence

Many individuals who have difficulty with ambivalence may believe that accepting ambivalence is undesirable, self-denying, invalidating, or settling for less. Some of these individuals may believe that they are entitled to having everything "right." Others may believe that gaining "an extra 10%" would be completely satisfying; they may be overpredicting their emotional response to an ideal alternative. Let's examine these roadblocks and their disadvantages.

First, viewing ambivalence as "undesirable per se" discounts any positives that might be experienced with a chosen alternative, and also discounts the costs of endless searching for the ideal. For example, taking a job that is 90% of what a person wants still provides considerable positives. Moreover, continuing to search may have significant costs—and in fact may eventually reduce the desirable alternatives. Second, refusing to accept ambivalence may deny individuals the opportunity to experience reward-ing benefits immediately. For example, a person who searches for a perfect partner—and then rejects the 90% alternative—will lose the immediate benefits of a current relationship.

Third, the belief that accepting ambivalence is invalidating is actually the opposite of the truth. One can say, "I do have mixed feelings, but I also believe that this is the best alternative." One can validate ambivalence while also pursuing a choice between two real alternatives in real time. Validating ambivalence implies finding the truth in mixed feelings—not equating mixed feelings with undesirable or unacceptable feelings. Fourth, the idea that one is settling for less is always true, unless one has the abso-lutely perfect choice with no cost. But cost-free choices do not exist. Rather, one can say, "I have decided on the best of the alternatives available at this time." To say that one is settling for less needs to be clarified: "Less than what alternative that is available?"

Fifth, the belief that one should not accept ambivalence because one is entitled to having everything just right can be examined in terms of the costs and benefits of insisting on entitlement and everything "just right." For example, the costs include continued dissatisfaction, continual demands that are never met completely, and the inability to live with real decisions in the real world. Since the world is not set up to reward entitlement, this belief is likely to result in frustration, disillusionment, conflicts with oth-ers, and the inability to get the best of the tradeoffs available. Sixth, the belief that going for the additional 10% will lead to everlasting bliss may be an illusion. For example, research on the so-called "hedonic treadmill" indicates that people soon adapt to their new, higher levels of attainment, with little or no stable increase in happiness (Brickman & Campbell, 1971; Mancini, Bonanno, & Clark, 2011). If the additional 10% will eventually lead to adaptation that reverts to the baseline level of happiness, then is it worth the extra search costs? If one can enjoy 90% now, why wait for the uncertainty of a probably unattainable 100% that, if achieved, might result in ephemeral benefits?

Let's return once more to the example of the man who felt ambivalent about his girlfriend and the idea of marrying her. He indicated that he loved his girlfriend, thought she was a good person, believed she would be an excellent wife and mother, and felt that she was very devoted to him. How-ever, he also indicated that there were times when he was not that interested in things she would talk about.

PATIENT: I do think Sarah would be a good wife. She has all the right qualities. But there are times that I am not that interested in things she says. So I have mixed feelings about getting married. I see her as 90%, but I wonder about finding the 100%—the one I wouldn't have mixed feelings about.

THERAPIST: What about having mixed feelings bothers you?

PATIENT: Well, I'd like to feel sure—I'd like to feel that there are no doubts.

THERAPIST: OK, so you seem to think you should not have any doubts. Why shouldn't you have doubts?

PATIENT: Well, when you plan to get married, you shouldn't have doubts. After all, if you have doubts, it must mean there is something missing.

THERAPIST: So are you saying that if there is something missing, then it is a bad choice?

PATIENT: I guess I am.

THERAPIST: Have you ever known anyone who had everything just right with their partner? Anyone who couldn't say, "Well, I like most things about her, but there are some things that bother me at times?"

PATIENT: I guess you have a point. But I wonder if I should wait for that perfect partner—someone I wouldn't have doubts about.

THERAPIST: Well, you've been single until now—and you are 37 years old. Do you think that this perfect person is out there? And, if she is, how long might it take to find her?

PATIENT: I haven't known anyone as good as Sarah. No, I never have.

THERAPIST: But perhaps there is someone out there.

PATIENT: Yeah, I don't know. Maybe I am dreaming. But it could take me years—if there is anyone like that.

THERAPIST: So that would be a cost for you—searching for years. And then you wouldn't be able to enjoy the relationship with Sarah and get on with your life in that way. But it is a gamble; it's a tradeoff. You could take 90% now or hope to get 100% later. But let's assume that someone out there never said anything that you weren't bored with.

PATIENT: That sounds impossible to me.

THERAPIST: Maybe so, but let's just imagine that—100% interesting all the time. Now how much happier do you think you would be with this person?

PATIENT: Maybe a little happier. I don't know. Maybe it wouldn't make any difference.

THERAPIST: You know, we often tend to adapt to what we have. So if your salary went up 10%, you might be happy for a month or so, but then you would get used to it. Maybe that's what happens when we look for that extra 10%. Even if we get it, perhaps the benefit lasts a short time. But then you have to think about what you give up to search for it, plus how likely you are to find it. And even if you found that person, would she want to marry you or someone else? There are a lot of uncertainties.

PATIENT: But let's say I decided on Sarah. Then that means I am settling.

THERAPIST: You could say that—but are you thinking that "I am settling for less than I can get or I deserve"?

PATIENT: Yeah, maybe I think I deserve more.

THERAPIST: Whether you do or do not deserve more, it might be that the world is not set up to give us what we think we deserve. We get what we get—what we decide on. What if you thought of this not as settling, but as "deciding"—that is, that you are deciding between the alternatives you are considering?

PATIENT: That sounds more realistic. Deciding is what I am doing.

THERAPIST: And if you decide, then you can try to make the best of what you decide on, whatever that is. An advantage of accepting the ambivalence is that you can actually make a decision. There are tradeoffs, no matter what you decide. Now one possibility is that you have mixed feelings because you are perceptive and have a lot of information. For example, imagine that you are 16 years old and you totally idealize your girlfriend. Is this because you are realistic or immature? Now that you are 37, you may have been around, known the ups and downs. Perhaps you are more perceptive. Is it possible that you are ambivalent because you are smarter now?

PATIENT: I never thought of it that way.


## SUMMARY

Intolerance of ambivalence, and the simplistic view of emotion underlying this intolerance, are responsible for a great deal of dissatisfaction, discounting of positives, negative filtering, and indecisiveness. These individuals are often driven by an illusion of emotional/existential perfectionism and pure mind; they refuse to accept uncertainty and imperfection in an imperfect world. Viewing tradeoffs as "sell-outs" or "settling," they are prone to fear of regret and rumination as they seek the perfect, no-cost alternative. Addressing the inevitability of ambivalence; relinquishing the maximizer strategy; embracing complexity; and taking the opportunity to accept contradiction, the occasional disappointment, and the imperfections of daily life can enable these individuals to make commitments to living in a real world that is not always the one they themselves. By encouraging such patients to accept ambivalence, to reframe it as awareness and honesty, and to work with what exists, the therapist can assist them in normalizing the nature of mixed feelings and in accepting the challenge to learn to love and accept what is imperfect. It may be easy to love the perfect, but it is the sign of wisdom to love the imperfect.

# CHAPTER 9

# Linking Emotions to Values (and Virtues)

Everything can be taken from a man but one thing:
the last of human freedoms—to choose one's
attitude in any given set of circumstances, to choose
one's own way.
—VIKTOR E. FRANKL, *Man's Search for Meaning*

The reason why we humans experience emotions is that "something matters" to us. We feel angry because we believe people do not respect us, they humiliate us, or they violate our rights—and respect, considerate treatment, and our rights matter to us. We think we should be treated differently. We are frustrated because we cannot accomplish an important goal, and achieving our goals makes a difference to us; we want to feel effective. We feel jealous because we believe our partners are more interested in someone else—and commitment and the centrality of intimacy are important values. A major objective of emotional schema therapy is to assist the patient in clarifying which values, goals, or personal qualities of character or virtue are important, and to link emotions to these purposes. Emotional schema therapy is not simply a therapy aimed at calming emotions or ridding one of uncomfortable feelings. Rather, it attempts to place emotions into a larger context of meaning, and to encourage an individual to accept the difficulties that emotions may lead, to in order to live a more complete life. The goal is not necessarily a "happy life," in the sense in which one might post a "happy face" after one's signature. The goal is not to live an easy life, free of frustration, anger, sadness, or loneliness. The

198

goal is not "feeling good," as if life were a hedonic calculus that involves weighing one feeling against another and always choosing the "happy feeling." Rather than aiming for "feeling good," the goal is to be able to live a life where one is willing to accept feeling *everything* in order to achieve a more complete, richer, and more meaningful life. If suffering is part of that life, then the goal is *to live a life worth suffering for.*

The importance of values in psychotherapy was advanced by Viktor Frankl in *Man's Search for Meaning* (1963). Frankl, an Austrian psychiatrist, was imprisoned in Auschwitz, and he observed that many of the inmates who died (before being executed) had given up on life. The few who seemed more likely to survive had hope—even if their hope was an illusion—that they would one day be reunited with their families and that their lives would continue after their release from the concentration camp. Frankl (1959, 1963) eventually rejected the psychoanalytic model, with its focus on the past and on the defenses against libido. He developed a new form of therapy called "logotherapy," which focuses on the meaning that one gives to one's actions and life. In several current versions of cognitive-behavioral therapy, there is a similar and growing emphasis on purpose and values: For example, both ACT and DBT stress the importance of values in "a life worth living" (Hayes, Levin, Plumb-Vilardaga, Villatte, & Pistorello, 2013; Wilson & Murrell, 2004; Wilson & Sandoz, 2008). This emphasis is long overdue. In addition, Gilbert's (2009) compassion-focused therapy centers on the important role played by the value and emotion of compassion in helping people find purpose, overcome anxiety and depression, and establish meaningful lives.

An iconic literary example of finding meaning in life is a short novella by Tolstoy (1886/1981), *The Death of Ivan Ilyich*. Ivan Ilyich has lived an appropriate, good life, but in a loveless marriage, without any meaning outside of conventional behavior. Now, at the age of 45, he suffers an injury while hanging curtains; after consulting with a number of doctors, he realizes that his death is imminent. As he lies on his deathbed, he reflects on whether his life has been of any value. One way of identifying the values that might guide us is to ask the question that Ilyich could have asked earlier in his life: "If you could go forward in time from this moment to the moment on your deathbed, what would you like to have experienced? What would you like your life to have been?" According to *Herodotus's History*, written almost 2,400 years prior to Tolstoy's novella, the Greek philosopher-king Solon told the Persian king, Croesus, that one cannot know whether one's life has been happy until the moment of one's death. Even the rich and powerful man can end his life in disgrace and humiliation, according to Solon. And the idea of reflection on what one's life has been is a central component of life review therapy, first advanced by Robert Butler (1963). The idea of reflecting on one's life—either Ivan Ilyich's imagined deathbed reflections, Solon's example of the final hours, or Butler's review of what one's life has meant—has been incorporated into ACT (Hayes, 2004). Clarifying meaning and finding purpose are also key elements of emotional schema therapy. Indeed, values constitute one of the 14 emotional schema dimensions discussed in earlier chapters and assessed with the LESS II.

This chapter presents 10 techniques for helping clarify the values that are essential to an individual—and for demonstrating how emotions may follow from those values. Values are central components in giving us purpose, meaning, and the ability to tolerate difficult emotions as a means to an end. I also discuss the characterological virtues that have from classical antiquity shaped ideas of what constitutes "happiness"—that is, the life worth living.

## NEGATIVE VISUALIZATION

The ancient Stoics proposed that one goal in life is to become happy or content with what we already have. The rationale is that we often get overly focused on what we do *not* have (goals we are trying to attain, which are often unreachable), and that this leaves us dissatisfied and frustrated. For example, a man described his frustration at not getting promoted at work, and ruminated and complained for weeks about the unfairness of his situation. While acknowledging that the situation might be unfair, his therapist suggested that he contemplate a number of simple exercises—each one focused on imagining that he did not have something that he already possessed.

Recognizing what we already have, but have failed to appreciate or notice, can often clarify that what is valued is already within our possession; the *sense* of possession simply depends on the ability to appreciate it. A woman complained that she wanted to lose weight, but felt "stuck" in her apartment in a large city. The therapist encouraged her to take more walks in the city or to join a health club, but the patient confided that she seldom did anything simply because it was good for her. She didn't feel important enough. The therapist suggested that she contact an organization that assisted blind individuals, and that she might consider taking a blind person for walks. A few weeks later, she reported that she had found the experience immensely meaningful:

> "I took this blind lady for a walk through the park. It was a really beautiful summer day, and we walked along, and I pointed out the birds and the landscape so that she could imagine what I was seeing. And I felt wonderful helping her. You know, I never realized that the park is so beautiful—I never saw it before until I described it to her."

The therapist reflected to her, "It's only from seeing through the eyes of the blind that you were able to see what was there."

A similar approach, although involving a purely imaginal experience, was taken with another patient:

THERAPIST: Now let's imagine some things that you take for granted. Perhaps we can consider your body and your senses. Let's take your legs. I noticed that you are able to walk, and you have told me that you jog on a regular basis. That's great. Now I want you to close your eyes. Try to let go of any tension. Just relax and concentrate on what I am saying. Imagine that your legs are paralyzed. Imagine that you could never walk again. What would you miss about walking?

PATIENT: My God. That's a horrible thought. I can't imagine it. It would be terrible.

THERAPIST: OK, it sounds like walking is important to you. Where would you miss walking?

PATIENT: Just simply getting up and going into the other room.

THERAPIST: That's something that you do every day. What else?

PATIENT: Walking through the city. I'd miss the freedom to go anywhere that I want to go.

THERAPIST: How often have you thought when you are walking around the city that you would miss being able to do this?

PATIENT: Never.

THERAPIST: So you haven't noticed that something very important to you is something that you are lucky to be able to do.

Negative visualization can be used for almost any experience that one could possibly value. For example, one can practice a visualization that one's partner is gone forever, or one's children do not exist, or that the sun never rises again, or that one has gone deaf. The purpose of negative visualization is not to make patients unhappy (although some patients may respond with that concern). Rather, its purpose is to help patients achieve satisfaction with and appreciation of what they already have.

Negative visualization is the antidote to the "hedonic treadmill," in which one attains something that is valued and then becomes habituated to it, since it is now taken for granted. By practicing momentary awareness of its absence, one renews the experience of its return. There is a value in missing something—and, ironically, an added value in being able to miss something that is already possessed.

## NEGATIVE EXEMPLIFICATION:
## "THERE BUT FOR FORTUNE GO I"

Another technique for enhancing the emotional significance of "what matters" is to observe the misfortunes of others. This is not a form of *Schadenfreude*, in which we take pleasure in the perception that people we envy are having difficulty. (*Schadenfreude* is discussed in more detail in Chapter 11.) Rather, we can use our appreciation of the misfortunes of others to remind ourselves of our better fortune—something that we can appreciate. Furthermore, it can be helpful to acknowledge that the misfortunes of others have a strong likelihood of resembling—or exemplifying—what we may suffer someday.

> THERAPIST: Now, when you walk through the city, do you ever notice an elderly person using a walker—perhaps someone who has suffered a stroke and has great difficulty?
>
> PATIENT: Yes, I feel sorry for them.
>
> THERAPIST: Could it be that you might also remind yourself how fortunate you are that you are able to walk and even run with great ease and comfort?
>
> PATIENT: I actually never think that way. I have to confess, I don't like seeing people who are disabled.
>
> THERAPIST: But what if you were to think of them as giving you the awareness of how fortunate you are? Perhaps you might even say, "How fortunate that I am reminded now of how lucky I am."
>
> PATIENT: Yeah, that's certainly better than not wanting to see them.
>
> THERAPIST: And you might also say to yourself, "Someday I will be old, I might need a walker. I might have a stroke." You might say, "There but for fortune go I."
>
> PATIENT: It's sad to think, but—you know—it's true. My father had a stroke, and he had real difficulty walking, and I felt sorry for him.
>
> THERAPIST: Well, then, you might look at someone who is having great difficulty to remind you of how fortunate you are. And it might also be an opportunity to feel compassion toward that person—as you do for your father—and to realize that our good fortune is temporary. And that it is up to us to appreciate it while we have it.

The therapist can suggest that patients observe examples in the news, people they meet or see, or events that they learn about that represent the misfortunes of others. The patients can then engage in directing compassionate thoughts toward these persons (including strangers), and then give themselves a reminder that "There but for fortune go I."

## POSITIVE EXEMPLIFICATION

Just as the painful and difficult conditions of others may remind us of our temporary good fortune, we can also recognize that the good fortune or excellence of others may exemplify qualities or experiences that we might value. Again, Chapter 11 discusses how the positive qualities of others might elicit envy—and the desire to see the more successful other persons fail. However, positive exemplification involves recognizing that the success of others can serve as a reminder of what we would like to achieve, or of role models that we might emulate. For example, observing the close and affectionate relationship between a husband and wife may elicit feelings of sadness and envy in a woman who feels lonely and hopeless in her life as a single person. This "trigger" for her recognition of what is lacking in her life can spiral her into a sense of hopelessness, filled with regrets about past relationships that have terminated. In contrast, she might use positive exemplification to perceive "loving feelings" as a positive goal to be pursued. The positive goal of "loving feelings" or "closeness" need not be limited to a marital relationship or even an intimate relationship. It can be embodied in any relationship where care, love, affection, and compassion are present. Indeed, it does not have to be between two people who know each other well; it can be directed toward strangers, toward colleagues, toward valued causes, and even toward animals.

THERAPIST: You felt sad when you saw Juan and Maria holding hands. What made you feel so sad?

PATIENT: I realized that I don't have anyone to express love toward—no one who loves me.

THERAPIST: So it sounds like loving and being loved are values that you want to pursue in your life. Those sound like excellent values. Let's see if there are ways of doing that now. You mentioned that you really care about your sister, Daniela. Can you think of ways that you have shown love and affection toward her?

PATIENT: Oh, yes, every time I see her I hug her and kiss her. I love her.

THERAPIST: OK, so there is love there, and you talk to her often, you told me. How about some of your friends? Are there people that you feel close to, people you care about?

PATIENT: Yes, my friend Xavier—he's been my friend since I was 8. We go back a long way. I haven't seen him for a while, but we always feel close when we do see each other.

THERAPIST: And I wonder about strangers that we see every day. Sometimes I think of looking for opportunities to show kindness toward strangers. I feel good when I help someone who has difficulties. I remember the other night walking home that I noticed an elderly woman who looked like she was having difficulty crossing the street, so I offered to help, and she said, "Thank you, God bless you." And I said to her, "No, thank you for letting me help you. It feels good to be kind, doesn't it?"

PATIENT: I never thought of it that way, but you're right.

The therapist can direct such patients to collect examples of kindness, affection, compassion, and love throughout the week. These can include memories of close and loving feelings toward a wide variety of people, and current examples of affection, kindness, and compassion toward people the patients see and interact with. The point to positive exemplification is that individuals can identify the emotions and values that they wish to pursue and find these in their everyday lives. These values need not be confined to a specific relationship (e.g., with a spouse or partner); they can be experienced in everyday life with a wide variety of people.

## "IT HAS ALL BEEN TAKEN AWAY"

It is an unfortunate irony that we often do not learn what was of value to us until it has been lost. A son realizes that he wished that he had told his father how much he loved him, but now the father has died suddenly, and that opportunity is lost forever. Or a friend moves away, never to be heard from again, and the friend left behind realizes at last how much he misses her. The technique—"It has all been taken away"—is a variation on negative visualization; it focuses on asking the patient to prioritize what seems most important.

A man complained about being cheated out of money in a business deal and said that he had been ruminating about it for weeks, complaining to his wife, and irritable at home with his kids. He had also been drinking more, since he realized he would likely never get the money that he deserved.

PATIENT: I'm really pissed off. They cheated me.

THERAPIST: You have every right to be angry. No one would blame you. And I can see it's eating away at you. But let's try something a little different today. Let's put the anger and the money up on a shelf—put it in a can—and you can take it down later. But right now I want you to imagine that everything has been taken away. You have no body, no family, no money, no existence. You have been reduced to nothing. Now, realizing that you are nothing and have nothing, I want you to think of the following. I will play God, and you can have one thing back at a time, but you will only get something back if you can convince me that you really appreciate it. And, also, you don't know how many things you will get back—maybe a few, maybe a lot. What do you want back first?

PATIENT: My two daughters.

THERAPIST: Which one do you want?

PATIENT: Do I have to choose?

THERAPIST: No, good answer. I will choose. Let's take your oldest first. What do you appreciate about her?

PATIENT: She's special to me. Even the difficulties we had last year made me realize how much I love her. [Patient goes on in detail about her, tears in his eyes. Then he discusses the second daughter.]

THERAPIST: OK. You've convinced me that you appreciate them, and you can have them back. What else do you want back, and why?

PATIENT: My wife. She puts up with me, but she's the best friend I have ever had. [Patient goes on, describing her good qualities.]

THERAPIST: OK, you can have her back. How about your eyes? Imagine that your eyesight has been taken away, and now you learn that you have 15 minutes when you can have your eyesight back. What do you want to see?

PATIENT: My family. I want to see them.

THERAPIST: Well, what's ironic and interesting is that you have these most important things right now, but since you have been mostly focused on the money, you haven't noticed what you already have.

PATIENT: I know. I know.

THERAPIST: Now tell me this. In what way are you the luckiest man that you know?

PATIENT: I have the people I love in my life.

THERAPIST: Yes, and so you can have a choice every day this week. You can either focus on the money, or you can focus on making your daughters and your wife feel loved.

This technique has the advantage of encouraging patients to prioritize what is most important to them. Imagining that everything has been taken away may seem to some like a fantasy, but the therapist can propose that it is not a fantasy, but an ultimate, inescapable reality:

"Everything will be taken away. Everything is impermanent. We will die, and everyone we love will die. It *will* all go away. So imagining that it will all be gone is really the ultimate reality. But the question we need to ask is this: 'What do I have at this moment that I have ignored, that I have not appreciated?' "

## CLARIFYING TEARS

Many years ago, shortly after my mother died suddenly from an unexpected brain hemorrhage, I told a friend about this terrible experience. As I spoke with him over the phone, I began to cry. He said to me—in a moment of his own self-reflection—"You know, I realize in speaking with you that I have never cried as an adult." I thought for a second, "What an odd thing to say to me," although I knew that he cared about me and my suffering. And then I thought later, "How sad not to have something worth crying over." We often believe that one of our emotional goals is to avoid crying: "I don't want to feel bad. I don't want to cry." We may often think (or may often have been told) that crying is a sign of losing control, being childish, acting unprofessionally, or even being a burden to others.

A man who for several months had been considering separating from and divorcing his wife began the session by saying that he had finally made the decision and moved out, but that he was now feeling overwhelmed and sad.

THERAPIST: It sounds like you are feeling very sad right now.

PATIENT: Yes. I know I shouldn't be upset because this is the right decision, but I am feeling really sad. I've been crying. I don't know what is wrong with me.

THERAPIST: What is making you cry?

PATIENT: I miss my daughter. I won't see her as much, and I miss her.

THERAPIST: Do you want to be the kind of man who doesn't miss his daughter?

PATIENT: No, I do miss her. I love her.

THERAPIST: So your crying reflects that you have something worth crying over. She matters enough that you are able to cry. And crying helps you understand how much she means to you.

PATIENT: That's true. Yes, very true. I miss her.

THERAPIST: When we cry, we are often seeing something is important. If she knew that you miss her so much that you cry, she would feel loved.

PATIENT: I guess that's true.

THERAPIST: It's hard enough feeling bad, but it's worse to feel bad about feeling bad. There are good reasons that we feel sad—reasons that say something about your love and your caring. Your tears come from a good place. They come from your heart.

The therapist can inquire, "Sometimes we understand how important things are if we can imagine crying over them. So I wonder, what has made you cry in the past? What could make you cry in the future?" Responses can vary from what most people would agree are major misfortunes (e.g., the death of a parent or child, the end or an intimate relationship, the loss of a job) to experiences that might not seem to others to "merit" tears (e.g., not getting invited to a party, losing money in an investment, feeling left out at a party). The therapist can then ask why the experience would make a patient cry. A woman who (like the patient above) was in the process of a divorce replied, "When the relationship broke up—when our marriage fell apart—I felt like I would never have that close home life that I always wanted. It's how I grew up." Her therapist responded, "You cry because it matters to you to have a close family life. You like the idea of being a mother, sharing your life with someone. So those are values that are very important to you—values that are worth crying over."

Sometimes the therapist may need to inquire more as to the meaning of why an event would lead to tears:

THERAPIST: I understand that you remember crying because you were not invited to a party. I wonder what it meant to you that you were not invited.

PATIENT: I guess it made me feel that people don't like me, that I never seem to fit in.

THERAPIST: So being included and cared about are very important to you and this triggered those thoughts and feelings for you. Perhaps we should be working on those values—feeling connected to others, feeling like you matter.

A rather successful single man, who seemed to have relationships with women with whom he hedged his commitment, complained that he couldn't understand why he felt numb, dissatisfied, and sad at times. He had been in therapy in the past regarding his decision to break off a relationship so he could "look for something better."

PATIENT: Everything is going well in my life—I have a good job, a nice place to live, I have friends—but something is missing, and I don't know what it is.

THERAPIST: I have known you for a while, and I can see that you are feeling sad right now. And I wonder how you might respond to this question: "Who needs you?"

PATIENT: (*Crying*) That's exactly it. No one needs me. You know, it's strange, but I don't recall crying since I was a kid. I have arranged my life so I am completely free of obligations. I have my freedom.

THERAPIST: It's also interesting that you haven't cried until just now. Maybe this is worth crying about. Maybe being needed by others matters to us.

PATIENT: I guess I saw my parents' marriage as a trap. My father would say, "Don't bother getting married; it's not worth it." So I have focused on being free—doing what I want to do.

THERAPIST: Having the freedom to come and go is not the same thing as having meaning. And when we know that we mean something to others, we have meaning.

PATIENT: I don't have that meaning.

THERAPIST: Maybe you might consider how you might be needed by other people. Maybe it might be important to know that someone misses you.

PATIENT: If I died right now, I don't think anyone would be affected that much.

THERAPIST: That might be worth crying over.

PATIENT: Yes, I guess it is. It is.

THERAPIST: And it might be worth doing something about that—that is, to live a life that matters to you, and to others.

As noted above, some people believe that their crying is a sign of losing control, of falling apart—a source of embarrassment. A single woman who was concerned that her "biological clock" was running out was pursuing a very frustrating course of *in vitro* fertilization. She attended an Easter service at her church and began to feel overwhelmed with her emotions as she saw young children with their parents.

PATIENT: I think I am losing control of my emotions. I began to cry at church on Sunday when I saw all these kids.

THERAPIST: What did that mean to you to see the children there?

PATIENT: It reminded me how much I want to have a child.

THERAPIST: So you were crying because you felt you were missing something that is important—something that you value.

PATIENT: Yes, but I shouldn't be crying. I'm an adult.

THERAPIST: Perhaps you were crying because, as an adult and as a potential mother, you recognized what you want, and it touched you very deeply.

PATIENT: But isn't that like being out of control?

THERAPIST: You could think of it that way. Or you could think of it as meaning that you were completely in touch.

## CLIMBING A LADDER OF HIGHER MEANING

Traditional cognitive therapy attempts to get at the deeper meaning of a thought through the technique of "vertical descent" or the "downward arrow." For example, with a patient who feels lonely and sad, a cognitive therapist might engage in the following exercise:

THERAPIST: OK, so you are feeling sad when you are in your apartment alone on Saturday night. Let's look at the thoughts that you are having. "I am feeling sad because I am thinking . . ."

PATIENT: I'm alone. No one loves me. I have no one.

THERAPIST: "And if no one loves me and I have no one, then I think . . ."

PATIENT: I must be a loser.

THERAPIST: "And if I am a loser, then that means . . ."

PATIENT: I will always be alone.

THERAPIST: "And if I am alone then I think . . ."

PATIENT: I will always be unhappy.

Vertical descent or the downward arrow is a useful technique for uncovering maladaptive assumptions and underlying core beliefs or schemas. But it necessarily focuses on the most negative, pervasive thoughts that a patient might have. The flip side of the downward arrow technique is what I call "climbing a ladder of higher meaning." With this technique, the therapist and patient look at the positive steps *upward* from the current situation: What would it mean or what would happen if the patient attained each step upward?

For example, a woman described in earlier chapters, whose husband had died a few years ago, would leave her office at the end of the day drinking from a small bottle in a bag. By the time she got to her apartment, she was intoxicated. She said she did this because it was so sad to return home.

THERAPIST: Now if you were not high when you got to the apartment, you would feel even more sad. What would you feel sad about?

PATIENT: I have no one there. I'm alone.

THERAPIST: That sounds like a sad thought for you. Now, if you had someone there, what would that mean to you?

PATIENT: It would mean that I could share my life with someone.

THERAPIST: "And the reason it would be good to share my life with someone is because . . ."

PATIENT: I like being close. I like loving someone.

THERAPIST: "And the reason I like loving someone is that . . ."

PATIENT: I am a loving person.

THERAPIST: So what I am hearing is that because you are a loving person—because that it the value that you cherish—it is painful to be alone and not have someone.

PATIENT: Yes, exactly.

THERAPIST: Now one consequence of having such positive values is that there is pain that comes when we don't have what we value at that moment. It is the cost of being a loving person. But don't you want to be a loving person?

PATIENT: Yes, I don't want to lose that. But it is so painful.

THERAPIST: It would be even more painful to lose the values that give meaning. Maybe we can think of ways to be a loving person. Let's take your daughter. Are there ways of being a loving person toward her?

The therapist then explored this patient's friendships and other relationships where she could express love, care, and closeness. The key to the technique of "climbing a ladder of higher meaning" is that patients focus on positive goals and values, many of which they can direct themselves toward in their current lives. A value is not reducible to any particular relationship; for example, patients can express love and affection even if they do not have an intimate relationship. It can be helpful to remind these patients that they may not have a relationship that they would ideally wish to have, but they do have the positive values that can direct them to other sources of significant meaning.

## LIVING A LIFE WORTH SUFFERING FOR

Many people will suffer losses that seem overwhelming and that challenge any sense of justice: a mother who loses a young child to an accident; a man whose wife dies after many years of suffering from cancer; or a friend who loses a friend to the ravages of war. After such losses, the survivors may be inconsolable. Life is filled with pain, with tragedy, with what feels truly horrible. Trying to look on the bright side of things only seems trivializing and invalidating. Taking a stoic position of indifference and claiming that one should not be too attached to anyone or anything feels invalidating and even inhuman. What can a therapist say or do when confronted with such tragic—but inevitable—losses of life?

A colleague told me that after more than 40 years of being together, his wife had finally died from a long, recurring, and painful cancer. "I know that it was the best for her to die—that her quality of life was now just terrible—but it has been over 8 months since she died, and I can't get over it. I can't get past it." I said,

> "I know this may not be what you might expect me to say, but I hope that you never get over it, and that you are always able to experience the sadness when you think about her dying. After all, you have lost your wife—the mother of your children, the center of your life. And that is something to feel sad about. But I also hope that you are able to build a life large enough, with enough meaning, enough love that it is large enough to contain that sadness. The meaning is not to live a life without suffering because when we love someone, we will suffer the loss of that person. If it matters to have someone, it matters to lose the person. *The meaning is to live a life worth suffering for.*"

He cried as I told him this, and then he hugged me. And I realized that suffering can be placed into a context of larger meaning. The idea of living a life worth suffering for is to have enough meaning—new meanings—that suffering can be allowed and contained.

Another man told me that he recalled the horrible loss of his father when he was 12: "I still remember how terrible I felt when they told me he died. I don't think that I have ever gotten over it." I suggested that he think about the possibility that we don't have to get over a loss; we need to contain the loss, use it, and put it into the context of what that person meant—and can still mean. I said, "Would you have preferred never to have known your father so that you would not have to suffer the loss?" As the patient cried, he acknowledged that he had loved him, and that was why the loss was so painful. I observed, "Sometimes our pain reminds us of what we have been fortunate enough to have had, even if it was only for what seemed like a short time. But suffering is part of a larger life—a life that you build, a life that contains the memories of that love, that reminds you that you were happy when you had him there and sad when you lost him."

Helping patients understand that they do not have to "get over it" and "move on" is often an immense relief to them. They can include their lost loved ones in their current lives; they can maintain the positive memories that are balanced against the sadness of the losses.

## A MONTH OF GRATITUDE

There is considerable empirical support for the value of gratitude in reducing the risk of depression and in enhancing physical and psychological well-being. In a study of college students, one group was asked to write a brief daily description of gratitude, while students in another group simply described what they did that day (Emmons & Mishra, 2011). Simply focusing on gratitude on a daily basis not only had significant positive effects on physical and psychological well-being, but was associated with greater effectiveness on working toward important goals.

One patient who was worried about his productivity and earnings in his sales job said, "When I focus on gratitude, it seems it's impossible to worry." Gratitude is the recognition that one is fortunate to have had positive experiences, and that one was not necessarily entitled to these experiences. Gratitude is a recognition that something mattered, that one is thankful, and that it did not have to happen that way. Many religions formalize rituals and prayers that commemorate gratitude; for example, morning prayers to give thanks to God are part of Judaism, Christianity, and Islam. There are prayers before meals, prayers during religious services—many focused on giving thanks. In both the United States and Canada, there are national holidays of Thanksgiving. In ancient Iran, prior to Islam, there were numerous holidays that expressed gratitude or giving thanks: for example, Noruz (thanksgiving for the new year), Mehregan (thanksgiving for love and justice), Tirgan (thanksgiving for water), Azargan (thanksgiving for fire), and Sepandgan or Espandgan (thanksgiving for women). In Christianity, the sacrament of the Eucharist literally means "Thanksgiving." We politely express gratitude when we say "Thank you" for rather simple things (e.g., holding the door) or for gifts that we receive. In fact, not to express simple gratitude is viewed as impolite and can sometimes elicit angry responses in others.

Gratitude exercises are a major focus in positive psychology (Seligman, 2002). A therapist can use this technique to help a patient affirm daily positive experiences that may go unnoticed:

THERAPIST: Sometimes we take things for granted. Let's consider eating a good meal. We may take it for granted and not even stop to think about what we are eating. We may be surfing the Internet or texting a friend or watching television. We don't stop to think about what we are eating, and we may seldom feel grateful that we have good food. I wonder if you might close your eyes and think for a moment that you are grateful that you are fortunate to have a decent meal.

PATIENT: (*Closing her eyes*) Yes, I just woolf it down. OK, I am thinking about the food. I'm actually feeling hungry just thinking about it.

THERAPIST: But I wonder, as you think about this food that is appealing, if you could say, "I am grateful that I have this food—grateful that I don't have to go hungry."

PATIENT: (*Repeats what the therapist says.*)

THERAPIST: Now imagine that you could think this about your partner: "I am grateful to have him in my life."

PATIENT: OK.

THERAPIST: Now, thinking about your partner, I wonder if you could just imagine that I am him and you are telling me why you are grateful.

PATIENT: "You put up with my craziness. You are warm. You listen. You are good to my mother. I am grateful for your laughter."

The therapist can suggest that such patients stop and think four times each day for a month of what they can be grateful for in their current lives. Writing down thoughts and feelings of gratitude can reinforce the awareness that simple—and not so simple—experiences can be points of gratitude. Gratitude can also be expanded to the past: Each day, patients can recall past experiences—people, events, or conditions—that they are grateful. The patients can even write brief notes of gratitude (often just a couple of sentences) directed toward the persons or situations that they are grateful for. In some cases, an individual can send a letter to a person or even arrange a visit. In other cases, where the other person may have died or is not available, simply imagining communicating the gratitude can be helpful. Role plays or imaginary letters can be used in such cases:

THERAPIST: If you were to write a brief statement of gratitude toward your grandmother who died many years ago, what would you say?

PATIENT: "I am grateful that I had you in my life. You were always so warm, so gentle; you took care of me; you always kissed me; I loved it when you cooked; I loved you. I am very grateful."

### "IT'S A WONDERFUL LIFE"

Some patients may think, "My life really is a failure. It doesn't amount to much. I don't have anything that matters. I am nobody." Such strings of self-negating thoughts can often spiral into a sense that these patients have no reason to continue to live—and perhaps that their lives have been completely devoid of meaning. Viewing one's life as a failure often implies that one has not achieved the goals one believes are essential—marriage, family, wealth, fame, power, or whatever else those goals may be. Life is viewed as a process of achievement. In contrast to this instrumental view of life—as achievement or acquisition or status—a therapist can direct a patient's attention to the connections that the patient has had throughout life: "How did you become who you are? Who contributed to your life? Who was affected by your life? What meaning have you had for others?"

The paradigm for this approach is the 1946 Frank Capra movie *It's a Wonderful Life.* Jimmy Stewart plays the role of George Bailey, a small-town banker who believes that his bank will fail; his guardian angel, Clarence Odbody, is played by Henry Travers. As Bailey contemplates suicide, Odbody asks him to consider what the town would have been like if he had never existed. As Bailey is taken through various fantasied scenes, he realizes that he has touched many people—and they have touched him.

I now address a direct question to therapists reading this: How would you apply this technique to yourself? Imagine what life for others would have been if you had never existed. Imagine if a depressed patient you helped who had contemplated suicide had never had your care. Imagine that someone with panic disorder whom you helped had never had a therapist like you. Think of the marriages you saved; the babies that were born because you helped people find relationships; all the other people who would feel grateful for your existence. Think about the people in your life—friends, family, or strangers—whom you helped. You would have been missed. You counted.

To extend the meaning of life to connections with others, you can reverse this process and ask, "Which people in your life have made a difference to me? Who has helped me?" For example, extending the meaning to these connections can include parents, siblings, teachers, doctors, friends, and other people who continue today to make a difference to you. Expanding your awareness to the connections that you are part of for others and that others are part of for you can help you to help your patients recognize that even if some things have gone badly, their lives belong to others and the lives of others have been affected by them.

> THERAPIST: If you were to look back on your life, I wonder if you could tell me which people have made a difference to you? It might be a small difference, it might be a big difference—but we can think of how people have touched us, affected us, and become aware of how we are connected to one another.
>
> PATIENT: Well, certainly my mother was the most important person when I was a kid. She still is.

THERAPIST: What stands out as something about her—perhaps a specific memory?

PATIENT: I remember when some of the kids at school teased me—I was about 9 at the time—and she told me that I would be OK, that these kids were just being stupid, and that all the other kids liked me. She put her arm around me and hugged me. I can still remember that.

THERAPIST: In what other ways did she make a difference?

PATIENT: She would play with me a lot. My dad was busy at work— he would come home late—and Mom and I would play and she would laugh, and sometimes she would walk around singing and it made me laugh. Sometimes I would sing with her.

THERAPIST: I wonder if you might reflect for the next week or two about other people who have made a difference—people who touched your life. These could be other members of your family, friends, teachers, strangers, or even people you saw in movies or television. Or people you read about. Just think about those people and how they affected you. I want you to think about how we are connected to others and how other people affect you.

PATIENT: OK. A lot of these people are people I haven't thought of for quite some time.

The therapist can suggest that patients keep a daily written record of short memories of people (or even experiences) who affected them in a positive way. As noted earlier, it is also helpful to write a short statement of gratitude—for example, "Thank you for playing with me when I was a kid," or "Thank you for being such an inspirational teacher." In the case of gratitude for experiences or situations, the individual can acknowledge, "Thank you to the sunsets that I see and that fill me with awe."

## VIRTUE AND FAIRNESS:
## BECOMING THE PERSON THAT YOU WOULD ADMIRE

The emphasis on values, of course, is not new. It can be traced to ancient Greek and Roman philosophers (e.g., Aristotle, Plato, Epictetus, Seneca, Cicero) who equated "values" with "virtues"—that is, character habits such as courage, integrity, and self-control. This line of thought is often identified with the Stoic tradition, but it has continued for over 2,000 years in Western philosophy and religion. Emotional schema therapy is not neutral about which values matter. Rather, it takes the position that the classic virtues (as described by Aristotle) and values of compassion, kindness, and fairness (as described by Rawls, 1971) can inform the moral and ethical choices that a patient considers. Aristotle (1984, 1995) viewed virtue as the qualities in a person that one would admire in another person, and so the goal is to become a person that you would admire yourself. I have found it helpful to ask patients to attend to this simple question: "What are the personal qualities in someone you would admire?", followed by "How could you become a person you would admire?"

The main virtues according to Aristotle are the following: courage, temperance, liberality, generosity, high-mindedness, right (i.e., appropriate) ambition, good temper, civility, sincerity, wittiness, modesty, and just (i.e., justified) resentment. According to Aristotle, the ideal level of a virtue is the "mean," or a balance that represents "excellence." Thus, one can have either a deficiency in a character trait or an excess of that quality. For example, the deficiency for generosity would be pettiness, and the excess would be vulgarity.

Patients can be directed to the qualities (or behaviors) that they do not like in specific other people:

THERAPIST: Can you tell me about someone that you strongly dislike? I think we can often learn something about what we value by observing what we do not like.

PATIENT: I don't like this guy Ned, who seems to be a bully. He teases people; he's a racist; he makes fun of people who are weaker than he is. I can't stand him.

THERAPIST: Can you identify the character traits in Ned that you do not like?

PATIENT: [Gives a description of Ned's negative qualities.]

THERAPIST: It sounds like Ned is lacking in a number of personal qualities that you value. He is not generous; he is not high-minded; he has a bad temper; he is not civil; and he seems overly resentful. So we can use him as an example of the *opposites* of qualities that are important to you.

Or patients can be asked to think more abstractly about the qualities they would like to have:

THERAPIST: One way of thinking of the values that might direct you is to consider the qualities in another person that you might admire. For example, would you admire self-discipline?

PATIENT: Yes.

THERAPIST: And if you admired self-discipline in someone else, would you value that quality for yourself?

PATIENT: Yes. I wish I had more self-discipline.

THERAPIST: Now one way we can think of the character quality of self-discipline is that it is something that requires practice. For example, the more that you practice self-discipline, the stronger that quality becomes. It's like exercise strengthening you. What could be some areas of your life where you might benefit from more self-discipline?

PATIENT: My eating—sometimes it seems out of control. And, of course, exercise. I keep coming up with reasons not to exercise: I'm too tired; I don't want to; it's too hard.

THERAPIST: So practicing self-discipline might be important in getting into better shape. How about self-discipline at work?

PATIENT: Yes, I procrastinate a lot. I waste a lot of time.

THERAPIST: So let's see if we can come up with a list of personal qualities that you can aim for, and see if you can keep track of them for the next week.

Figure 9.1 is a sample form (not intended to be reproducible) that can provide guidance for a therapist and patient in the patient's efforts to "become the person I would admire."

Patients facing moral dilemmas can benefit particularly from work on values and virtues. For example, a patient who is considering acting out a fantasy of infidelity can examine the choice in terms of the virtues of integrity and self-control, and in terms of the implicit social contract of fairness and reciprocity underlying the primary relationship. The tension that underlies the choice helps clarify the commitment to these virtues and values, and may clarify the patient's identity and the problems and strengths of the relationship. In emotional schema therapy, therefore, values are not arbitrary or neutral, but are examined in the light of virtue and implicit social contracts of fairness and justice. Indeed, the concept of fairness has been extended by Nussbaum (2005) to recognize that compassion and protection of the very "weakest" (e.g., young children, persons with disabilities) may necessitate expanding the concept of "social contracts" to focus more on kindness, compassion, and universal suffering than on effective methods of determining justice. It is far beyond the scope of this chapter to examine the implications of virtue, justice, compassion, and other moral sentiments, but it is worth emphasizing that emotions often have an evaluative and even moral component implied in their evaluations. Helping patients realize that values and virtues can have emotional costs may help some tolerate—or even grow as a result of—the difficulties that arise in life.

**Instructions:** Keep track of examples of each of these personal qualities during the course of the week. List examples of your behavior or thoughts that represent each of these qualities. For example, if you are supportive to a friend, list that as compassion. If you persist in your work and get it done, list that as self-discipline. Are there additional personal qualities that you would like to develop? If so, list those in the blank spaces at the bottom of the first column, and keep track of them.

|  | Mon | Tues | Wed | Thurs | Fri | Sat | Sun |
|---|---|---|---|---|---|---|---|
| Self-discipline |  |  |  |  |  |  |  |
| Courage |  |  |  |  |  |  |  |
| Temperance |  |  |  |  |  |  |  |
| Liberality |  |  |  |  |  |  |  |
| Generosity |  |  |  |  |  |  |  |
| High-mindedness |  |  |  |  |  |  |  |
| Right ambition |  |  |  |  |  |  |  |
| Good temper |  |  |  |  |  |  |  |

| Civility | | | | | | | | |
|----------|--|--|--|--|--|--|--|--|
| Sincerity | | | | | | | | |
| Wittiness | | | | | | | | |
| Modesty | | | | | | | | |
| Just resentment | | | | | | | | |
| Compassion | | | | | | | | |
| | | | | | | | | |
| | | | | | | | | |
| | | | | | | | | |

**FIGURE 9.1.** Keeping track of work on virtues and values. (Do not reproduce.)

## SUMMARY

The emotional schema model is not "value-neutral." Indeed, it proposes that emotional processing, emotion regulation, and adaptation are all part of establishing meaning in life. People will tolerate great difficulty, endure considerable pain, and face what seems like insurmountable obstacles if they believe that doing so is part of a meaningful life. For instance, if childbirth is the most excruciating physical pain for a woman, it is also one of the most meaningful experiences in life. Similar to ACT, which suggests that finding a purposeful life is a key part of therapy, emotional schema therapy proposes that not only goals should be clarified, but character strengths, virtues, and ethical principles. Perhaps there are some patients who would rather forgo these considerations—and that is a value in itself—but the model advanced here enables therapists to make these considerations available. Indeed, the clarification of meaning in life opens new possibilities for behavior and new relationships. Losses are not as complete as they may seem. For example, an elderly woman whose husband died after a long illness came to realize that this loss made new possibilities necessary—such as new friendships, new community activities, and new meanings. Moreover, the loss of the husband was not as complete as it initially seemed: "You never lose someone completely, as long as you realize that the memories are forever."

# PART IV

## SOCIAL EMOTIONS AND RELATIONSHIPS

# CHAPTER 10

# Jealousy

O, beware, my lord, of jealousy;
It is the green-eyed monster which doth mock
The meat it feeds on; that cuckold lives in bliss
Who, certain of his fate, loves not his wronger.
WILLIAM SHAKESPEARE, *Othello* (Act 3, Scene 3)

Jealousy is an emotion that people kill other people (or themselves) over. In its less dramatic forms, jealousy leads to psychological and physical abuse, stalking, constant interrogations of the partner, testing the partner's intentions, and continual worry and rumination. I define "jealousy" as the emotion experienced by an individual who believes that his or her relationship is threatened by another individual who is gaining favorable attention or affection from another person. Jealousy is often characterized by anger, anxiety, sadness, and a sense of helplessness. A man who feels jealous because his wife is talking with another man who is perceived as attractive may believe that the security of his relationship is threatened, that his honor is insulted, and that he must get revenge. He may respond by derogating his supposed rival, or he may badger his wife with insults, or he may seek reassurance that he is the more attractive person. People kill other people or kill themselves over jealousy.

As indicated above, jealousy is associated with increased partner aggression for both men and women (O'Leary, Smith Slep, & O'Leary, 2007) and with abusiveness (Dutton, van Ginkel, & Landolt, 1996). Indeed, jealousy is one of the leading reasons that men kill women in marital relationships

(Daly & Wilson, 1988). Findings on the gender differences in jealousy are mixed, with some studies showing greater jealousy in men (Daly & Wilson, 1988; Mathes & Severa, 1981), others showing greater jealousy in women (Buunk, 1981; Kar & O'Leary, 2013), and still other studies showing no difference (Hansen, 1982; McIntosh, 1989). Morbid jealousy is dramatically increased with alcohol abuse (Dutton et al., 1996).

White has suggested that jealousy can be understood in terms of cognitive appraisals, behavior, and emotion activated during the development of a relationship (White, 1980, 1981; White & Mullen, 1989). According to this model, during the earliest stages of a relationship, there is little investment—so jealousy should be minimal. In a well-established, long-lasting relationship, there is less uncertainty—so jealousy should also be less. The model predicts a curvilinear relationship between extremes of investment (very low, medium, very high) and jealousy. Knobloch, Solomon, and Cruz (2001) have expanded this model to include the negotiation of "relationship uncertainty": They attempt to integrate the development of commitment, relationship uncertainty, and attachment issues into a model suggesting that attachment anxiety interacts with relationship uncertainty to determine jealousy.

Jealousy has also been linked to supposed deficits in self-esteem (Guerrero & Afifi, 1999), higher dependency (Ellis, 1996), and serotonergic effects (Marazziti et al., 2003). Cognitive-behavioral approaches to jealousy have focused on correcting or modifying the dysfunctional interpretations or assumptions that give rise to jealousy (Bishay, Tarrier, Dolan, Beckett, & Harwood, 1996; Dolan & Bishay, 1996; Ellis, 1996). However, these approaches are limited to traditional testing or challenging dysfunctional thoughts, and have not included recent advances in cognitive-behavioral therapy. An exception is my colleagues' and my work on an integrative cognitive-behavioral model of jealousy, which views jealousy in terms of traditional Beckian cognitive theory, metacognitive models, acceptance, mindfulness, and emotional schemas (Leahy & Tirch, 2008).

Psychologists have often viewed jealousy as an irrational, negative, destructive emotion that is a result of low self-esteem and problematic attachment history. Although jealousy may be a consequence of problematic self-esteem, I argue for a more inclusive model of jealousy as an emotion that also reflects positive values of commitment and is linked to the adaptive value of protecting parental investment.

Similarly, envy has been described in surveys on emotion as one of the least acceptable emotions. When we are envious, we believe that others have more desirable qualities than we do; as we compare ourselves with these idealized others, we may feel inferior, think of ourselves as "losers," resent the "fact" that the other persons' success is making us feel bad about ourselves, and feel an urge to belittle the other persons (or, at the least, to avoid them). Although envy is another "disparaged" emotion—one about which people often feel ashamed or guilty—I argue in Chapter 11 that envy is a universal emotion and an emotion that may be directed toward positive behavior rather than problematic strategies for coping.

Although the words "jealousy" and "envy" are often used interchangeably, there are significant differences between these two emotions. Jealousy is defined in the *Oxford English Dictionary* as being "troubled by the belief, suspicion, or fear that the good which one desires to gain or keep for oneself has been or may be diverted to another; resentful towards another on account of known or suspected rivalry," with examples referring to love, success, God, or general suspiciousness. Thus a man may be jealous that another man is attracted to his wife, or a woman may be jealous that her success might be diminished by actions taken by her boss. Jealousy focuses on threat, distrust, suspiciousness, and the belief that one's interests will be taken away by another. The word "jealousy" is most commonly used in connection with romantic relationships—that is, to describe jealousy focused on a threatened attachment. "Envy," on the other hand, refers more to the threatened loss of status due to the advantage or superiority of another person. The OED defines "envy" as "the feeling of mortification and ill-will occasioned by the contemplation of superior advantages possessed by another," which includes malicious feelings toward the other. Thus envy is the result of a perception of social comparison where the self falls short of the standard; another person's success exemplifies the inferiority of the other; and the individual harbors negative feelings and may seek to undermine the other. Individuals who experience envy are often focused on their status within a social system or hierarchy, believing that the increased success of another person must lead to a drop in status for themselves. We can distinguish between depressive envy ("I feel like a loser compared to her") and hostile envy ("I think that she manipulated her way up"), although many individuals experience both depressive and hostile envy.

Jealousy can also entail envy, since the object of jealousy may possess perceived advantages or superiority that the self lacks. For instance, a man may be jealous of another man who has great success and good looks, believing that he himself lacks these qualities and that the other man exemplifies his own inferiority. This perceived inferiority may then be related to the perceived threat (romantic or otherwise) that the other man occasions. Jealousy and envy also differ to the extent that jealousy is often experienced as a more intense emotion with a more immediate threat, whereas envy is experienced less intensely with less urgency.

In this chapter, I provide an integrative emotional schema model of jealousy. Both here and in Chapter 11, I link jealousy and envy to evolutionary adaptation. Jealousy is a manifestation of parental investment strategies, while envy is an essential component of dominance hierarchies.

## MODIFYING EMOTIONAL SCHEMAS OF JEALOUSY

### Normalizing Jealousy

As emphasized throughout this book, a key aim of emotional schema therapy is to help normalize difficult emotions. Some individuals believe that their feelings of jealousy are a sign of a serious psychological disturbance, and that they should never feel jealous. For example, a young woman indicated that she felt jealous that her boyfriend had dinner with his ex-girlfriend: "What's wrong with me? I got so jealous, I was bitchy. He says it means nothing that he saw her—they're just friends—but I know that she has her eye out for him. I don't trust her. Why does he have the need to see her?" She then went on to invalidate her own feelings: "I don't want to be that crazy girlfriend that guys talk about—you know, the jealous one who goes around feeling insecure." Her beliefs were that only insecure, low-self-esteem women who are out of control are jealous; that there is no rationale for being jealous; and that she should be sophisticated and accepting all the time.

> THERAPIST: So it sounds like you think that there must be something wrong with you that you feel jealous, and that your jealousy doesn't make sense.
>
> PATIENT: Yeah, what's wrong with me? But, still, I don't see why he had to have dinner with her.
>
> THERAPIST: I wonder how many of your women friends would feel jealous if their boyfriends had dinner with an ex-girlfriend.
>
> PATIENT: Oh, yeah. Like, all of them. My friend Janine said, "What the hell is wrong with him? She's the past. I'd be pissed."
>
> THERAPIST: So your ex-girlfriends would be jealous, too? So your feelings are the feelings that a lot of people have?
>
> PATIENT: Yeah, maybe. But what am I supposed to do—not feel what I feel?
>
> THERAPIST: No, you can feel what you feel. Those are your feelings. Those are the feelings a lot of people have. But maybe we can try to make sense of jealousy, and then see if there is another way to look at it and see if there are *things* that you can do when you are jealous that won't create problems.

Thus this patient became able to recognize that other people would feel jealous in the same situation, and that jealousy was not an emotion unique to her. In fact, jealousy may be a universal emotion under a variety of conditions. Evolutionary psychologist David Buss has observed that when he was in college he thought, "If my girlfriend wanted to have sex with other people, that is her decision; she is the one in control of her body—what right do I have to tell her that she shouldn't do that?" And then he realized that his feelings changed when he got a girlfriend (Buss, 2000; Buss, Larsen, Westen, & Semmelroth, 1992; Buss & Schmitt, 1993). An evolutionary model of jealousy is based on "parental investment theory." That is, a person is going to be more committed (to sharing resources, taking care of the young, etc.) if there is a high genetic investment in the other person (Trivers, 1971, 1972). For example, we are more committed to taking care of our biological children than the children of strangers. We have an investment in passing on those shared genes. Jealousy is a strategy that has evolved to protect this genetic investment. If a man's female partner is having sex with many others, then—from the male's point of view—there is complete uncertainty as to who is the biological father of her children. His parental investment is threatened. If the male is promiscuous, then the female may doubt that he will commit his resources or protection to the offspring. Each member of a dyad thus has a parental investment in maintaining the commitment of the other party. Third parties are a potential threat, and they may be driven off by the jealous partner, and/or the "cheating" partner may be punished.

In therapy, therefore, jealousy may be normalized by describing how early humans who were not jealous and who tolerated promiscuity in their partners were less likely to pass on their genes and more likely to "waste" resources taking care of the genes of competitors. Jealousy is part of the natural competitiveness of genes and parental investment. Indeed, some evidence suggests that jealousy is not associated with relationship instability, and in some cases may even communicate the greater commitment of the jealous partner (Sheets, Fredendall, & Claypool, 1997). Thus sometimes an individual might elicit jealousy from the partner in order to assure the partner's commitment. Finally, individual's behavioral responses to their own jealous feelings may be more predictive of outcome than simply the feelings themselves. Thus an individual may feel jealous but may be able to refrain from denigrating the competition, accusing the partner, or withdrawing affection. It may be such behaviors are the problems, not simply the feeling of jealousy.

Jealousy need not be limited to romantic relationships; it can also be seen in friendships and even professional or collegial relationships. That is, one can be jealous that one's friend is spending more time with another friend, that a colleague gets more attention from another colleague. In each case, the jealousy may reflect a belief that the primary relationship with the friend or colleague is threatened, and that the enjoyment that one gets from this friend or colleague will be diminished if the other person becomes more interested in others. For example, a college student became jealous that his male friend was spending more time with another male in the college; he feared that he himself would end up with no one to spend time with. This is different from a parental investment model, but it does reflect the idea that jealousy may be activated when one believes that resources and rewards will be lost to another person. Whether the jealousy arises from romantic, friendship, or collegial relationships, the emotional schema approach can be applied to each domain of jealousy.

One way to normalize jealousy is to find examples in popular culture or in music, literature, or even mythology. For instance, a patient can collect examples of jealousy in the lyrics of popular songs, television or movie plots, or even tabloid headlines. Classical examples of jealousy include Shakespeare's *Othello* or the jealousy of Greek gods and goddesses (e.g., Hera's jealousy that Io was the focus of Zeus's interest). Indeed, in the Judeo-Christian tradition, even God is jealous—since He abhors the idea that one can worship other gods. "If God can be jealous, why can't you?" might be a question to ask.

## Validating Jealousy

Rather than approaching a patient with the idea that his or her jealousy is entirely due to dysfunctional and irrational thoughts, the therapist might first start with validating the feelings and the perceptions. For instance, the therapist might have said to the jealous woman described above, "I can see why you might feel uncomfortable and jealous with your partner's seeing his ex-girlfriend. It sounds like you were feeling that it was a sign that he might be interested in someone else, and I know that commitment and monogamy are important to you. So, looking at it this way, you might very well have those feelings." Or: "A lot of people would feel uncomfortable in that situation." Moreover, the therapist can encourage the patient to validate his or her feelings are important: "It may be important to recognize that your own feelings of jealousy are important, rather than criticizing yourself for these feelings." Validating the jealous feelings is not equivalent to justifying the tendency to ruminate, worry, criticize, or act on the jealousy.

## Emotional Schema Dimensions and Jealousy

Many of the dimensions of emotional schemas described in earlier chapters may be related to jealousy. As just mentioned, validation of the emotion is important. In addition, the individual may believe that the jealousy will last indefinitely, that it is out of control, that the jealousy needs to be eliminated completely, that it does not make sense, that it is unique to the self, and that it cannot be accepted. Some individuals feel guilty about or ashamed of their jealousy.

Similar to other fears that are exacerbated by the belief that "If I am afraid, then it is dangerous," the jealous individual uses the intensity of the emotion as evidence that the threat is real. This kind of emotional reasoning often perpetuates the jealousy, magnifying its intensity as the emotion and the jealous thoughts escalate together. However, just as such individuals use their emotions to evaluate reality, they may have a corresponding conviction that they cannot tolerate uncomfortable emotions (Leahy, 2002, 2007a). This may include beliefs that their jealousy is escalating out of control or is a "bad sign." It may also include the belief that ambivalence about a partner—or a partner's ambivalence about the self—cannot be tolerated. These emotional schema dimensions may be addressed as follows.

• *Duration*: "Is it possible that your jealous feelings rise and fall, and that they sometime go away on their own? Or if you are doing something different, does your jealousy go away? If you knew that your jealousy might be temporary, would you be less upset?" For example, individuals may notice that their jealousy is less when they are working or talking with friends about other topics—or when they are engaged in rewarding activities with their partners.

• *Control*: "You may think that your jealousy is out of control. Many individuals believe their jealous emotions will escalate unless they do something, such as interrogate their partner or demand reassurance." The therapist can then ask, "Is there a difference between feeling a jealous feeling and acting in a problematic way? For example, could it be possible to acknowledge that you are feeling jealous but not seek reassurance, cross-examine your partner, or punish your partner? Aren't feelings different from actions? Do you have to act on the feeling, or can you act in other ways that are more adaptive?"

• *Consensus*: "If jealousy is a universal emotion and if jealousy is related to evolutionary adaptation, then doesn't it seem that you are not alone with your jealous feelings?" As noted earlier, knowing that jealousy is a universal emotion helps to validate and normalize it, and to reduce the sense that one's emotions are incomprehensible.

• *Acceptance*: "If you accepted that you sometimes feel jealous—rather than criticize yourself or try to eliminate the jealousy—would there be any advantage? What if you said to yourself, 'Yeah, sometimes I have jealous feelings. Sometime they come, sometimes they go'?" Again, acceptance is not equivalent to saying that the feelings are pleasant or desirable—only that they are "here for now" and can be gone at a later time.

## Core Beliefs, Assumptions, and Schematic Processing

In some cases, jealousy is related to core beliefs about the self and others. Problematic core beliefs about the self include thoughts that one is unlovable, flawed, doomed, or entitled to special treatment. Beliefs about others may include thoughts that others are not trustworthy, rejecting, abandoning, manipulative, or inferior. For instance, individuals with a core belief that they are sexually undesirable may be more likely to be jealous (Dolan & Bishay, 1996). Or the individual may have core beliefs about others that "Men can't be trusted," or "Women are manipulative." Or they may have a series of assumptions or rules about a relationship: "My partner should never find other people attractive," "I need to know everything that my partner is thinking and feeling," "If things between us are not perfect, then my partner will leave me," and "I could never survive without this relationship."

As a result of such beliefs, an individual's thinking (and consequent feelings) is driven by selective, schematic processing. Thus the jealous individual is likely to misinterpret neutral information as a threat to the relationship and to engage in cognitive biases—for example, mind reading ("She is interested in him"), personalizing ("He is reading the paper because he no longer finds me attractive and interesting"), fortunetelling ("She is going to leave me"), and overgeneralizing ("He's always doing that"). Selective negative thoughts about the self may add to insecurity: "I sound boring," "I am getting old and less attractive," "I am a burden."

Traditional cognitive therapy techniques can be used for automatic thoughts, assumptions, and core beliefs (Leahy, 2003a). These include identifying the content of the thoughts, categorizing the distortions, examining the costs and benefits, evaluating the evidence, role playing against the thought, asking what advice one would give a friend, and developing more balanced and rational responses (Leahy, 2003a; Leahy, Beck, & Beck, 2005; Young et al., 2003). For example, mind reading and personalizing can be examined by asking the patient whether there is any evidence that the partner is interested in what the third party says or does, whether there is any evidence that there are no rewarding aspects to their relationship, whether the patient has engaged in fortunetelling about abandonment or cheating before (and, if so, how many times the patient has been wrong), and whether there is any evidence that the partner has no commitment to the relationship.

## Developing a Case Conceptualization

Similar to other cognitive treatment models, the emotional schema model begins with a case conceptualization on which the therapist and patient may collaborate (J. S. Beck, 2011; Kuyken, Padesky, & Dudley, 2009; Needleman, 1999; Persons, 1993). Figure 10.1 provides a general template for such a case conceptualization. The general outline suggests that evolution has led to the emergence of jealousy as a protective strategy that is universal and adaptive *in certain situations*. This evolutionary model serves the purpose of "depathologizing" the experience of jealousy, thereby providing some validation for the "right" to have jealous feelings. Significant early and later relationship issues may be identified (e.g., threatened or actual separation of parents, or infidelity/betrayal in adult relationships), as well as cultural values associated with sexuality, gender roles, and romantic idealization. Core beliefs about the self may include thoughts that one is basically unlovable, ugly, defective, or vulnerable to being manipulated. Core beliefs about a relationship may be examined, such as "Women [men] should never have male [female] friends" or "The only quality that counts is physical attractiveness." Situational triggers may vary from neutral (attending a party) to nonexistent (insecurity when the partner is at work) to provocative (the partner's having dinner with a former lover). All these factors may give rise to cognitive, emotional, behavioral, and interpersonal coping strategies to face potential threat to the relationship—for example, interrogating, seeking reassurance, searching through emails and phone messages, criticizing the "competition," stonewalling, complaining, threatening to

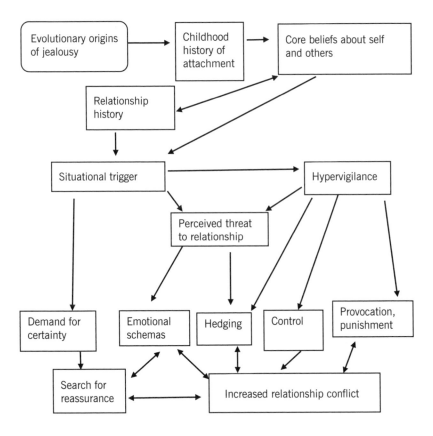

**FIGURE 10.1.** Case conceptualization of jealousy.

leave, physical intimidation, and other unhelpful behaviors. The therapist will explore the rationale behind hypervigilance, attempts to find certainty, reassurance seeking, emotional coping strategies and beliefs, hedging, control, and attempts to punish the partner and devalue perceived competition. For example, what does the individual hope to gain by stonewalling or criticizing the partner? What could be the potential costs?

A case conceptualization of jealousy was used with a woman who was concerned that her partner was losing interest in her. The therapist explained the evolutionary adaptiveness of jealousy as a protection of parental investment, thereby linking jealousy to a universal strategy of self-protection. Core beliefs about self included the ideas that "I am boring," and "I don't bring that much to the relationship," along with core beliefs about the partner that "He is such a winner," and "He is almost perfect." Her family history revealed that her mother and father had a committed relationship, but that her mother was continually concerned about whether she was losing her looks and often sought reassurance from others, including the patient. The underlying assumptions in the family—ones that the patient held—were that "The woman has to do everything to hold onto the man," and that "A woman is nothing without a man." Her problematic coping included scolding her boyfriend, criticizing other women, and pouting.

The value of case conceptualization is that it addresses a number of emotional schema dimensions and targets areas for intervention. For example, case conceptualization helps "make sense" of jealousy, normalizes jealousy, helps the individual realize that he or she is not alone, links jealousy to specific triggers and automatic thoughts, identifies vulnerable schemas about self and others, distinguishes between jealous emotion and jealous (compensatory) behavior, identifies jealousy as a form of agitated worry, and illustrates how jealous behavior can undermine the interests of the patient in the relationship that appears threatened. Let us now examine specific elements of this conceptualization and how interventions can address each concern.

## Linking Jealousy to Values

One way to view jealousy is that the individual values commitment and monogamy: "If you didn't value the relationship, you might not have any feelings of jealousy."

> THERAPIST: Sometimes jealousy is related to the positive values that we have, like the values of monogamy, commitment, honesty, and closeness. Are these values that you have?
>
> PATIENT: Yes, of course.

THERAPIST: So one way of looking at your jealousy is that things matter to you. You are not a superficial person when it comes to a relationship. You take things seriously.

PATIENT: Of course I do.

THERAPIST: What if your partner said to you, "You know I think everyone should be free to do what they want to do, so if you wanted to go out with other people—and have sex with them—that would be OK with me"? If your partner said that, what would you think?

PATIENT: I would think that he wants to screw around with other people. I wouldn't trust him.

THERAPIST: So, in a sense, you would want your partner to be capable of jealousy because it would be a sign of commitment and would indicate that things matter to him.

PATIENT: Yes. If he weren't jealous, I would think he couldn't be trusted. I would also think that I didn't really matter to him.

THERAPIST: So, just like any emotion, perhaps jealousy has a positive side and a negative side. I think it's important to recognize that jealousy not only makes sense, but may be a capacity of commitment and trust.

PATIENT: That makes me feel a lot better about who I am.

## Linking Jealousy to Problematic Coping

The therapist can help the patient distinguish between feeling jealous and acting in problematic ways: "Is it possible to have a feeling of jealousy without acting on it? What if you were to disconnect having a feeling from taking an action, so that you didn't always act on that feeling?" Jealous individuals believe that they must take action, gain control, and find out "what is really going on." Consequently, they activate problematic interpersonal coping strategies, which often lead to even greater insecurity (Borkovec, Newman, & Castonguay, 2003; Erickson & Newman, 2007). As noted earlier, these may include reassurance seeking, degrading competitors, attacking the partner, controlling the partner, keeping the partner under surveillance, deferring to the partner, threatening to leave, hedging through infidelity, or substance misuse.

THERAPIST: I understand that you have those feelings of jealousy, but I also wonder what you do when you have those feelings.

PATIENT: Well, sometimes I try to test him out, see how he might feel about someone else. I might ask him, "Do you think she's attractive?" Or I might look for reassurance: "Do you still find me pretty?"

THERAPIST: So you are looking for evidence that you are still attractive to him, and that the other woman is not as attractive? Are there other things you do to cope with your jealousy?

PATIENT: Well, it might sound hypocritical, but I sometimes flirt with other men. Like, there was this guy at work who seemed interested in me, and I encouraged him. I know it's not fair of me to be jealous and then flirt, but I did.

THERAPIST: Could it be that you are trying to protect yourself, so that if things didn't work out, then you could have a fallback position? Or maybe you are trying to get reassurance that you are attractive?

PATIENT: It's a little bit of both.

THERAPIST: Anything else that you do?

PATIENT: Yeah, sometimes I pout. I'll act like I'm not talking, but then when he says, "Is there anything wrong?", I tell him "No."

THERAPIST: I guess that you can punish him—try to make him concerned, maybe feel guilty—but then also test him out: "If he were interested in me, he would ask me how I am feeling."

PATIENT: Yeah, that's what I do.

The therapist can examine with the patient how these coping strategies are working. Do they strengthen the relationship? Do they contribute to arguments? Does the individual get the validation and support that he or she is seeking? Ironically, jealous feelings are often the result of insecurity about the relationship, but problematic coping actually is the real threat to the relationship. If the jealous partner is pouting, punishing, testing, and berating, the other partner may conclude that the relationship is too costly. Jealous behavior can become a self-fulfilling prophecy that the relationship is really in danger.

## Characterizing Jealousy as Angry, Agitated Worry

Jealousy can be characterized as a form of worry or rumination. That is, the individual is threat-oriented, gets stuck on a repetitive thought, believes that his or her threat detection and coping strategies will prevent being surprised or harmed, and feels that these thoughts need to be attended to and answered (Leahy, 2005d; Leahy & Tirch, 2008). Similar to the worrier, the jealous individual believes that uncertainty about the partner's real interests is intolerable, and consequently attempts to eliminate this uncertainty through looking for clues, seeking reassurance, or "testing" the partner. This seldom results in a satisfactory resolution, thereby fueling more demands for certainty (Dugas, Gosselin, & Ladouceur, 2001).

Like all worry, jealousy involves a search for certainty, and the individual equates uncertainty with bad and uncontrollable outcomes. The patient can practice self-flooding with the uncertainty message (e.g., "I can never be sure if my partner will betray me") (Dugas et al., 2004; Leahy, 2005d). By habituating to the jealous thoughts (or becoming bored with them), the patient may come to realize that the occurrence of a thought need not require hypervigilance, questioning, or punishing.

Further similarities to worry and rumination may include heightened cognitive self-consciousness, the belief that jealousy is protective, the view that jealous thoughts are potentially out of control and require suppression, and the belief that negative consequences will result from these thoughts. These beliefs are similar to metacognitive beliefs and strategies for worry, rumination, and anger (Papageorgiou, 2006; Papageorgiou & Wells, 2001b; Simpson & Papageorgiou, 2003).

As with other forms of worry or rumination, the therapist can approach jealousy with a variety of cognitive and behavioral techniques (Leahy, 2005a, 2009a; Leahy, Holland, & McGinn, 2012). These include examining the costs and benefits of jealous worry and rumination, setting aside specific times to engage in worry ("worry time"), examining whether the jealousy will lead to productive behavior, and evaluating the legitimacy or rationality of automatic thoughts. For example, a woman may recognize that her jealousy is making her angry and anxious, and that it is leading to frequent arguments, but she may also believe that jealousy has advantages: She will not be surprised; she will be able to keep her partner from straying; and she can hedge her bets by finding an alternative partner. The therapist can help the patient evaluate whether the jealousy is really paying off, or whether it is actually adding to her difficulties. One distinction that some patients find useful is to examine whether the jealousy can lead to productive action: "Is there any action today that can lead to a better relationship or a more secure relationship?" If the patient is concerned about the security of the relationship, then a "to-do list for today" can suggest some positive and productive actions. For example, being more rewarding to the partner or, alternatively, engaging in self-care (seeing friends, volunteering, other positive activities) may take the pressure off. However, in many cases no specific productive action may be possible at the moment, so the patient may need to consider that the jealousy is unproductive: "Worrying about this will not lead to any productive action." In this case, the therapist can suggest that there are three elements of acceptance—accepting uncertainty, accepting some lack of control, and accepting the emotion.

Acceptance of existential uncertainties is often equated with danger and defeat in the mind of a jealous individual. The therapist can ask the patient what the costs and benefits are of accepting uncertainty. For example, the benefits might include less worry and jealousy, greater ability to enjoy the present moment, fewer arguments, and less self-doubt. However, some individuals believe that if they accept uncertainty, something terrible will happen that could have been foreseen. The therapist can indicate that nothing can be guaranteed and that bad things could happen, but can also inquire how worry and jealousy will lead to certainty. Moreover, the therapist can indicate many aspects of daily life for which the patient already accepts uncertainty (e.g., meeting people, eating food, taking on new tasks, traveling). Similarly, the therapist can examine the costs and benefits of accepting less control, and can indicate current behaviors and situations where the patient already accepts less control. Finally, the therapist can suggest that the patient accept having the emotion rather than attempt to eliminate the emotion, and that such acceptance might help reduce the sense of anxiety and frustration.

THERAPIST: You seem to be upset that you feel jealous, and you want to either act on the jealousy or get rid of it. What if you decided, for the time being, to accept that you have a jealous feeling for the present moment? For example, you might say, "I have a jealous feeling right now. There it is."

PATIENT: But the jealousy bothers me.

THERAPIST: Yes, but it could be it might bother you less if you accepted that you had it for the moment.

PATIENT: How do I do that?

THERAPIST: Well, let's imagine you had a little indigestion, but you knew it wasn't going to kill you. You might say, "I guess I will feel uncomfortable until things settle for me."

PATIENT: I guess I can try. But it seems hard to do.

THERAPIST: Now accepting that you have an emotion does not mean that you act on the emotion. In fact, if you accept that you can tolerate the feeling of jealousy—"I am having a jealous feeling at the moment"—you can also say to yourself, "I don't need to act on it."

PATIENT: That can be hard. I just want to say something when I am jealous.

THERAPIST: Yes, I know, and then you have to ask whether saying things to your partner will help you. If you don't say something hostile, what is the worst thing that will happen?

PATIENT: Actually, it would make things better.

THERAPIST: You can distinguish between having a jealous emotion and choosing to take action. Standing back and observing and waiting—rather than acting—might be in your best interest.

Some jealous individuals believe that they need to say or do something in order to control a partner and prevent infidelity. The rationale is "I need to make my partner aware of the consequences." On closer evaluation, however, such patients can recognize that the partner already knows these potential consequences, and that further attempts to control (through punishing or cajoling) may make the relationship more insecure. Other individuals may believe that they need to express their emotions—a kind of expressive compulsion ("I need to tell him [her] what I am feeling")—without considering the style of communication or its possible impact. Such expressions of jealousy often involve accusations or attacks on the partner; they are not confined to stating, "I am feeling jealous." Thus these expressions can lead to counterattacks or withdrawals, which further jeopardize the security of the relationship, leading to additional jealousy. Of course, none of this is meant to discourage patients from legitimate assertions about boundaries or agreed-upon appropriate behavior. If a partner really is pursuing infidelity, then the jealousy is merited, and an individual needs to consider taking action to protect his or her rights.

## Defusing Jealous Thoughts and Feelings

Like many other intense emotions, jealousy often involves a fusion of thoughts, feelings, and beliefs about reality. For example, as noted earlier, a jealous individual may use an emotional reasoning heuristic: "I am feeling jealous; therefore, something must be going on." This form of reasoning can have profound effects on maintaining and escalating jealous emotions and behavior. Emotional schema therapy utilizes both metacognitive and acceptance approaches to disentangle and defuse the thoughts and emotions that constitute jealousy (Hayes, Strosahl, & Wilson, 2003; Wells, 2009). And, again, jealousy is similar to worry and rumination in many respects: Jealous individuals often believe that their jealous hypervigilance will prevent any surprises, prepare them for the worst, or allow them to catch things before they fall apart (Wells & Carter, 2001; Wells & Papageorgiou, 1998). These individuals also have high cognitive self-consciousness, continually scanning their minds for jealous thoughts or memories. Like worriers, they are caught in a dilemma—believing that their jealousy protects them, but also believing that the jealousy is out of control. Consequently, they attempt to control the jealousy by suppressing, seeking reassurance, or avoiding the situations that give rise to jealousy (Wells, 2004).

The therapist can indicate that thoughts are not the same thing as reality, and that an intrusive thought (e.g., "My partner is interested in someone else") need not be treated as a signal of the truth about what is going on. Moreover, helpful techniques from metacognitive therapy can be used for jealous emotions and thoughts (Wells, 2009). For example, mindful detachment techniques can assist the patient in standing back, observing an emotion (or thought), letting it happen, and observing that it passes along. These include thinking of the occurrence of jealousy as a telemarketing call that one does not take, viewing jealous thoughts and emotions as cars on a train that passes through a station (but that one does not board), or viewing the emotions and thoughts as clouds drifting in the sky (see Wells, 2009). The point to recognize is that one can have an emotion or thought, but simply observe that it exists separately and transiently—and that nothing need be "done" but to observe. This is an important part of defusing jealous thoughts, emotions, and behaviors, since many people who experience jealousy believe that they must do something immediately. The detached mindfulness that one can take toward jealousy also reflects that one need not engage with the jealous thoughts and feelings, and need not get rid of them (Papageorgiou, 2006; Papageorgiou & Wells, 2001b; Simpson & Papageorgiou, 2003). Jealous thoughts and feelings can coexist with thoughts, actions, and emotions focused on other meanings and goals in life. They may be viewed as parallel rather than entangling.

Defusing jealousy can also include distinguishing jealousy from how one defines the self. For example, statements such as "I am jealous," or "I am a jealous person," involve a conflation of one's identity with one's emotion. Distinguishing oneself from one's emotion can be facilitated by pointing to the emotion as an event: "There is a jealous feeling," or "I noticed a jealous thought." The advantage of disentangling one's identity from one's jealous emotion is being able to recognize that jealousy is one of many possible emotions toward another person, and that one has the freedom to step away from this emotion to engage with other emotions.

> THERAPIST: When you say that you are "a jealous person," it sounds like a very general and global way of viewing yourself. I wonder what it would be like if you thought of yourself as having a wide range of emotions, thoughts, and behaviors at different times— and kept in mind that these thoughts and emotions and behaviors are continually changing. For example, you might say, "There is a jealous feeling at this moment," rather than "I am jealous."
>
> PATIENT: I am not sure if I understand.
>
> THERAPIST: Are you a jealous person, or are you a complex person who sometimes feels jealous?
>
> PATIENT: I guess I am complex. I feel a lot of things.
>
> THERAPIST: OK, so you are not reducible to a single emotion. You have a lot of emotions. Would it be fair to say that you have emotions of happiness, curiosity, boredom, excitement, sadness, and appreciation—at different times?
>
> PATIENT: Yes, I have a lot of feelings.

THERAPIST: So, imagine that you experienced a feeling of jealousy and you said (*pointing*), "There is that jealous feeling." It's "there," it's not "you." Here, try pointing over there while saying, "There is a jealous feeling."

PATIENT: (*Pointing*) "There is a jealous feeling." It feels strange doing this.

THERAPIST: OK, it's there, outside me. It's not me. I am not one emotion; I have a lot of emotions. Let's try the opposite: Point to yourself and say, really loud, "I am a jealous person."

PATIENT: (*Pointing to self*) "I am a jealous person."

THERAPIST: How did that feel?

PATIENT: I felt really bad doing that. Like I was criticizing myself.

THERAPIST: Which felt better—pointing "there" or pointing at yourself?

PATIENT: Pointing over there.

THERAPIST: You are more than just your feeling.

This and other defusion techniques can assist the patient in detaching from an emotion. Through the immediate experience of observing that the emotion occurs as a single event that the patient need not engage with, the patient can come to see it as an event that is separate from his or her identity. By experiencing an observing or "pointing to" role with the emotion, the patient can take a meta-emotional stance toward the jealousy—that is, stand above and separate from it. This will be an essential component in separating the experience of jealousy from problematic behaviors. Emotions do not have to lead to behaviors. The patient has a choice.

## Decastrophizing Potential Loss

Jealousy is often an anxious appraisal that the loss of a relationship would be devastating. For example, the individual may believe that the loss of a relationship would lead to permanent misery—an example of affect forecasting. Or the person may believe, "If I am betrayed, I could never trust anyone again." Eliciting the automatic thoughts and assumptions that accompany the fear of loss can be an important part of putting jealousy into perspective. The patient can examine the meaning of the feared loss: "If this ended, I would be humiliated," "I could never trust anyone," "This confirms I am unlovable," and "I would not be able to take care of myself." Each of these beliefs can be evaluated via traditional cognitive therapy techniques—for instance, evidence for and against the thought, giving advice to a friend, role playing against the thought, and the continuum technique. Beliefs about the essentiality of a specific relationship for one's life can also be tested by examining alternatives available for a meaningful life independent of the relationship, including how life had meaning prior to the relationship.

Here is an example of examining the evidence for and against a thought about potential betrayal:

> THERAPIST: Of course, anything can happen, and we never know for sure. But what would it mean to you if Brian did betray you?
>
> PATIENT: It would be humiliating. I would feel like a loser.
>
> THERAPIST: That sounds like a difficult thought. How would his dishonesty make you a loser? Why should you feel bad about yourself if he lies and cheats?
>
> PATIENT: Well, I guess I never thought of it that way. I don't know. I would have lost the relationship.
>
> THERAPIST: Yes, that's true; the relationship would be over. But are you a loser? Did you fail if he lied and cheated? Isn't it possible that you might think that *he* failed?
>
> PATIENT: I guess that's true.

Another way of looking at the potential loss of a relationship is to examine the costs and benefits of *not* having the relationship. This is not meant to trivialize the relationship, but rather to address the mitigating factors that might arise as a result of moving on after its end. For example, the therapist can ask:

> "Would there be any new opportunities if the relationship ended? What would they be?"
>
> "Is the relationship so close to perfect that nothing else would be worthwhile?"
>
> "What rewarding and meaningful experiences have you had prior to this relationship?"
>
> "How have you coped with other relationships that ended?"
>
> "What could be some new sources of reward and meaning in the future?"
>
> "Do you know of any people whose partners have cheated, but who have moved on to rewarding lives?"

Coping with potential loss is a combination of problem solving and affect forecasting. Problem solving might involve examination of new behaviors that might be useful in the event of the relationship's ending— for example, networking, renewing friendships, becoming more outgoing, taking on new work, or even moving. The therapist can also ask the patient whether he or she has a tendency to overpredict the extreme of emotions for problems that might arise: "You seem to be predicting that you will be miserable indefinitely if the relationship ends, but I wonder if this tendency to predict that your negative feelings will be permanent is something that you do at other times." Affect forecasting about loss adds to a sense of helpless and hopelessness, augments the threat of loss, and contributes to the intensity of jealousy.

## Decreasing Coercive Control and Increasing Adaptive Relationship Skills

As noted at the start of this chapter, jealousy is often followed by destructive spousal or partner behavior. For example, a jealous individual may utilize coercive control by punishing the partner, interrogating, spying, stalking, devaluing the competition, and threatening self-harm. The idea that one can keep a partner from straying through coercion and continual interrogation may actually lead the partner to leave the relationship. And attempts to derogate the competition can add to the perception that the jealous person is out of control and unpleasant to be around. The irony is that the jealous partner fears the loss of the relationship, but the consequence of jealous behavior is that the relationship may end because of the jealousy. Some jealous partners may even terminate their relationships because they can no longer tolerate their own jealous feelings—even if there is no sufficient evidence of betrayal.

Many jealous partners follow an emotion–behavior fusion paradigm: "I feel jealous, so I must take action." This fusion can lead to impulsive responses to the feeling of jealousy and preclude any flexibility in adaptive behavior, as in this case:

THERAPIST: I notice that when you have the emotion of jealousy, you seem to believe that you have no choice as to what you do. It's as if your emotion and behavior become the same: "I feel jealous, so I interrogate, accuse, and attack." Does the emotion have to lead to the behavior—or do you have a choice?

PATIENT: I never thought of having a choice. It just overwhelms me.

THERAPIST: Yes, I can see it feels that way. It's like you have to act on this emotion. But is it possible to have a feeling and not act on it? For example, have you ever been angry at someone, but chosen not to criticize them or not to take action?

PATIENT: Oh, yes, many times. Even with my husband.

THERAPIST: OK, that's good to know. What would be the advantage of stepping back from the emotion—taking a few minutes to think it over—and choosing not to act on it?

PATIENT: I guess we would have fewer fights.

The therapist can then direct the patient as to how to handle the emotion of jealousy and the action tendencies that often accompany the feelings. For example, unlinking jealous emotions from behavior can be achieved by asking the patient to consider the specific actions under consideration (e.g., accusing), the costs and benefits of that action, the alternatives (e.g., gentle inquiry, skilled assertion, or distraction), and alternative interpretations of events. By illustrating that an emotion (jealousy) does not necessarily lead to an action (accusation), the patient can address the emotional schema of control ("My emotions are out of control"). The therapist can also inquire what the patient predicts will happen if he or she does not engage in coercive control. For example, if the jealous partner does not accuse or interrogate the partner, does this mean that the partner will actually cheat? What actually happens? It may be that the individual's coercive control serves the function of a "safety behavior": The preservation of the relationship is attributed to the coercive control, rather than to any intrinsic commitment the partner has to the relationship.

Modifying emotion–action fusion helps the patient experience a sense of control. If the patient is willing to consider abandoning coercive control, then attention can be directed to introducing more positive and rewarding interpersonal behaviors into the relationship. In relationships in which jealousy has become a significant factor, a considerable focus may be on the problematic jealous behavior, or (in some cases) on the fact that the object of the jealousy becomes more secretive so as to avoid further arguments, thereby fueling even more jealousy.

THERAPIST: It may not be possible to maintain a good relationship by coercing your partner and accusing and threatening. However, those are some of the feelings and behaviors that seem to be the focus of the relationship. One way of looking at relationships is that they rise and fall on their own merits—not necessarily because someone else has interfered. If the relationship is working for both of you, and you both have a commitment, then why would anyone want to leave? If they want to leave, then maybe it's not the right relationship. So how do we make it more rewarding to stay?

PATIENT: But there are times I don't trust him.

THERAPIST: That makes sense that you have those feelings at times. But coercing your partner will not gain you the feeling of trust. The question is, what would make it more rewarding for the two of you?

PATIENT: I guess if we had fewer fights.

The therapist can then assist the patient in decreasing destructive behaviors (e.g., withholding, contempt, stonewalling, criticizing, labeling, and mind reading) and increasing positive behaviors (e.g., positive tracking, reward, active listening skills, shared activities, and validating the partner's sense that the jealousy has been damaging). Targeting unhelpful behaviors, and monitoring when one has a desire to engage in them but chooses *not* to engage in them, can facilitate a greater sense of genuine control and allow the individual to test the idea that the partner needs to be coerced in order to be "kept in line." As with many emotions, this focus on improving the relationship may involve "opposite action"—that is, doing the opposite of what the patient desires to do. For example, rather than criticizing the partner, the jealous individual can praise the partner, show affection, or engage in rewarding activities with him or her. The therapist can suggest setting up "experiments" of opposite action for a few weeks, to see whether this increases the individual's sense of security in the relationship and how this affects the intensity of jealous feelings.

## Promoting Self-Care

In many cases, a jealous individual's sense of identity has been submerged in the relationship, and the threat of loss of the relationship has become overly threatening. Jealousy tethers the individual's feelings to the partner's actions and thoughts in an angry, struggling dependency: "I don't know what I would do without her," or "My whole sense of who I am is wrapped up in this relationship."

THERAPIST: It seems that your emotions are almost completely tied up with what your partner says, does, feels—or might do. It's as if you believe that you have lost your sense of yourself in the relationship, so the possible loss of the relationship might mean the loss of who you are.

PATIENT: Yes. It's like I feel that I don't have a sense of myself.

THERAPIST: That may make your jealous feelings even more difficult for you. What we might want to examine is how you can take charge of other positive feelings that are not dependent on the relationship. You might think of it this way: "Emotions come from lots of different experiences. Which experiences can I have that will give me the emotions that I like having?"

PATIENT: Well, I haven't been seeing my friends as much, so I can do more of that. And, you know, I actually do like my work, so there are some good feelings there.

THERAPIST: That's a start. I wonder if you might consider thinking of other sources of good feelings—other behaviors, experiences, opportunities—maybe things that you are doing now, things you did in the past, things that you have dreamed of doing. It's good to have a good relationship, and it's also good to have a good life that you call your own.

As in this example, the therapist can focus the patient on personal goals and values that are *independent* of the other person. The patient can be encouraged to develop supportive friendships, independent activities and interests, involvement in community activities, and valued work. This can reduce the sense of desperate dependency and overfocus on the relationship. The belief in the "essentiality" of the other—or of the relationship—feeds into the angry, desperate dependency and jealousy. "If I lose this relationship, I lose everything" often underlies jealous desperation. By diversifying sources of reward, interpersonal support, and meaningful goals, the individual can unlink positive feelings from the absolute necessity of the other, thereby decreasing the fear of losing the relationship.

## SUMMARY

Jealousy is an emotion that people will kill others—or themselves—over. Yet it is an evolved emotion, based on the evolutionary value of protecting one's parental investment and thus the survival of one's genes. People may differ as to the situations that might elicit jealousy or jealous behavior, but jealousy appears to be widespread, even universal. The emotional schema model attempts to normalize jealousy, while distinguishing among jealous thoughts, emotions, and behaviors, and to assist the patient in choosing behaviors that are in the interest of the self and (if possible) the relationship. Conceptualizing jealousy within the framework of this broader cognitive-behavioral model may help the individual understand the innate predisposition toward jealousy; the earlier attachment and socialization experiences that might confer greater vulnerability; the recognition of thought–action–reality fusion; and the possibility that one can choose to act in a manner that is not determined by jealous emotions, but rather by self-interest. Decastrophizing potential loss and developing plans for self-care can help the individual decrease his or her agitated dependency on a partner whose commitment is doubted. In the next chapter, I turn to envy, another emotion that can lead to destructive behavior.

# CHAPTER 11

# Envy

Hatred is active, and envy passive dislike;
there is but one step from envy to hate.
——JOHANN WOLFGANG VON GOETHE

A man who has been working in a large corporate firm has recently been passed over for promotion. He feels resentful that his accomplishments have not been fully recognized, but also wonders what he has done wrong. As he comes into contact with a colleague who was promoted, he feels sad, defeated, hopeless, and angry. To him, his colleague's success exemplifies his own "failure," and reminds him that he has been "publicly humiliated." Although he knows his colleague to be quite competent, and although he has always liked him personally, he notices that now he has angry feelings toward him. Realizing this only makes him feel ashamed and guilty, and he recognizes his own sad and anxious feelings when around him—so he now avoids him. Feeling awkward around others at work, he interacts much less at the office, while ruminating about his "defeat." His wife has commented about his lack of attention to his three children and to her, and he finds himself dwelling on the sense of defeat at work while he is with his family.

In this chapter, I describe an emotional schema approach to envy, and I suggest some strategies that may help reverse the negative effects of this often misunderstood emotion. Although the terms "jealousy" and "envy" are often used interchangeably, there are significant differences between these two emotions, as I have described at the beginning of Chapter 10. The model of envy advanced here (like the model of jealousy outlined in the previous chapter) is an integrative cognitive-behavioral model that incorporates elements from evolutionary theory, in which envy can be viewed as adaptive. The model encompasses the role of dominance hierarchies; perception of scarcity of resources; overfocus on need for approval; problematic status seeking and overidentifying self-esteem with perceived status; overfocus on upward comparison; viewing the self as the product of acquisition versus experience; the metaphor of life as a ladder or race; and the desire to devalue others. In short, envy is angry, agitated rumination based on status anxiety.

## THE NATURE OF ENVY

As noted above and at the start of Chapter 10, we tend to feel envious of people when their success, in our minds, exemplifies our defeat or inferior status. Envy may take the form of "depressive envy" (in which we feel sad and defeated as we compare ourselves with others who seem to be doing better) or "hostile envy" (in which we desire the downfall of others who seem to be doing better). Our envy is usually directed at someone who is somewhat similar to us in the performance of a desired quality, and the achievement that we envy is one that we highly value for ourselves. For example, a college professor may be envious of a colleague who has recently published a book because she views herself as similar to this colleague and she values professional advancement. She may harbor the view that her colleague's success reflects on her own lack of publications. She may mobilize her attributional biases and theories to undermine or discount the success of her colleague, pointing out that the work is not original and lacks empirical rigor. She may argue that her colleague is undeserving or that the colleague has personal qualities that detract from an appearance of professionalism. Or she may think that she herself has not received the recognition for her work that it deserves, and that, with time, she will show everyone what really outstanding scholarship looks like.

As indicated, we are generally not envious of people whose accomplishments are outside our sphere of social comparison. For example, I will not feel envious of whoever won the Most Valuable Player award in Major League Baseball because I do not play professional baseball—and even if I did, I would never be in the major leagues. This is outside my realm of comparison. However, I might feel envious of a colleague who is getting a lot of positive publicity for new psychological ideas because I see the two of us in the same sphere of comparison. We generally envy what we see as a possibility for ourselves.

One aspect of envy is *Schadenfreude*, or pleasure in the downfall of people whom we envy. For example, the envious professor will take pleasure in hearing that her colleague's work has been refuted by recent research showing that the findings are not replicated and can be more easily explained by a new variable. Research on envy and *Schadenfreude* indicates that where there are hostile feelings associated with envy, there is a much greater likelihood of *Schadenfreude* (Brigham, Kelso, Jackson, & Smith, 1997; Smith et al., 1996), and that *Schadenfreude* is much more likely when the target of envy is viewed as similar to the self (van Dijk, Ouwerkerk, Goslinga, Nieweg, & Gallucci, 2006). Envy may also lead to selective attention—for example, greater attention directed toward the behavior of the targeted person who is envied (Hill, DelPriore, & Vaughan, 2011). This may have an advantage, in that observing more successful individuals may convey information that can be used to improve one's own skills. However, greater memory for the target's behavior is associated with a decrease in performance on an anagram task, suggesting that envy can have depleting consequences. It may be that recollecting the performance of a "more successful" individual may undermine one's own confidence and interfere with one's own performance. This is consistent with a model of depressive envy.

A distinction has also been made between "benign envy" (where one wishes to improve one's own position) and "malicious envy" (which is aimed at pulling the superior other down) (Salovey & Rodin, 1991; Smith & Kim, 2007). Benign envy (admiration) can lead to increased performance (i.e., it motivates the individual to work harder toward desired behavior), whereas malicious envy (angry and hostile feelings toward an individual performing better than the self) can lead to decrements of performance (van de Ven, Zeelenberg, & Pieters, 2011). van de Ven and colleagues (2011) found that malicious envy was more common when individuals perceived themselves as unable to attain the higher goals exemplified by the target person.

Moreover, although both men and women were found to be envious of target persons with greater wealth, only women reported greater envy of more physically attractive targets (Hill et al., 2011). Although, as just noted, envy can motivate one to try harder to move up in a status hierarchy (van de Ven, Zeelenberg, & Pieters, 2009), it is more often associated with depression, anxiety, resentment, and anger.

Envy is also affected by the perception of whether positive outcomes are deserved: In another study, benign envy was associated with the view that positive outcomes for the other were deserved and controllable whereas malicious envy was more often expressed when positive outcomes were viewed as undeserved (van de ven, Zeelenberg, & Pieters, 2012). Furthermore, envy is more likely to be experienced as unpleasant when upward comparisons are associated with deficits in emotional and behavioral self-control, impeding the ability to use upward comparisons to motivate behavior for self-improvement (Crusius & Mussweiler, 2012).

Hill, Buss, and their colleagues have viewed envy within an evolutionary framework. They see it as a consequence of "positional bias" (i.e., valuing the relative position that one holds in a hierarchy, rather than the absolute level of one's position). For example, individuals will prefer a lower compensation, as long as it is higher or equal to that of others, over an alternative higher compensation that is lower than that of others. Concepts of fairness or distributive justice appear to prevail over absolute level of consequences (Hill & Buss, 2006). The purported evolutionary advantage of envy is to motivate individuals to notice the behaviors that confer relative advantage and rank, and to become highly motivated to acquire those behaviors (Buss, 1989; Gilbert, 1990, 2000b)—or, alternatively, to modify the distribution matrix that is employed. Emotional schema theory draws on evolutionary models of envy to help normalize envy and assist in making sense of this emotion.

Envy can be found even in young children. In a study of responses to competitive outcomes, Steinbeis and Singer (2013) found that children between the ages of 7 and 13 felt better about winning if another child lost and felt worse about losing if another child won. Preferences for equal outcomes increased with age, and there was a decrease in spite with increasing age. Finally, envy is more common among youth endorsing materialistic values, whereas gratitude is associated with lower levels of depression and envy (Froh, Emmons, Card, Bono, & Wilson, 2011). Fiske (2010) has proposed that "envy up" is associated with anger, shame, humiliation, lowered self-esteem, and a sense of unfairness, whereas "scorn down"—which is often associated with contempt—focuses more on the self and decreases the ability to understand or have empathy for those of lower status. These "power perceptions" are often part of the ongoing process of social comparisons, which underpin status concepts, outgroup stereotyping, and the deactivation of mental concepts about others. As Fiske aptly notes, "Power corrupts." As we gain more power over others, it may activate scorn, contempt, and—ultimately—dehumanization of others.

Let us now examine how envy can be addressed from the perspective of an integrated emotional schema model. As noted earlier, this larger case conceptualization model draws on elements of evolutionary theory; it also focuses on the "value" of benign envy, the overemphasis on social comparison, and the emotional schemas that underlie this challenging emotional experience.

## MODIFYING EMOTIONAL SCHEMAS OF ENVY

The realistic goal is not to eliminate envy, since envy is viewed as an emotion that is universal and part of almost any social grouping. Rather, the goal is to modify the effects that envy has on the individual—for example, to reduce the guilt and shame over envy, decrease confusion about envy, overcome the tendency to avoid envied others, reduce or eliminate complaining and undermining, and reduce the tendency to ruminate about the unfairness or nefarious comparisons that underlie envy.

## Normalizing Envy

Although most people experience envy, they usually also feel considerable shame and guilt over having this emotion. Envy is often a disparaged emotion—one that an individual is hesitant to acknowledge to others. Indeed, one of the motivations behind criticizing more successful people that one envies is the reluctance to acknowledge that one's driving emotion is envy. Ironically, this universal emotion is often not shared as "I am feeling envious"; rather, it is more favorably reframed as "They don't deserve that." However, envious individuals may feel alone and embarrassed about their envy. When I have given workshops and discussed envy, I have asked participants to raise their hands if they have ever felt envious, and almost all of them raise their hands. Perhaps therapists are more willing to acknowledge their envy than other people are, but this almost unanimous acknowledgment suggests that envy is a universal emotion.

One can ask, from an evolutionary perspective, "What is envy good for?" One way of viewing envy is to examine the role of dominance hierarchies in the lives of animals who live in groups. What is the advantage of being higher in a dominance hierarchy? An early model of dominance hierarchies in humans was advanced by Price (1967), who proposed that increases in dominance behaviors occur with instability in a hierarchy, increased emphasis on competition, insufficient resources, and overcrowding. Among group-living animals, higher social rank among males is associated with much higher rates of impregnating females, greater access to females, preferential choice for food, better nesting sites, and greater survivability. Thus individuals in a dominance hierarchy have significant motives to increase their position in the hierarchy, and they may often "test" the ability of higher-status individuals to maintain the favored position.

Stevens and Price (1996) and Sloman, Price, Gilbert, and Gardner (1994) have advanced a model of depression based on social rank. They propose that loss of social rank leads to depressive behavior (avoidance, deference, loss of sexual interest, decreased aggression, passivity), which reduces the risk of competition with individuals higher in rank and thereby "protects" those of lower rank. Presumably, an individual who has already lost the competition with more dominant figures would be "wise" to show appeasement rather than aggression, by subordinating the self to others. Research supports the social rank model of depression (Gilbert & Allen, 1998; Johnson, Leedom, & Muhtadie, 2012), suggesting that loss of status in groups does lead to depression for some individuals. In rats experiencing subordinate status, stress was associated with weight loss and early mortality, as well as with decreased aggression, copulation, feeding, and overall activity (Blanchard & Blanchard, 1990). As position in the dominance hierarchy changes, levels of serotonin vary in vervet monkeys (McGuire, Raleigh, & Johnson, 1983). And increasing serotonin levels through the use of Prozac leads to individual vervet monkeys' rising in the hierarchy

(Raleigh, McGuire, Brammer, Pollack, & Yuwiler, 1991). Similarly, Tse and Bond (2002) found that humans treated with selective serotonin reuptake inhibitors were perceived by others in their groups as engaging in more dominant eye contact, more affiliative behavior, and less submission in general.

Thus social rank theory suggests that perceived loss of status may lead to more depressive affect. One way of coping with this loss of status may be to delegitimize the perceived greater status of others by claiming that they do not deserve their higher rank and that "the game is rigged." That is, envy—particularly angry, resentful envy—may be an attempt to defend against depressive subordination by psychologically undermining the legitimacy of higher-status individuals. On the other hand, many individuals experience depressive envy, probably as result of the social rank loss that they experience. Some individuals experience both depressive and angry envy, depending on their appraisal of the legitimacy of an envied individual's position. Envy may be adaptive if it motivates one to challenge the dominance hierarchy, and thereby to improve one's position regarding resources and genetic advantage. On the other hand, envy may also be adaptive, from the perspective of social rank theory, if the consequent depression reduces unwinnable challenges by the envious individual. These evolutionary and social rank conceptualizations are important components of the emotional schema model, and discussing them in session can help the therapist and patient conceptualize envy within the broader context of these processes.

Of particular relevance are the triggers for the patient's envious feelings. For example, does the professor described earlier feel more envious when she hears about the success of her colleague? Or when her work goes poorly, does her mind shift to thinking of how well the colleague is doing? The triggers for envy lead to social comparisons, often at the expense of the self. This then leads to anxiety, sadness, and anger. In many cases, the temptation is to devalue the other person, so that the comparison between self and others appears less invidious. Figure 11.1 illustrates this cycle.

The therapist can then help the patient identify maladaptive coping strategies in response to envy. These include complaining to others about the unfairness that one is experiencing (if this complaining will sabotage one's own standing); attempts to undermine the envied target; rumination; avoidance of the envied person; withdrawal from others; and overdrinking, binge eating, and other self-destructive behaviors. Some individuals believe that criticizing themselves for their envy will help them get rid of it. Of course, this only adds to their depression and makes them even more vulnerable to envy. The emotional schema model proposes that a therapist and patient accept (for the moment) feelings of envy, normalizes those feelings, and validate the difficulty in having those feelings. Of course, acceptance does not preclude change, as we will see. Let us turn now to specific interventions that are relevant to coping more effectively with envy.

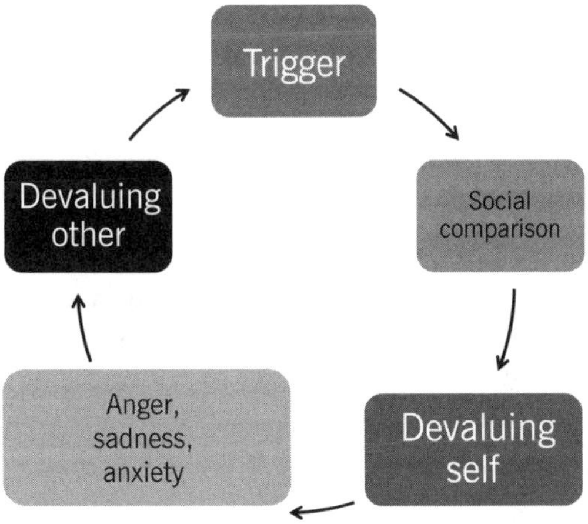

**FIGURE 11.1.** The cycle of envious feelings.

## Validating Envy

An essential part of working with envy in emotional schema therapy is to validate the painful and confusing feelings that accompany envy. The therapist can begin by saying:

> "It sounds like you are struggling with some feelings of envy that make you feel uncomfortable. Since all of us experience envy at times, it is one of those emotions that we all know about—but many of us feel uncomfortable with these feelings. Are there other feelings that go with the envy?"

The therapist can then explore with the patient the nature of these other emotions, such as sadness, anxiety, anger, confusion, resentment, and hopelessness. It is important for the therapist to convey an accepting, non-judgmental stance toward the envy, since many people feel embarrassed and humiliated over their feelings. The therapist can validate that envy may activate sadness, anger, anxiety, and shame—and that these emotions are often the "normal experience of envy." In particular, the sense of shame, accompanied by the feeling that the success of another is humiliating to the self, can be directly examined by pointing out that almost everyone feels envy, but that "we are taught that we should not have these feelings"; we thereby become reluctant to acknowledge them as "envy," and instead focus on whether others deserve their success. Acknowledging that "I feel envious" redirects the patient's attention to reconsidering a response to the situation of the success of another; it encourages the patient to examine the choices for the self. Envy must come out into the open to be examined if it is to be used constructively.

## Identifying Envious Emotions and Separating These from Behavior

Envy is a difficult emotion for people to accept, since it often conveys the sense that one begrudges the success of others and that one wants to sabotage someone who may have achieved success fairly. It is often experienced as the "sore loser" emotion—one that envious individuals are reluctant to admit to. As indicated above, validating and normalizing envy are important steps in getting such individuals to accept that the emotion is not unusual and does not set them apart from others. Expressing envy may be difficult in social interactions, since an individual may then be confronted with the judgments of others (e.g., "You sound like you are envious of her"), which may lead to further marginalization and criticism. But if envy is a universal emotion, based on the dynamics of dominance hierarchies and competition, then recognizing the envy for what it is may be an important step in coping with it. The individual who believes, "I am a bad person because I feel envious," can recognize that envy is part of human nature—perhaps an emotion that can, in the right circumstances, help him or her acquire greater skills and even come to use the envied person as a role model rather than an enemy. Moreover, it is not the envy per se that causes problems, especially if one accepts that emotion. It is not separating the emotion of envy from the problematic actions that follow, such as avoidance, criticizing, and sabotaging others.

Envy is often accompanied by a variety of negative and positive emotions, although the individual who ruminates may focus excessively on the negative. Thus envy can include anger, sadness, anxiety, regret, helplessness, and hopelessness, which can lead to complaining, rumination, worry, reassurance seeking, self-criticism, avoidance, and suicidal ideation. But the individual focused on envy can also examine whether any positive emotions are possible, such as curiosity, appreciation, challenge, excitement, gratitude, or contentment. Often envious individuals will have mixed feelings toward the person they envy—especially if that person is a friend. They may feel sad, resentful, and bitter, but still find that there are qualities they like about that person. These mixed feelings can lead to guilt, rumination ("What is wrong with me?"), and avoidance.

Decoupling an envious feeling from envious behavior is an important step in helping individuals cope with their feelings of envy. Choosing not to act on envy—but rather on important values and adaptive strategies—may help reduce the sense of being overwhelmed with envy and the worry that envy will return. Recognizing that the emotion of envy can be accepted, normalized, and tolerated—along with taking effective action toward positive goals—may lead to *less anxiety about feeling envious.* Realizing that "I can feel envious, but can choose behaviors that are in my real interest" can be a liberating experience of flexibility and decoupling from the sense of being compelled by the envy. A patient can eventually say, "Just because I feel envious doesn't mean I need to act like an envious person. I have a choice."

## Examining Core Beliefs, Assumptions, and Schematic Processing

Envy is often linked to core beliefs about self, others, and the nature of competition. The envious person may endorse core beliefs that "I am not lovable, capable, important, or effective," and that "I must compensate for these inadequacies by getting approval, climbing a status hierarchy, and defeating others." Envious individuals endorse the full range of automatic thought distortions: personalizing ("He got ahead, which reflects badly on me"); mind reading ("People think I am inferior now that she was promoted"); labeling ("He's a winner, and I am a loser"); fortunetelling ("She will continue to advance, but I will fall behind"); dichotomous thinking ("You either win or lose"); discounting positives ("The only thing that counts is getting ahead"); overgeneralizing ("Nothing works out for me"); and catastrophizing ("It's awful not to be ahead of others"). Since envy entails schemas about self (e.g., "unwanted") and the nature of the competitive world, the mode of envy drives schematic processing of attention. For example, hostile envy focuses attention and memory to information related to falling behind and to others' doing better. It selectively ignores the many other sources of reward and meaning that are present, but devalued in the envious mindset.

There is a logic to both hostile and depressive envy—that is, a string of negative implications about the relevance for the self of the success of others. For example, consider the following as examples of the logic of depressive envy:

> "He is more popular than I am."
> "If he is more popular, then I am not popular."
> "I will be marginalized."

And consider these examples of both depressive and hostile envy, and responses to these:

> *Depressive envy:* "I must be a loser. I will never be accepted. I have no future."
> *Response:* Withdrawal, rumination, self-criticism.

*Hostile envy*: "He is a phony. People don't know what a fake he really is. He doesn't deserve to be popular."
*Response*: Sarcasm, sabotage, passive–aggressive behavior, pouting, avoidance.

The basic assumptions—or "rule book" for envy—include the following beliefs:

"You have to evaluate everything you do."
"It's important to compare yourself with others."
"If someone does better than I do, then I am inferior."
"If I am inferior, I am not worthwhile."
"I can't stand the idea of unfairness."
"If I devalue people who are more successful, I can feel better about myself."
"The world should be fair, and I should be rewarded for everything I do that is good."
"Some people are worth more than others."
"There are winners and losers."
"It's terrible to lose. If you lose, then no one can love you or respect you."

Each of these beliefs can be examined by using standard cognitive therapy techniques. For example, the assumption "The world should be fair, and I should be rewarded for everything I do that is good" is a common belief underlying just-world illusions. The costs and benefits of this belief for the individual can be examined ("Is this really helping you, or is it making you more resentful?"), as can the evidence that there are any organizational systems that are consistently fair or even ideally efficient. An alternative belief that might be helpful is the following: "Many unfair things happen in life—or in any game that I play. But does that mean that I cannot play the game?" The goal is to help the patient function effectively in a world where unfairness is ubiquitous.

## Evaluating the Need to Compare and Judge

Many people who struggle with envy assume that they must compare themselves with others—especially those doing "better"—and then form judgments about themselves and these others. This focus on judgments leads to status anxiety, with individuals becoming frustrated and feeling a sense of personal defeat when they "fall short" of those above them, while either disdaining those below them or fearing that those below will overcome them. Theories of social comparison suggest that people may compare themselves with others in order to motivate themselves, learn which behaviors to use to gain rewards, learn about social norms, or build their self-esteem, although social comparison can also lead to a decreasing sense of self-worth (Ahrens & Alloy, 1997; Festinger, 1957; Suls & Wheeler, 2000; Wood, 1989). Generally, people will engage in upward comparisons to motivate themselves and downward comparisons to build their self-esteem (McFarland & Miller, 1994). The therapist can inquire, "What do you hope to gain by comparing yourself with others?" For example, one patient indicated that he thought that by comparing himself with others on his team at work, he would be motivated to work hard and "not let myself off the hook." There might have been some value in observing which behaviors were rewarded, but his excessive focus on comparisons and negative personal appraisals led him to become more depressed, ruminative, avoidant, and reluctant to interact with his team. The therapist suggested that he might focus more on working effectively with the team, getting his work done, and "managing upward" to make clear what his added value was. The choice was between productive work and negative comparisons.

Similarly, the idea that a patient can feel better by devaluing others can be examined:

"What is the evidence that you feel better? Or do you feel angry, anxious, and even depressed when you indulge your envy? Can you feel better by focusing on positive goals rather than negative goals? What are some constructive things that you can do now that might be rewarding?"

The importance of social comparison can be evaluated:

"What is the disadvantage of comparing yourself with others? What do you hope to gain? If you chose to focus on positive goals and values rather than comparing yourself, what could you do? How would that help? Is there any downside to focusing on positive goals rather than social comparisons?"

The therapist can help the patient focus on *observing and noticing*, rather than engaging in evaluative judgments. For instance, the patient can say, "I noticed that the boss complimented Sarah," rather than "Sarah is getting ahead of me," or "I must be failing." Or the patient can expand the observation to notice that "many people, including myself, are doing good work." Even evaluations such as "Sarah's work is better than mine" can be relinquished and replaced by "Sarah got the report in, and I met with a client." The therapist can ask the patient to monitor every evaluative judgment that he or she makes. In place of evaluations, the patient can record behavioral observations: "Spoke with a client," "Asked Tom about his weekend," "Participated in a meeting." By shifting to observations, behavioral descriptions, notes on specific situations, and nonevaluative statements while refocusing on productive action, the patient can collect information to test the idea that he or she needs social comparisons and judgments to be motivated.

## Developing a Case Conceptualization

Figure 11.2 illustrates a case conceptualization of envy that can help the therapist socialize the patient to the therapeutic model and identify targets for change. The case conceptualization begins with the evolutionary model of dominance hierarchies, selective fitness, and the advantages of dominant status. In addition, the evolutionary model assumes scarcity of resources in the original emergence of dominance. The question is whether current conditions merit following a model that assumes scarcity. What does the individual assume are the current advantages of dominance?

In addition, the therapist and patient can examine the emphasis on status (and how it was defined) in the family of origin. For example, did the patient's parents emphasize status in sports, physical beauty, intellectual achievement, aggressiveness, or popularity/social standing? What were the status dimensions in the peer group when the patient was a child or adolescent? Did the patient occupy lower status during childhood than peers or siblings? If so, how did the patient attempt to compensate for this status—for example, by avoiding, working exceptionally hard, forming other alliances, or rebelling? Whose approval did the patient attempt to secure? What core beliefs about self and other did the patient develop? For

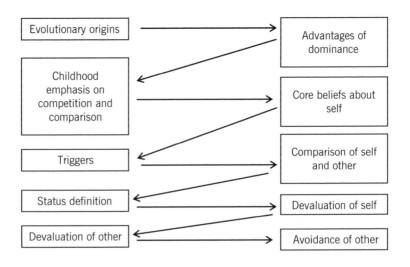

**FIGURE 11.2.** Case conceptualization of envy.

example, did the patient learn to see the self as inferior, defective, marginalized, unattractive, strange, helpless, or special—and others as judgmental, rejecting, aloof, competitive, humiliating, nurturing, or accepting?

What are the patient's triggers for anxiety about status and envy of others? Does the individual feel envious and threatened when he or she hears about the success of others? Does the patient feel envious when frustrated with his or her own progress, and then engage in comparisons with others? Who are these other people? Does the patient ever compare downward, or primarily upward? Is self-worth defined in terms of status (e.g., "I am falling behind. I am losing. I am a loser")? Does the patient view the social world primarily as a hierarchy or a ladder to climb? Is the concern for status so great that other aspects of a meaningful life are sacrificed? For example, is the concern for success affecting family life, relationship with friends, loss of sleep, health, and stress? Does the patient believe that someone's higher status at the moment necessarily means that he or she must devalue the self? Is the individual able to describe other aspects of self-concept or self-worth that are independent of status? How does the individual respond to the success of others—avoidance, criticism, sarcasm, reassurance seeking, self-criticism? Does the individual devalue people who achieve higher status, while seeking the reassurance of others that the "more successful" persons are undeserving?

A case conceptualization was used with a patient who became anxious, angry, and despondent when he was around colleagues who had achieved higher status in his company. The therapist indicated that dominance and status are part of most groups, that evolution selected out a preference for dominant status, and that these evolutionary pressures were based on conditions of severe scarcity in the evolutionarily relevant environment. However, such severe conditions no longer exist, so these tendencies to be concerned about status are less relevant today. The patient described how his mother had emphasized status and achievement, and how she had been overinvolved in his life, often trying to make decisions about his play activities and friendships. He felt marginalized by other children, who treated him as something of an outsider, leading him to withdraw more to seek out his mother's approval. Status was defined for him by academic achievement, which he pursued relentlessly; however, he still harbored the feeling that he was an outsider that others thought boring, not fun to be with, and "not one of us." He viewed his lack of belongingness to his basic defect of "lacking a personality," which then made him more avoidant and socially anxious. This hesitant interpersonal style kept him from forming alliances and working toward social inclusion at his job, since he engaged in continual mind reading that he was unwanted, was being rejected, and would never succeed in "reaching the top." He believed that only by reaching the top could he feel secure. Triggers for his envy were learning about the success of others or hearing that a colleague was included on a project.

He interpreted their success or inclusion as indicative of his marginalized status. His envy was more depressive envy, characterized by helplessness, regret, self-criticism, and sadness—although he expressed anger toward the "unfairness of the system," which he believed did not recognize his "true merit." This led to excessive depressive rumination: "Why me? I can't believe that I am not included. Do I have any future here? I will continue to be marginalized and never get ahead." The case conceptualization was extremely valuable in implementing many of the techniques described in this chapter.

## Linking Envy to Values

Envy implies that one is falling behind along a valued dimension of performance. For example, if one does not value being a great tennis player, then hearing that someone is a better player will not activate envy. However, if one views financial success as a measure of "being worthwhile"—or as a measure of "success or failure"—then one is vulnerable to envying those who are more financially successful. Self-evaluations are also related to values: For instance, an individual who values being popular above all else may be vulnerable to feeling marginalized. The therapist can inquire as to which values are being threatened by the perceived success of others. Is the individual overly focused on a specific value—for example, popularity, financial success, recognition, or physical attractiveness? What other values does the patient have? What is the patient's hierarchy of values?

> THERAPIST: You seem to be focused on the value of your title in the firm, as if this title would define your worth as a human being.
>
> PATIENT: I know. But it's important to me.
>
> THERAPIST: It's good to have goals and to be conscientious. But I wonder about what other values you might have. For example, where would you put the welfare of your family and your relationship with your wife and kids in your value system?
>
> PATIENT: They should be more important, but I have been so busy with work and so depressed about not getting ahead.
>
> THERAPIST: Where would you put your physical and mental health in your value system?
>
> PATIENT: They've suffered. I haven't been working out, and I overeat. My wife thinks I drink too much; maybe I do.
>
> THERAPIST: Where would you put being a good friend in your value system?
>
> PATIENT: I've lost contact with my friends.

The therapist can affirm that doing well at whatever value the patient is focused on can be important, but can also examine whether a focus on that performance or status has crowded out other values:

> "What if you tried to focus on other values, in addition to the one that you are concerned about? If you had a better relationship with your family, and valued that, or if you connected with friends, and you valued that, then perhaps you can achieve other values that mean something to you. If you are focused on one thing to the exclusion of all else, you may lose your perspective."

In addition, the patient's value of success at work can be reframed as "conscientiousness" or "doing a good job." This can be separated from status: "Is it possible to take some pride in the work that you do each day—on the tasks that you accomplish—rather than measuring yourself simply in terms of status?" For example, the patient whose case conceptualization is described above was able to shift from status concerns to focusing on getting his work done and looking for opportunities for challenge. Similarly, overfocusing on looks as status can be reframed as "being rewarding to other people."

## Deconstructing Success and Failure

An envious person is likely to view success or failure as categorical—that is, in all-or-nothing terms: "Either I am a success or I am a failure." Success is viewed as a trait quality that the individual possesses—one that perhaps cannot be modified. In contrast, the therapist can propose that a person succeeds or performs to various degrees on a variety of tasks at different times. The therapist can use the continuum technique to evaluate success along a number of dimensions for different behaviors at different times:

> THERAPIST: It seems that you view success and failure in all-or-nothing terms. And you also label yourself as a "success" or "failure." I wonder if that makes sense. Imagine that you go to see your doctor, and she says, "Your lab tests are fine and you seem very healthy, but we discovered from our examination that you are a failure as a human being." Would that make sense?
>
> PATIENT: (*Laughs*) No, I guess that sounds absurd.
>
> THERAPIST: But you are saying that about yourself at times. What if we gave you a grade from 0 to 100 on 10 different tasks or classes of behavior? For example, have you worked with clients and had some success?

PATIENT: Yes, I have done well. Some of the clients like me.

THERAPIST: OK, so if we looked at how you did with the last five clients that you worked with, what kind of grade would someone give you for each one?

PATIENT: It might vary between 80 and 90. I guess I do pretty well. I'm not perfect.

THERAPIST: And I imagine that there are a lot of behaviors that you engage in with a single client, and that you might rate yourself along this scale for each behavior for each day. Would you conclude that your performance varies with the day, the client, the behavior, and the task?

PATIENT: Yes. Some clients are easier to work with, and some of the projects are very complicated.

THERAPIST: So if your performance varies so much, then does it make sense to give anyone a blanket label of "success" or "failure"?

PATIENT: No, I guess that's going too far. It depends on what you are doing.

THERAPIST: And if we examined the performance of this person that you label a "success," you might also find a lot of variability too?

PATIENT: Yes, there are some things that he doesn't do as well on. In fact, there are some things that I do better on. But, again, it depends.

THERAPIST: Perhaps we can keep in mind what you just said—"It depends."

Just as various degrees of success can be viewed along a continuum, emotional responses to failure on a task can evoke emotions other than frustration and a sense of personal defeat. The therapist can suggest that outcomes on tasks can be viewed as learning experiences that can elicit feelings of curiosity, a sense of challenge, and an opportunity to learn.

## Examining Envy as Depressive or Angry Rumination

Envy is seldom an emotion that is fleeting. Individuals who are envious are prone to ruminate, to dwell on the sense of "unfairness," to focus on their own resentment, and to think about the negative implications of someone else's success for their own "lack of success." For example, the man who was passed over for promotion (as described at the start of this chapter) would spend part of each weekend ruminating about his envy of his colleague. Moreover, the nature of the rumination is both depressive and angry. Focusing on his sense of "defeat" and "humiliation," the passed-over man would dwell on how he was falling behind, how he was trapped, and how he had failed. Alternatively, the rumination can also activate feelings of anger—even the desire for revenge. Trapped in recurring negative thoughts, and isolated from others, the envious person may detach from more rewarding possible aspects of life.

As with any form of worry or rumination, an integrative cognitive-behavioral approach can be helpful. This includes the following steps: (1) identifying and tracking examples of rumination to increase self-awareness of problematic coping; (2) evaluating the costs and benefits of rumination; (3) asking whether the rumination is productive (e.g., "Does it lead to making progress on valued goals?"); (4) if it is unproductive, then asking whether there is some unfairness, uncertainty, or inequality that can be "accepted" as outside of the patient's control; (5) setting aside rumination time (at which time the patient can use cognitive-behavioral techniques); (6) asking, "What thoughts are triggered as a result of the other's success?"; and (7) asking, "How would you challenge these thoughts?"

For example, some individuals believe that others' success means that they themselves have failed, that these others (and others in general) are thinking less of them, or that they cannot be happy if others are doing better—especially if the others' success is seen as undeserved. These thoughts can be examined for costs–benefits and for supporting evidence, and alternative interpretations can be offered. For instance, the idea that "I have failed if someone else has succeeded" can be tested:

"Would that mean that nothing that you do is of any value? What are some positive behaviors that you engage in? Are you looking at success and failure in all-or-nothing terms? What if you were to look at different behaviors that 'pay off' and keep track of those behaviors every day?"

The thought that "Others are thinking of my failure" can also be tested:

"Are you engaged in mind reading? How do you know what people are thinking right now? Are you always thinking of other people and how they are doing? What are you thinking about if you are not thinking of everyone's status? Are you personalizing what others achieve? Could it be that others' success is irrelevant?"

The thought that "I cannot be happy if others are doing better" can be evaluated:

"Does it mean that no one else can have any pleasure if someone does better? Do you know of other people who were not promoted who are engaged in pleasurable behavior—who are happy? Is it the other person's success, or is it your tendency to personalize, mind-read, judge yourself, and ruminate that makes you unhappy? Keep track of your pleasure and mastery every hour of the week, and see if there is any pleasure or mastery that you experience."

One alternative to depressive rumination is to engage in mindful awareness of the present moment. For example, rather than ruminate about past injuries or current sense of unfairness, the patient may practice mindful awareness of the breath or mindful observation about the current environment. In addition, as described in earlier chapters, metacognitive techniques of "detached mindfulness"—such as observing a ruminative thought as a phone call that is not taken or a train that one chooses not to get on—can help decouple the individual from entanglement with intrusive thoughts (Wells, 2009). Moreover, the individual can focus on other productive action or pleasurable behavior during the present moment. For example, rather than focus on the success of another person, the individual can direct his or her energy toward pleasurable activities, such as exercising, playing with the children, reading a book, or going for a walk. Or the individual can work on other projects that may or may not be related to the issue of success or status. The occurrence of an intrusive thought of envy does not necessitate continued engagement with that thought.

## Turning Envy into Admiration and Emulation

As noted earlier in this chapter, "benign envy" can be used as a motivating force to make oneself better. That is, rather than ruminating on envy, an individual can acknowledge the feeling, normalize it, validate it, and then use it constructively. For example, an individual who observes that someone else is promoted might acknowledge feeling envious *at the present moment*. The emphasis is on "at the present moment," since the argument here is that emotions are transitory; they lessen as other experiences or emotions occur. The next step can be to reframe part of envy into admiration of the skills and success of the other person: "I can admire how he [or she] was able to be productive and form valuable alliances." Admiration is a central element in effective role modeling and developing a sense of personal competence; one can look for others whom one admires. "Admiration" has a more positive connotation than "envy," in that it acknowledges that others' skills can be valuable for oneself, and that one can observe (admire) them without the negative affect entailed in "envy." The third step can be emulation: For example, one can ask oneself, "How can I strategize to achieve these skills so I can enhance my position?" This would be a productive use of envy.

For example, in the case of the individual who ruminated about someone else's promotion, he was able to change his focus to identifying the skills and alliances that the other individual exemplified. These then became targeted behaviors for him, turning him into one who would avoid interactions with the envied target to one who wanted to observe and learn from him.

## Putting Status into Perspective

Envy is often the result of the tendency to overvalue status within a specific hierarchy. Status hierarchies are almost always "local"; that is, generally only those within a small reference group even know what the hierarchy is (De Botton, 2004). However, individuals experiencing envy may believe that their particular hierarchy is known by everyone and somehow reflects their ultimate value as human beings. The passed-over man commented, "If someone is ahead of me and gets promoted, then it means that I am a failure—I am nothing. Then I think, 'There is no sense in going on.'" He continued, "I feel that when I am at work, everyone is thinking that I was passed over—that I am a loser." Status is usually viewed in all-or-nothing terms—"Either you have it or you don't"—and is also viewed as something people are thinking about all the time.

An approach to this is to examine what "status" means—and what it does not mean. For example, status within an office culture may mean the kind of office a person has, the compensation the person receives, or the responsibilities that are assigned to him or her. However, even an individual who does not have "higher status" can still do a competent job, still interact with others, still receive compensation, and still have a life outside the office. The therapist can ask:

> "Does it make sense that people are always thinking of your status? What else might they be thinking of? Before [the specific event that triggered envy], were there things other than status that you were thinking about? Is status generalizable across situations? For example, if you have higher status within a group of coworkers, do you have higher status in all interactions in life? When you are with friends and family, are there aspects of these interactions that are enjoyable that do not involve status?"

The therapist can also ask, "If status failed to exist, would you still be able to be effective at work, have friends, have intimacy, or have fun?" The patient who is envious of perceived status of others might examine when he or she is experiencing pleasure and mastery, and whether all or any of this is related to status. For example, the therapist can inquire: "When you are playing with your children, talking with your friends, enjoying a sports event on television, eating a delicious meal, or having sex with your wife, are you deriving pleasure because of status or something else?"

Many people who experience envy view life as a race ("I am falling behind") or as a ladder to be climbed ("She's higher up than I am"). These metaphors for "success" and "competition" often give the individual a belief that there is a real race or real ladder, and that it is necessary to "get ahead." The implication would be that anyone who is not in the front of the race or on the top rungs of the ladder would have to be miserable. The therapist can help the patient identify these metaphors, and examine the costs and benefits of viewing the self and life in these terms:

> "If we go out on the street, will we be able to see a race going on? Are different people in different races? If someone is standing still, are they falling behind? Does everyone see it that way? Doesn't this metaphor lead to undue pressure, a tendency to discount important parts of life, stress over not getting everything done, excessive concern about the opinions of others, and self-criticism? What if the metaphor were replaced with a view that there are many different kinds of behaviors that are rewarding, and many different kinds of experience that are meaningful? For instance, what if the metaphor were one of a team working together to accomplish a goal?"

## Shifting Emphasis from Status to Experience

Erich Fromm, in *To Have or to Be* (1976), contrasts two modes of existence: One mode focuses on achievement, control, acquisition and domination (the "having" mode), and the other focuses on experience and connection (the "being" mode). The having mode focuses on competitiveness and defining one's meaning through status hierarchies and winning–losing. This contributes to dissatisfaction, concern about loss of status, and envy. Individuals who are overly focused on this mode can be encouraged to shift (at least in part) to the being mode, with its emphasis on having meaningful experiences, staying in the present moment, connecting, appreciating, and having mindful experiences with what is simple and universal. For example, the therapist suggested to the patient overly concerned with his position in the status hierarchy that he might consider other forms of being:

> THERAPIST: There are two ways of approaching life. One is focused on achievement and acquisition, and the other is focused on experiencing and connecting. For example, if you focused on experiencing, you might be listening to music, sharing a memory with your wife, playing with one of your children, swimming in cool water, or walking along a path in the woods. I wonder how you are doing with experiencing these things in your life.

PATIENT: Not too well, I guess. I am so focused on work and feeling resentful.

THERAPIST: OK. That might be something to consider. For example, what if you focused on playing with one of your children? What would that experience feel like?

PATIENT: I guess a lot of the time, I am too preoccupied with work. I love to play with my daughter. She's 6 and she can really have a lot of fun just being silly and kicking a soccer ball. And laughing. She laughs a lot.

THERAPIST: So, as you recall this at this moment, how does that feel?

PATIENT: It feels good—but it also makes me feel a little guilty because I just don't spend enough time with her. Or the other kids.

THERAPIST: Well, that might be an experience to have more of, don't you think? I wonder, if you were able to see the world from your daughter's point of view—to be in the present moment, to take the job out of playing, to imagine seeing something for the first time—what would that be like for you?

PATIENT: See something for the first time? What does that mean?

THERAPIST: Well, you like music. Imagine that you were listening to your favorite piece of music for the first time, that you had never heard it before. You might feel a sense of appreciation. You might listen carefully. You might have a sense of awe.

PATIENT: I used to feel that way.

## Differentiating Self-Concept from Status

Envy and the preoccupation with status often entail equating one's self-concept with a particular rank or status. For example, the statements "I am a managing director," "I am a principal," and "I am a foreman" all convey a sense of equating self with title or status. The patient who believes that "I am nothing because I was not promoted" has equated his self-concept with the new rank. The therapist can help examine this belief as follows:

> "If you are nothing because you were not promoted, then it means that even if you were promoted, then you had been a nothing the moment before the promotion. Does that make sense? They promoted a 'nothing'? Was the person who was promoted a 'nothing'?"

The therapist can inquire further about this dichotomous view of self by asking the patient to describe all the different roles and experiences that the patient has occupied in the last 2 years:

THERAPIST: I wonder if you can you describe the roles that you have in your life. For example, aren't you a husband, father, brother, friend, member of the community, coach for your oldest kid's team, someone who learns, someone who enjoys sports, someone who reads, someone who exercises, someone who has a spiritual life?

PATIENT: Those are a lot of roles. I don't know where to start.

THERAPIST: Let's start with your family. What are some things that you do with them?

PATIENT: I play soccer with my son. We go bike riding on the weekends. I don't know, we watch films together, we talk, and we laugh together. I help all the kids with their homework.

THERAPIST: So if we expanded this discussion to describe all the other roles that you are in—all the experiences that you have—would all of these be related to status?

PATIENT: Not really. It's more part of being a human being.

THERAPIST: Let's keep that in mind when you think of yourself as a "nothing" because you were not promoted.

## Universalizing Humanity

Envy relies on beliefs about dividing people into higher and lower status, and often relegating those of lower status to perceived qualities of being less worthwhile. The envious mind views people as divided in this way; some are seen as less deserving, others are seen as entitled. In contrast to the division of people into hierarchies, the envious person can be invited to consider the possibility of the universal nature of human beings. Challenging a hierarchy involves finding the commonalities of humans:

"Do you know any people who have less money, less success, or less status than you? Let's think of some people like that. Do they have parents? What do you think they did when they were kids? How do they relate to their friends? Are there holidays that they celebrate? When they talk with their children, what do they talk about? What do they laugh about? What do they cry about? What do you have in common with them?"

The therapist can then help the patient think of ways that one can respect and love people who have lower status in the particular hierarchy that the patient is concerned with. For example, a highly educated individual who was concerned about his status in his university reflected on the people whom he loved from his childhood: "I grew up in Brooklyn, before it was so cool to live in Brooklyn. We were poor; my parents were immigrants who escaped from the Nazis. I remember my grandfather, who seemed to have more time for me than my father did. Yeah, I loved them." Feeling connected to people from different educational levels, income levels, races, and cultures can help the individual put "status" in its place.

In further extending the idea of universal humanity, the therapist can suggest that the patient direct kindness and compassion every day to people of lower status. Since status divides and alienates, while compassion unites people, the patient can experience the feelings in him- or herself and others after directing kindness toward strangers. For example, one patient who was concerned about losing status was directed to give money to homeless people every day, to look into their eyes, and to wish them well. She indicated that this was an extraordinarily emotional experience for her, helping her recognize that she was much better off than many people, but also even much better off when she could give something to someone else. The emotional schema model proposes that certain emotions can "trump" other emotions; in this case, kindness and appreciation for what one has can trump status envy.

## Practicing Appreciation and Gratitude

As just mentioned, appreciation and gratitude for what one already has can offset feelings of status envy, which are generally focused on something one lacks or has never had. These positive emotions broaden one's thinking and enhance cognitive functioning and a sense of well-being (Fredrickson, 2004). "Appreciation" is a conscious recognition that one is lucky to have what one has and gives thanks for it in a general sense. "Gratitude" entails directly thanking someone for the good fortune that one has experienced. A patient may be directed to aspects of life he or she currently appreciates (work, friends, children, partner, physical wellness, etc.). In addition, the patient can reflect on the people he or she would like to thank for their contributions in the past—beginning with parents and childhood teachers and friends. Each day the patient can write a brief statement of gratitude to one of these people, even if some of them have died. Again, since envy often entails a focus on something one is missing or never had, gratitude refocuses attention on what one is fortunate to have. It is difficult to entertain emotions of gratitude and envy at the same time. The clinician can utilize the gratitude interventions described in Chapter 9 on values. Gratitude moves one away from social comparisons and a sense of falling behind in a never-ending race. It replaces these comparisons and competition with awareness of what one has, what one experiences, and what one has lived through.

## Practicing Opposite Action

The DBT technique of acting in opposition to one's current emotion (Linehan, 1993, 2015; Linehan et al., 2007) is a powerful intervention that can modify how one responds to envy. For example, rather than responding to feelings of envy by derogating self or others, the individual can direct "loving kindness" toward the envied target. This is a form of the Buddhist practice of *mettā bhāvanā*, whereby one directs feelings of loving kindness toward self, friends, strangers, enemies, and all sentient beings. In the case of envy, reaching the point of wishing an envied person well may seem like an insurmountable task—perhaps one that may be unnecessary. However, refocusing from anger and depressive envy to empathy, compassion, and kindness can allow an individual to relinquish these troubling emotions and experience greater psychological and physical well-being (Ameli, 2014; Fredrickson, 1998, 2013; Fredrickson, Cohn, Coffey, Pek, & Finkel, 2008; Hawkley & Cacioppo, 2010).

THERAPIST: I can see that you feel caught up in these emotions of anger, sadness, and resentment. It must be hard carrying all that around with you—hard on you, I would think. One technique that we have found useful in getting unstuck from these feelings is to focus on loving kindness toward self and others. When we are feeling compassion and kindness, it's hard to be sad and angry. Let's start, if you are willing, with directing some loving kindness toward yourself. Close your eyes and imagine that you are saying, "May I be happy. May I be well. May I be safe. May I be peaceful and at ease."

PATIENT: "May I be happy. May I be well. May I be safe. May I be peaceful and at ease."

THERAPIST: Now stay with that thought and notice your feelings. Notice where you have those feelings.

PATIENT: This feels calm, peaceful.

THERAPIST: OK. Now think of a friend or a family member that you care for. And repeat slowly, "May you be happy. May you be well. May you be safe. May you be peaceful and at ease."

PATIENT: OK, I am thinking of my husband. OK. "May you be happy. May you be well. May you be safe. May you be peaceful and at ease."

THERAPIST: Now let's try focusing on this person that you feel envy toward. Let's get her face in your mind, and now repeat slowly, directing your feelings of kindness toward her, "May you be happy. May you be well. May you be safe. May you be peaceful and at ease."

PATIENT: Oh, this is going to be hard. OK. "May you be happy. May you be well. May you be safe. May you be peaceful and at ease." OK.

THERAPIST: Now stay with that feeling of loving kindness toward her. Notice your breath as it goes out, and breathe out kindness toward her. Feel the kindness flowing toward her.

PATIENT: I am trying.

THERAPIST: OK. That's good. Now, as you are feeling loving kindness, bring that back toward yourself, repeating, "May I be happy. May I be well. May I be safe. May I be peaceful and at ease."

PATIENT: Yes, I feel that.

## Dealing with Resistance to Relinquishing Envy

Some patients believe that they cannot or should not relinquish their envious thoughts, feelings, and behaviors. As indicated earlier, some individuals believe that envy motivates them to try harder. Others believe that envy will give them an edge of competitiveness and dissatisfaction that will help them become more competitive. Yet others believe that envy is simply the way that they feel, and that they cannot or will not change their feelings. Some believe that giving up their envy is "letting themselves off the hook too easily"—that they should feel uncomfortable about not measuring up to others, and that their envy is realistic. Others resist giving up envy because they equate modifying their envy with saying that the unfairness is acceptable—that they are allowing themselves to be treated unfairly. And, finally, still others believe that envy will provide the motivation to get back at others who are undeserving or who are perceived as depriving them of their rightful position in the status hierarchy.

We have already examined the claim that envy motivates. Of course, there are many cases in which this is true, but it also assumes that one would not have motivation without envy. One can imagine working very hard because one takes pride in doing well, because the work is intrinsically interesting, or because one is paid a bonus for performance. None of these involves envy. Indeed, if one is only motivated by envy, then it is possible that one can do well but be miserable and anxious in the process. And, of course, if one works hard but others do better, relying primarily on envy to motivate will result in a sense of humiliation and personal defeat.

The claim that "I must be envious because that is simply the way I feel" would suggest that no feelings can ever be changed. In such a case, the therapist can inquire: "Have you had other negative feelings in the past, and have any of those changed? Similarly, have any positive feelings changed? What would be the advantages of feeling less envy?" In regard to letting oneself off the proverbial hook, envy seems only to act as a hook into depression and anger. The therapist can ask: "What is the advantage of being on a hook? Rather than being on a hook, can you imagine being more productive, having a wide range of sources of meaning and reward, and letting go of the rumination that keeps you on a hook?"

The desire for retaliation or sabotage is a strong feeling for some people who struggle with envy. Taking pleasure in the failings of others—*Schadenfreude*—may be a universal phenomenon, as noted earlier in this chapter. But ruminating about others' misfortunes may not be the most rewarding way to go through life. Focusing on negative goals—such as viewing the competition as the "enemy"—may deprive one of the intrinsic enjoyment of the work itself. Letting go of retaliatory goals does not mean saying that everything is fair or that one does not deserve better treatment. Rather, it allows one to step away from competing against others in order to engage in more productive goal setting. For example, it might be less anxiety-provoking to focus on getting work done or engaging in positive interactions with one's family than fantasizing about the failure of others. Even a humorous suggestion may be helpful: "Which holiday card would you like to receive: 'I hope that you and your family have a lot of wonderful times' or 'I hope you spend a lot of time fantasizing about other people failing'?"

## SUMMARY

Envy can be either benign or malicious, and can be either depressive or hostile. Many individuals experience envy but feel ashamed to admit that their emotion is envy; they either focus on the unfairness of others' success, brood on their own sense of failure and helplessness, or (in many cases) refuse even to mention the emotion that they harbor in agitated silence. Often associated with rumination, bitterness, avoidance, helplessness, and the desire to avenge, envy can lead to self-defeating behaviors that alienate friends, family, and colleagues, and can even endanger the envious individuals' position in the work environment. The integrated emotional schema model assists patients in making sense of envy, universalizing the experience of social comparison and envy, and distinguishing between the productive and unproductive experience of envy. Therapists can utilize the emotional schema model, together with cognitive, metacognitive, ACT, and DBT models, to help patients cope with these intrusive and difficult thoughts and experiences.

# CHAPTER 12

# Emotional Schemas in Couple Relationships

Let me not to the marriage of true minds
Admit impediments. Love is not love
Which alters when it alteration finds,
Or bends with the remover to remove . . .
—WILLIAM SHAKESPEARE, Sonnet 116

A married man described in Chapter 4 came to therapy "because my wife thinks I have an anger problem": "You know, if she would just pay attention to what I say, we wouldn't have these problems. I mean, how many times do I have to ask her to do something? I know I shouldn't yell at her, but it seems that's the only way to get her to pay attention." How did he respond when she spoke to him? "I wish she would just get to the point. I'm the kind of guy who gets things done. You tell me a problem, and I'll find the solution." This individual illustrates a number of problems in communication and in his understanding of emotion that fueled his anger, made him feel cut off from his wife, and made his wife feel humiliated and controlled.

The emotional schema model proposes that couple relationships entail awareness and respect for the emotions of both parties. This particular individual endorsed several dimensions of problematic beliefs about his wife's emotions—or her communication of emotion: duration ("Her emotions will go on and on"); control ("She just starts getting upset and can't control the way she feels. She should control herself more"); lack of comprehensibility ("She doesn't make sense. She should be happy"); lack of

271

consensus ("Her emotions are different from other people's emotions"); rationality ("She should be rational, logical, and factual"); blame ("She's the problem—she shouldn't be so difficult"); lack of acceptance ("I can't stand her moodiness"); lack of validation ("I don't want to hear these complaints. They don't make sense to me"); and expression ("She wants to talk and talk; I want to get problems solved").

Such beliefs and styles of interacting in an intimate relationship are significant contributors to discord and increase the risk of depression in both partners. In our research, we used the 14-item Relationship Emotional Schema Scale (RESS; see Chapter 4, Figure 4.2) to collect data from over 300 adult patients who were cohabiting or married. This simple questionnaire assesses how a patient views a partner's response to the patient's emotional difficulties. A composite score on this short questionnaire accounted for almost 36% of the variance on the Dyadic Adjustment Scale (DAS), thus proving to be a better predictor of relationship satisfaction than either depression or one's own emotional schemas.

In this chapter, I describe how implicit theories of emotions of others may lead to unhelpful responses to emotional distress in couple relationships, such as contempt, dismissive responses, stonewalling, or overcontrol. I review strategies for assessing theories about emotions in others, modifying beliefs about emotions in others, and implementing adaptive strategies for emotional interaction. In addition, I examine resistance to utilizing "helpful" strategies, such as beliefs about fairness and turn taking; assumptions that validation will only perpetuate complaints; beliefs that one has to fix the problem rather than share the problem; and beliefs that one cannot tolerate listening to the emotions of another person. I review the value of acceptance, mindfulness, and compassionate-mind techniques, as well as examining emotional schema beliefs about the emotions of partners—such as overgeneralization, excessive demands for rationality, labeling of defectiveness, and overreliance on problem solving and winning the argument.

## EMOTIONAL SCHEMAS AND DYSFUNCTIONAL STYLES OF RELATING

As the example of the married man illustrates, an individual can endorse a wide range of negative beliefs about emotion, and these beliefs are related to relationship dissatisfaction. How are these beliefs manifested in behavior? How do beliefs about emotion lead to contempt, sarcasm, stonewalling, criticism, withdrawal, and refusal to engage in validation, mutual problem solving, or encouragement to share feelings? Individuals who are focused primarily on problem solving, rationality, and facts often view emotions as a distraction, a waste of time, and a selfish indulgence. Consequently, a person with these negative beliefs about a partner's emotions will not only fail to empathize, but will often openly criticize or limit the partner's expression of emotion. Ironically, individuals may view their own emotions as the only important issues, and thus may view the emotions of others as depriving them of the opportunity to get their emotional needs met. In fact, this particular individual's case illustrates this problem. On further inquiry, his major complaint was that his wife did not validate him ("just like my father never validated me"), and he believed that she was too focused on her needs and not on his. Such asymmetrical beliefs about validation are not uncommon.

The therapist and patient reviewed the patient's specific problematic emotional schemas regarding his wife's emotions and communication style, and evaluated how these specific beliefs led to other negative beliefs and to behaviors that attempted to control or suppress the wife's emotional communication. For example, his belief in the durability of his wife's frustration and complaints ("Her emotions will go on and on") led him to believe, "I can't stand her constant complaining—it will go on indefinitely. If I don't do something right now, there will be no end to it." He viewed his wife's frustration as a fixed trait rather than a temporary and situational occurrence, and labeled her as a "complainer," thereby discounting the significant contribution she was making to family life and to solving problems. Moreover, his beliefs in the durability of her emotion made him feel helpless about "changing" her and hopeless about the future ("I will have to listen to this forever"). These feelings of helplessness led to his anger and his attempts to assert power over her to "end this complaining." His belief that she had no control over her emotion, and that she should suppress her complaints ("She just starts getting upset and can't control the way she feels. She should control herself more"), led him to believe that he had to control her or force her to control herself. Again, his recurrent belief was that he had to "do something," or the complaining would escalate and overwhelm him. Since he also believed that he had to solve her problems and get her to feel better immediately, he became infuriated when he thought she was putting problems forward and then rejecting his "well-intentioned" solutions. He believed that listening and validating would only further the reinforcement of her complaining, and that control needed to be implemented immediately. Many of their arguments originated in these attempts to control, suppress, or solve problems.

Because the patient believed that his wife's emotions were incomprehensible ("She doesn't make sense," "She should be happy"), he responded to her with condescension, contempt, sarcasm, and patronizing lectures, which further frustrated her and led to complaints about his response. Moreover, he thought that if he acknowledged that her frustration made sense and was warranted, he would be accepting blame for her problems, and that doing so would be intolerable and humiliating. In fact, he believed that her frustration with the children, homemaking, and getting things done was a veiled criticism of him and "the life I provide her," and a direct rejection of his "well-meaning advice." He believed that her emotions were different from other people's emotions (lack of consensus), leading him to invalidate her, dismiss her, and treat her emotions with contempt: "Other wives in this situation would be appreciative. It's not like she is wanting for anything." By marginalizing her feelings as a sign of her personal defects and irrationality, he contributed to her belief that he would never hear her needs, leading her to alternate between complaining more and withdrawing. Moreover, his belief in the power of rationality ("She should be rational, logical, and factual") led him to believe that listening, validating or accepting her emotions would only reinforce an "overly emotional" and "inefficient" style of coping, and that he had to insist that she comply with his rules for rationality. He maintained that rationality and problem solving were the only legitimate ways of thinking and communicating, and that anything else needed to be dismissed immediately.

As a result of his beliefs about duration, control, and rationality, he also viewed her emotions with an indifference and contempt for validation ("I don't want to hear these complaints. They don't make sense to me"), and the expression of her feelings ("She wants to talk and talk; I want to get problems solved"). Similar to many people with a negative view of emotion in close relationships, he believed that encouraging her to express her feelings and validate them would only lead to an endless stream of complaints, loss of control, and failure to solve problems, and would provide a bad example for the children. In fact, he believed that directly invalidating her ("You don't make any sense") would get her to see things more realistically and lead to an end to her complaining. Finally, all of these beliefs about her emotion "logically" led him to conclude that he could not accept her complaints and feelings, since to do so would be to tell her she was right; this, he believed, would result in his accepting fault for her feelings and would lead to an endless pattern of complaints and emotional dramatics. His beliefs made sense to him and, on the surface, had an element of logic and consistency. However, they were also contributing to the partners' mutual discord and their belief that they lived in a parallel universe, never connecting. When his attempts to control or suppress her feelings failed, he "doubled down" on his strategies of dismissing and repudiating her feelings, which led to further escalation of conflict, further confirming his belief that she was "out of control."

Each of the emotional schema dimensions illustrated in this man's beliefs about his wife can be addressed by using cognitive therapy techniques. For example, such a patient can examine the costs and benefits of believing that the partner's emotions are out of control, last indefinitely, do not make sense, are completely different from the emotions of others, or are shameful. Usually beliefs in durability lead to feelings of helplessness and hopelessness; beliefs in incomprehensibility lead to confusion and dismissing the partner; and beliefs about lack of consensus with others leads the partner to pathologize and label the other partner's expressions of emotion. What could be the advantages of such beliefs about the partner's emotions? In some cases, if the judging partner believes that the other's emotions are durable, out of control, and incomprehensible, this will allow the judger to withdraw and not engage, thereby (from his or her perspective) avoiding an argument. Or, conversely, these beliefs may lead the judger to suppress, eliminate, attempt to persuade, or distract the partner, so that the partner's emotions can be changed and the "problem" can be solved. The therapist can ask the dismissive partner to look at the evidence that these beliefs are useful—that they are achieving the goals of getting the partner to "stop feeling that way." In addition, the judging partner can examine the evidence for and against the belief that the partner's emotions are durable ("Do they ever change? What other emotions does your partner have?") and are out of control ("Is your partner in control of anything in life? Does your partner accomplish tasks? Is your partner insane? How do other people see your partner?"). Beliefs that the partner's emotions are different from everyone else's emotions can be examined in terms of the evidence ("Are there other people who feel sad, angry, anxious, confused? Do you partner ever have these feelings? Indeed, what emotions are you having in discussing this topic?"). The idea that one's partner should be rational rather than emotional can likewise be examined in terms of costs–benefits and the evidence. Is the judging partner always rational?

An individual may also believe that relationships should always function smoothly, without conflict, and with efficient and clear communication, and that the partner should not have enduring problems or "be a burden." The consequence of these perfectionistic beliefs about emotion is that emotional expression, disagreements, and "irrational" statements are judged and rejected, and the partner is verbally dismissed. In such cases, I have found it useful to "normalize the abnormal":

THERAPIST: You complain that your husband "has baggage" and is often very emotional, and then you try to get him to change his feelings. What about his emotions bother you?

PATIENT: Well, he says things that are irrational—sometimes just plain stupid. I don't know; he seems to have a lot of baggage.

THERAPIST: Don't we all? Sometimes I hear people say that they are looking for someone who doesn't have any baggage. I have found that we all have baggage, and what we should be looking for is someone who will help carry our baggage.

PATIENT: (*Laughs*) Yeah. I guess I have my issues, too, right?

THERAPIST: We all do. What do you think of this idea? There was a book years ago that was very popular, called *I'm OK, You're OK*.

I don't know; maybe I have seen too much of human nature to buy into that. I would suggest a different way of looking at it: "I'm not OK, you're not OK, but that's OK."

PATIENT: (*Laughs*) That sounds like our marriage.

THERAPIST: Yeah, but you're not OK with things not being OK. Sometimes we get a lot further in accepting that we are all a little crazy. In other words, we can "normalize the abnormal," so we can accept what truly is. Who wants "normal" when you can have alive and authentic and real—all filled with warts and bumps, and embraced by understanding and acceptance?

PATIENT: Now that would be something that might make a lot more sense.

THERAPIST: So accepting that no one ever completely lives up to our expectations—and that we don't always live up to them—makes room for accepting, forgiving, and putting things in perspective. Maybe the baggage you are carrying can be carry-on bags, rather than five suitcases filled with demands and resentments.

We can look at emotional schemas in relationships as reflecting a wide range of automatic thought categories and underlying assumptions or conditional rules. For example, the man described in Chapter 4 and above engaged in fortunetelling ("Her emotions will go on forever"), labeling ("She's a complainer"), personalizing ("She doesn't appreciate how hard I work"), catastrophizing ("Her complaining is intolerable"), overgeneralizing ("She just complains and complains"), discounting the positives ("Yeah, she does a lot, but I have to listen to the complaints"), all-or-nothing thinking ("All she does is complain—she is always complaining"), and "shoulds" ("She should not complain so much"). These automatic thoughts fueled his underlying assumptions about emotions and complaining: "If she complains about things, then she doesn't appreciate what we have and what I do," "I need to put a stop to it," "Wives who have husbands who support the family should never complain," "If she complains about me, I should defend myself," and "My wife should be rational and efficient all the time."

The particular emotional philosophy endorsed by this individual failed to include emotions as a way of connecting to important needs. In fact, he viewed emotional expression as interfering with problem solving, and placed instrumental, task-oriented functioning in a privileged position: "If we are not solving a problem, then it is a waste of time." Individuals may vary in their views of the purposes of communication, with some people (who are often, though not always, men) believing that the purpose should be to solve problems, while others (who are often, but not always, women) may emphasize sharing experiences and emotions (Tannen, 1986, 1990, 1993). This contrast of communication and functioning was first described by Talcott Parsons, who distinguished between two roles in the family (and in groups)—the "instrumental" and "expressive" roles—with the former focused on task accomplishment, and the latter on emotional expression and connection (Parsons, 1951, 1967; Parsons & Bales, 1955). Although this distinction may be biased toward particular cultures, individuals often engage in communication by adapting one of these two styles. In the present context, one person's emphasis on the instrumental (problem solving, tasks, facts, logic) with another individual who focuses on the expressive (connection, emotion, experience) will lead to misunderstanding and conflict. Of course, both functions are important, and the ability to shift from one to another as demands change is a key element of adaptation.

Moreover, informal communication often involves turn-taking, as well as an exchange of anecdotes or comments unrelated to problem solving or collecting facts that can be viewed as a form of "mutual grooming behavior" ("I will listen to you and you will listen to me, and we will feel connected"). An overemphasis on information, problem solving, and getting to the point leads an impatient listener to devalue emotional expression, sharing of anecdotes, reports of experience, and other "noninstrumental" discourse. The difference between two individuals in communicative purposes often involves a belief that communication is either about facts or about experiences and feelings. Research on the actual content of informal communication indicates that an overwhelming amount of the content has nothing to do with facts that have any utility (Dunbar, 1998).

Such informal communication, in fact, is an important aspect of couple attachment. The emotional schema model draws on models of attachment across the lifespan. These models emphasize the evolutionary adaptiveness of maintaining close relationships for purposes of mutual protection, reward, procreation, inclusion within the group, socialization, shared child rearing, and mutual nurturance (Bowlby, 1973, 1980). The attachment system activates oxytocin, which has a calming, comforting, and almost sedating antianxiety effect in the brain (Olff et al., 2013). Research on oxytocin levels in a variety of species ranging from voles to humans indicates that this hormone is associated with attachment behavior, pair bonding, lactation, touching, and other affiliative and parental behaviors (Love, 2014).

Also of importance to the emotional schema model of close relationships (and couple relationships in particular) is the role of touch. Research by Tiffany Field and her colleagues indicates that touch has pervasively positive effects on the development of preterm infants, and that in adults it reduces pain, increases attentiveness, diminishes depression, and enhances immune function. In an initial study on the effects of touch, Field observed that preterm infants isolated in incubators received little tactile stimulation from mothers or staff. Drawing on the observations of earlier researchers on the nature of attachment and touch, she and her colleagues introduced daily "touch therapy" for such infants, with a mother or nurse reaching through an aperture in the incubator to massage an infant. Those receiving the touch therapy gained 47% more weight and required 6 days less in the hospital (Field et al., 1985; Scafidi et al., 1990). A year later, these infants still showed higher weight gain and better abilities on tests of behavior and cognition. Touch therapy has also been found to reduce the experience of pain in people with arthritis or those undergoing surgery. Massage therapy reduced anxiety levels for HIV-positive males and had a positive effect on stress hormones and immune functioning (Ironson et al., 1996). Women with breast cancer also benefited from massage therapy, with levels of dopamine, natural killer cells, and lymphocytes all increasing over a 5-week course of treatment (Hernandez-Reif, Field, Ironson, et al., 2005). Positive results for massage therapy for children (32 months old) with cerebral palsy have also been found, including reduced spasticity and improved motor functioning (Hernandez-Reif, Field, Largie, et al., 2005).

Moreover, touch is an important component of communication. We can actually tell what emotions other people are trying to communicate simply by the way that they touch us. We can tell whether it is anger, fear, disgust, love, gratitude, or sympathy that these other persons are trying to convey—with their touch. And when we observe someone touching someone else, we can tell what emotion this touch communicates (Hertenstein, Keltner, App, Bulleit, & Jaskolka, 2006, p. 531): "Sympathy was associated with stroking and patting, anger was associated with hitting and squeezing, disgust was associated with a pushing motion, gratitude was associated with shaking of the hand, fear was associated with trembling, and love was associated with stroking."

Accordingly, the emotional schema therapist will evaluate the extent of touching, kissing, stroking, and hugging between partners in intimate relationships, as well as each individual's response to receiving affection or touch and willingness to initiate this behavior (Dunbar, 2012). In the evaluation of social communication and relationships, the therapist will inquire about the experience of touch: Was the patient touched and held during childhood? How does he or she respond to being touched and to touching others? Since touch has such powerful emotional implications for many people, it is an essential component of experience to be discussed. This directly relates the emotional schema model to models of child and adult attachment systems.

## MODIFYING INTERPERSONAL EMOTIONAL SCHEMAS AND MALADAPTIVE COPING

The underlying emotional schemas and assumptions about emotion and emotion control described to this point will continue to support an individual like the "logical" married man in maladaptive coping—which, ironically, can become a self-fulfilling prophecy confirming these negative beliefs about emotions in close relationships. Thus an individual who has a negative belief about the partner's emotions will be more likely to engage in contempt, sarcasm, dismissive behavior, ignoring, stonewalling, attempts to suppress the partner's emotions, overrational disputation of the partner's emotions, and unwanted problem solving. These strategies then become "the problem" in the relationship and lead the other partner either to escalate expression of emotion, to prolong the expression, to reject help, to counterattack, or to withdraw.

## Responding to the Partner's Emotions

Each relationship has its own points of difficulty, misunderstandings, possible differences in emotional styles, problematic strategies and behaviors, and conflicting belief systems about emotion. One partner may view talking about emotion as essential while the other may view it as a waste of time. One partner may place considerable emphasis on rationality, facts and logic, while the other partner places emphasis on closeness, sharing emotions, and affection. Understanding these differences and focusing on reaching some common ground for communication and relating is a key factor in the emotional schema approach to intimate relationships.

### The Values-Based Relationship

One of the first considerations in developing a plan of treatment is to determine the values and goals that the partners are committed to. In many cases, individuals respond to situations that trigger negative automatic thoughts, maladaptive assumptions, and their own personal schemas (of inadequacy, unlovability, special status, or abandonment). The therapist can pose a series of questions to each partner that can help both of them clarify how they want their relationship to function: "How do you want your partner to feel and think about this relationship? Is it important that your partner feel respected and cared for, that he [or she] is a priority, that your partner's contributions are appreciated, and that he [or she] can feel secure and can trust you?" Of course, other values can be suggested by either the therapist or the partners, but identifying values and goals in terms of emotions, respect, appreciation, gratitude, and other positive qualities can direct the couple toward enhancing their relationship rather than defending their past behavior or taking positions.

### Mindful Awareness

Taking an observing, detached, aware, nonjudgmental, and noncontrolling relation to the partner's feelings, thoughts, and behaviors allows each individual to step away from the immediate "trigger" or situation and notice what is happening currently. Each person is thus given an opportunity to consider listening, accepting, and using the information about the partner's experience while considering a range of adaptive alternatives. For example, rather than "automatically" responding to the partner, practicing noticing and stepping away while being completely present allows the individual not to be "hijacked" by the partner's expression or behavior, while considering responses that are congruent with valued goals.

## Identifying Triggers for the Self's Emotions

Emotion regulation skills depend on knowing which situational triggers evoke one's emotions and on identifying the emotions that are experienced as "problematic" for the self. For instance, if a woman believes that her anger is the most problematic emotion for her, then identifying situations that elicit this anger can help her develop a strategy in anticipation of difficulties that might arise. For example, is anger elicited when the partner is dismissive of her career, overly preoccupied with his own needs, unwilling to share child care, or controlling of her behavior? Knowing in advance what will trigger their problematic emotions may help partners develop strategies for understanding how misinterpretations arise and how problematic responses to emotions only perpetuate the problem.

## Identifying Triggers for the Other's Emotions

Similar to identifying the situations that trigger "problematic" emotions in the self, the individual can identify what triggers such emotions in the other. For example, if jealousy is a problem in a marriage, the partner who is the target of the jealousy (e.g., the wife) can identify that when she goes on business trips, this elicits jealousy in the husband. The couple can anticipate that these emotions will be elicited, and that the husband will have a variety of automatic thoughts (e.g., fortunetelling, catastrophizing, mind reading, personalizing) and problematic behaviors (interrogating, reassurance seeking, withdrawing). The wife can then identify her typical responses to the husband's jealousy—for example, defending, labeling ("You're neurotic"), counterattacking, and apologizing—and evaluate whether these strategies are working. In the likely event that they are not working, the couple can develop strategies that might work (for this example, see Chapter 10 on jealousy) and carry out their plan.

## Understanding Different Emotional Styles

As discussed earlier, individuals have different emotional styles: Some prefer discussion of feelings, affection, and closeness, while others may prefer more "matter-of-fact" discussions, limited affection, and more independence. It is not uncommon for one partner to personalize the other partner's emotional style when it differs from his or her own, in the belief that deviations from the preferred style are signs of trouble, marginalization, rejection, or manipulation. For example, if one partner takes more time or has more difficulty in describing feelings, it may be helpful for the listener to be more patient. The listener who says, "Get to the point," may only create greater anxiety in the speaker. For example, a couples can determine whether one partner prefers expanding on expression, while another partner prefers being more concise and pragmatic in discussing emotion. Rather than personalizing and judging each other's styles, the partners can negotiate acceptance and some modification, as described in more detail later in this chapter.

## Giving Time and Space

Emotions take time to access in the self, time to express, and time to validate. As just suggested, speakers and listeners often have different assumptions about the amount of time that is needed, with one partner attempting to rush the other while discussing emotion. Some listeners believe that the speakers should "get to the point" as quickly as possible and fear "wasting time," reflecting a belief in extreme efficiency in communication of the "essentials." Others view emotions as experiences that one should "get over," insisting that the speakers "snap out of it" and "move on." An alternative view would be to allow emotions sufficient time and "space" in the relationship, so that one partner can, for example, experience his or her jealousy until the jealousy diminishes on its own. This is a recognition that emotions are largely ephemeral and situational and do not have to be controlled or constrained in their duration.

In addition, partners can view the larger context of their lives as capable of containing the emotions. For example, a woman who is communicating about the loss of her father may seem to perseverate about her feelings, and the partner may urge her to "move on," which only adds to her sense of being dismissed and criticized. Rather than suggesting that she move on, the therapist can observe:

> "Right now at this time, this is where you are, and your life is filled with so many other meanings and connections that maybe you can find enough space and meaning in your life to contain this sadness. When you reflect on the loss of your father, it will always make sense to have that sadness, but also to have a life large enough to contain it and hold it."

The idea of a life large enough in meaning to contain sadness can be compared to a vessel that contains water: "Imagine your life as an ocean that is now open to new water coming from a new river, and that river is this sadness, and the ocean takes it in. Rather than resisting it, you might think of letting it in, to mix with everything else there is in your life." Recognizing the ability to expand in experience, and opening to what is the experience at the moment, will allow the partners to let go of struggling to let in what the feelings are.

## Focused Compassion

Gilbert (2009) has proposed that one can activate a "compassionate mind" toward others (and toward the self). This state of mind is characterized by nonjudgmental, accepting, loving kindness, with the intention to wish another well or soothe the pain that the other is feeling. Compassion activates the oxytocin system and is reflective of other calming effects of the attachment system. When one is being criticized, of course, it is difficult to activate this loving kindness toward the person who is criticizing. The therapist can illustrate the compassionate-mind approach by asking the individual to recall a memory of someone who was loving and soothing in his or her life—focusing on the details of the face, hair, body, voice, and eyes of the compassionate image—and then to imagine this compassion being felt by the self. While keeping in mind the experience of receiving compassion (the soothing and calming feelings), the individual who is angry at the partner can imagine directing a compassionate wish toward the partner, and thus can act against the anger by activating an opposing system of functioning. This can be extended further to writing a kind and compassionate note to the partner, in which the individual wishes the partner to feel better and to achieve peace of mind. Although some individuals may be reluctant to engage in compassionate thought and feeling, for fear that they will therefore be giving up, being "phony," or making themselves more vulnerable, the activation of compassion can shift them away from intolerance and judgment.

An example of a parent–child rather than a couple relationship demonstrates the power of a compassionate mind. A man in his 40s reported considerable anger toward his mother for her history of manipulation and what he perceived as her self-centered thinking. The therapist inquired about the mother's early years and learned of her troubled history growing up—how she was denied the opportunity to advance in education and how she had to defer to her brothers. The patient also indicated to the therapist that his mother's mother had committed suicide when his mother was 12, and that she had to focus thereafter on taking care of the family, further limiting her own opportunities for education. As he spoke about his mother, he realized that even though he had his difficulties, she also had a sad tale to tell, and he began feeling sorry for her. In the session, the therapist played the role of the mother and the patient described his newly compassionate thoughts and feelings about her, based on his recognition of her struggles; he finally forgave her. Although they continued to have intermittent difficulties, he reported that seeing his parents over the holidays went much better than it had before. Using a compassionate-mind focus allowed him to take things less personally and activated his feelings of care, rather than judgment, toward his mother.

## Flexible Response Set

Many people become hijacked by the emotions of their partners, replaying old patterns of response that have continually proven to be failures. The therapist can suggest that one can have a wide range of responses to the emotions of others, and not be limited to the one response that gets repeated. The discussion can begin as follows: "When your partner is sad and complains about his sadness, what do you tend to do?" The initial response may be rather innocuous ("I try to listen"), but then this is followed, on further inquiry, with a problematic response ("I tell him he's repeating himself"). Just as patients are often surprised that they have a choice in how they respond to their own intrusive thoughts, they can also have a choice among many alternatives in how they respond to their partners' feelings. In this example, the therapist can say:

> "From what you told me, it seems that you have a habit of responding with telling your partner to stop complaining about his sadness. But I wonder if there might be a lot of other possibilities in how you can respond. What would it be like if you were more flexible in how you responded to his emotions? For example, what if you had a number of different techniques that you could use to respond, such as not taking it personally, putting it in perspective, validating, looking for direction together on solving problems, accepting the feelings for now, refocusing to other positive qualities, or being compassionate? I'm not saying any one of these is necessary, but would it help to have a range of responses so that you could choose?"

Simply knowing that they can choose how to respond is often a new experience for many people, since they sometimes believe that their partners' behavior automatically elicits their negative responses. Being flexible opens up the possibility of being more effective.

## Modifying Specific Dimensions of Emotional Schemas

Emotional schema therapy for a couple can address each of the problematic emotional schema dimensions mentioned earlier in this chapter, via psychoeducation, cognitive evaluation, role plays, and behavioral experiments. In particular, the therapist can use standard cognitive therapy questions for each of these dimensions by asking each partner about the costs and benefits of a particular belief, or the evidence for and against this belief. The examples from the case of the married man described in Chapter 4 and at the start of this chapter are used.

**Duration:** "Her emotions will go on and on."

THERAPIST: I understand that you believe that your wife's emotion will go on and on. How does that make you feel when you think that?

PATIENT: I guess I have a lot of feelings—primarily frustrated, I guess. But I also feel sad and then I feel angry. She just doesn't have to feel this way.

THERAPIST: It sounds like you care a lot about how she feels and it really has an impact on you.

PATIENT: Yeah, I care about her, but it's hard to listen to this stuff every day.

THERAPIST: So it's frustrating to you that you listen to this, and you believe that her emotions go on and on. When she starts complaining, what do you say to her?

PATIENT: I tell her that she's complaining again, but she just goes on again, and then she complains that I don't listen to her.

THERAPIST: So I guess telling her that she complains doesn't work. Let's take your thought that her emotions go on and on and there is no end to them. Let's look at the advantages and disadvantages of that belief. What do you see as the disadvantage of your believing that her emotions go on and on?

PATIENT: It makes me frustrated and angry, and I feel like no matter what I do, nothing will change.

THERAPIST: So it adds to some feelings of helplessness and hopelessness. Is there any advantage in believing that her feelings go on and on?

PATIENT: Probably not. I don't know. Maybe I can get her to change.

THERAPIST: OK. Now let's take the thought that her emotions go on forever. Is there any evidence that her emotions come and go and that she has a wide range of emotions?

PATIENT: I guess you have a point. She has a lot of feelings, and a lot of the time she's really upbeat and fun to be around.

**Control:** "She just starts getting upset and can't control the way she feels. She should control herself more."

THERAPIST: It sounds like you believe that your wife's feelings are out of control. What do you think will happen if her feelings go more out of control?

PATIENT: I guess I fear that she will get more and more emotional, and it will just get out of hand.

THERAPIST: What does that look like, in your mind, if her feelings got out of hand?

PATIENT: I don't know. I haven't thought it through.

THERAPIST: OK, so when you think she is out of control, what do you do next?

PATIENT: I try to get her to change the way she deals with things. I try to talk some sense. I want to solve problems, and she wants to complain.

THERAPIST: So when you try to solve problems and get her to change, what happens next?

PATIENT: She gets more upset and tells me I'm not listening.

THERAPIST: What if you didn't try to control her and change her, but just set aside some time to listen and validate her?

PATIENT: That's what she wants, but won't that just feed into more complaining?

THERAPIST: I don't know. Have you tried that?

PATIENT: No.

THERAPIST: So trying to control her when you think she is losing control hasn't worked, but you think that letting her be and have her feelings and express them is something that you haven't tried— probably because you think it will make things worse.

PATIENT: Yeah, I haven't tried just listening.

**Lack of Comprehensibility:** "She doesn't make sense. She should be happy."

THERAPIST: You seem to think that your wife's feelings don't make sense. Why is that? How do they not make sense?

PATIENT: Well, she gets upset about trivial things, like the amount of housework that she has to do. And I just don't understand why she needs to complain about it. "Just get it done," that's what I think.

THERAPIST: Well, it sounds like you don't understand why the housework is so frustrating for her, and you don't understand why she needs to complain. If I were to ask her why she needs to tell you about this, what would she say?

PATIENT: (*Hesitating*) I guess she wants me to understand why she feels the way she feels.

THERAPIST: So her purpose is to be understood. But it sounds like you think that when you and your wife are talking, simply being understood is not a good enough reason.

PATIENT: I know it sounds crazy. I know.

THERAPIST: There are a lot of reasons that couples talk about things. What if you accepted that it was OK just to be understood, to share experiences, and to just be known by each other?

PATIENT: Maybe if I thought that way, I'd be less angry.

THERAPIST: Are there times that you just want to be understood?

PATIENT: Yeah. A lot of the time.

THERAPIST: Do you feel understood when we are talking?

PATIENT: I do.

THERAPIST: And how does it make you feel—to be understood?

PATIENT: Good.

**Lack of Consensus:** "Her emotions are different from other people's emotions."

The belief that the partner's emotions are unique to him or her contributes to labeling, personalizing, blaming, dismissing, and invalidating the partner. These beliefs about "how other people feel" are often based on an idealized view of how intimate relationships should function, and they serve to marginalize the other person.

THERAPIST: It sounds like you believe that your wife's feelings are somewhat unusual, compared to those of other people in this situation. I wonder which of her emotions you see as specific to her and not in other people.

PATIENT: Well, this sense of dissatisfaction that she feels about things. I mean, she seems to get frustrated about trivial things.

THERAPIST: Yes, I can see that she is frustrated and dissatisfied at times. But I wonder if it might be part of human nature to feel those feelings. I mean, it seems like you might be feeling those feelings when you talk about her.

PATIENT: I guess you're right. Yeah, I'm dissatisfied. But she gets frustrated about the smallest things.

THERAPIST: Have you noticed that little hassles—what we call "daily hassles," like noise, being stuck in traffic, waiting for an elevator, and other things—sort of annoy a lot of us?

PATIENT: That's true. I feel really frustrated even waiting for an elevator.

THERAPIST: What if you viewed your wife's frustration as part of the bigger picture about all of us—that all of us are a bit frustrated, irrational, and sometimes neurotic?

PATIENT: I guess I'd be less frustrated.

**Rationality:** "She should be rational, logical, and factual."

The belief that a partner should be rational all the time is not consistent with the role of emotions, or even with an important role of communication. As noted earlier, communication often involves "mutual grooming," sharing anecdotes, and talking about experience and feelings.

THERAPIST: You told me that you get upset when your wife says something that is irrational or illogical. Why does that bother you?

PATIENT: I thought that this was cognitive therapy and you are supposed to be rational. She'll say things that don't make sense to me.

THERAPIST: Yes, I know I also say things to my wife that don't make sense and are irrational. Don't we all do that?

PATIENT: OK, you're right, I do, too. But shouldn't she be rational?

THERAPIST: I don't know. A lot of communication is reporting experience and simply connecting. Maybe it's the nonrational—just being who you are at the moment. But what does it mean to you if she says something that is irrational?

PATIENT: I guess my first thought is that there is no sense in talking.

THERAPIST: Maybe when someone is emotional and talking about things that are irrational the best thing to do is to listen. And show you care.

**Blame:** "She's the problem—she shouldn't be so difficult."

The belief that "the problem is my partner" is a significant predictor of couple discord and only adds to selective focus on the negative, feelings of helplessness, and a dismissive attitude.

THERAPIST: I can see that you blame her at times, calling her "irrational" and "too emotional," and that this upsets you. Is there any advantage that you can think of in blaming her?

PATIENT: Not really. But she is a problem.

THERAPIST: I imagine that all of us can seem like a problem to other people at times. But it depends on what your demands are and what your goals are. So if you demand rationality and compliance, then she will be the problem. But what if you thought of her as a human being with a wide range of thoughts, feelings, and behaviors, and that you could simply accept that sometimes she won't live up to your expectations on everything?

PATIENT: I would be less angry. But she does say things that really annoy me.

THERAPIST: Yes, that happens at times. Maybe we need to find out what leads her to say those things so she might consider saying something else. But will blaming her make it better?

PATIENT: No.

## Lack of Acceptance: "I can't stand her moodiness."

Some people believe that accepting their partner's emotions will indulge the patient, lead to more emotional problems, or be viewed as a sign that "I am saying it is OK." Acceptance, though, can simply be the first step in acknowledging that the other person has the feelings he or she has, without judging or attempting to change them: "If I accept that you are sad, I am recognizing and hearing the sadness. I am recording it in my mind without attempting to change you." Acceptance can be an experience about the other's emotion that is momentary or ongoing.

THERAPIST: I wonder what it might mean to you to accept that your wife will say things that are irrational or emotional, and that this is simply how she is feeling at the moment.

PATIENT: I have a hard time with that. I guess I want to get her to feel better.

THERAPIST: That's supportive to think that way, and it comes from your love for your wife. You probably wouldn't think that about a stranger, so your difficulty in accepting her feeling at the moment is that you care about her. But another way of caring about her is to meet her where she is, accepting for the moment that she is having the feeling she is having, and see what both of you can learn and share.

PATIENT: I guess my fear is that if I accept her feeling, it won't change.

THERAPIST: Maybe the first step in change between two people who care about each other is accepting both persons where they are at this moment in time and then see what the other person needs and wants. So accepting that she is feeling frustrated might then lead the two of you to talk about what she needs from you at the moment. Maybe what she needs from you at the moment is that you simply accept her, listen to her, and show an interest.

PATIENT: I think she would agree with you.

THERAPIST: You know they say you should always give the customer what they want.

PATIENT: (*Laughs.*)

**Lack of Validation:** "I don't want to hear these complaints. They don't make sense to me."

In our RESS research, the perception that one's partner validates—cares about, wants to hear—one's feelings was a significant predictor of relationship satisfaction. However, other dimensions of emotional schemas interfere with validation. For example, the belief that the partner's emotions do not make sense, that they are different from those of others, or that they are out of control and will last a long time may contribute to the reluctance to validate. Later in this chapter, I discuss specific reasons that keep individuals from validating their partners. Let's examine how the therapist addressed the patient's reluctance to validate in the case of the "rational" married man.

THERAPIST: I wonder if your wife is looking for a sympathetic ear from you—just a chance to share her feelings, feel like you respect her and care about the way she feels, and just be there as a good listener at times.

PATIENT: Yeah, but won't that just feed into her complaining?

THERAPIST: I can understand your logic—it's that "If I listen to her and show I care this will reinforce her complaining." But isn't she complaining that you don't seem to care about her feelings and don't listen?

PATIENT: That's true. But that's why it's so confusing to me, because I don't want to just feed into her negativity.

THERAPIST: One of the interesting things about complaining to someone is that it is a form of *wanting to be heard.* So if someone is complaining and they believe that you are not validating them, then they will complain until you hear them. For example, sometimes kids will throw a temper tantrum because they think you don't hear them.

PATIENT: You know, that's interesting. I guess I shout at her because I think she doesn't hear me.

THERAPIST: Think of it this way. What if she validated you and said, "I know that I complain a lot and it's hard to listen, but I really appreciate the efforts that you are making to be a good listener"?

PATIENT: I'd feel a lot better.

THERAPIST: So maybe each of you needs to be validated by the other.

**Expression:** "She wants to talk and talk; I want to get problems solved."

Simply expressing emotion is not necessarily productive, since intense and accusatory expressions of emotion can lead to greater conflict. Later in this chapter, I provide some guidelines for more effective expression of emotion in intimate relationships, but continually trying to suppress the expression of emotion in a partner contributes to the partner's perception that the suppressor does not care about his or her emotion and is simply marginalizing the partner.

THERAPIST: When your wife starts to talk about her emotions, you seem to get frustrated and annoyed. What is the first thought that you have when she starts talking about her feelings?

PATIENT: That she will go on forever.

THERAPIST: That would be hard if that happened. And what do you say to her when she does start talking?

PATIENT: I get pissed off. I say, "This again? Why don't you stop complaining? You have it better than most people do."

THERAPIST: And then what happens?

PATIENT: She gets angry with me, and sometimes she just keeps going on, and I get more pissed off.

THERAPIST: What if you set aside some time and space for her to share her feelings—kind of like "listening time"—and said, "It sounds like you have some things on your mind. Maybe you can tell me about how you feel, and I can try to understand what is going on for you."

PATIENT: I guess she'd like that. But I wonder if she would go on and on.

THERAPIST: Yeah, that would be a problem, I can see. What if the two of you worked out some guidelines for talking and listening? Let's say that the guidelines went something like this: She can talk uninterrupted for 10 minutes, and you can just listen and, if necessary, just rephrase what she says so that she feels like you have heard her. Ten minutes to start?

PATIENT: Yeah, but she blames me.

THERAPIST: OK, that must be hard to hear for you, and that can also be a guideline for talking. She can talk about what she wants you to do—for example, help out with your daughter—but she can't label you as selfish.

PATIENT: I guess we can try.

## Winner–Loser Scripts and Emotional Schemas

Couples often engage in pointless arguments that focus on who will win and who will lose. Partners treat communication as a form of prosecution and defense, trying to establish who is right and who is wrong, often taking roles of who is the more innocent victim or the bigger martyr. These interactions are often based on a negative view of each other's emotions ("You don't have any right to be disappointed [frustrated, angry, sad, etc.]"); a rejection of validation ("If I validate her, I will admit that she is right," or "If I validate him, he will go on forever with his complaints"); the view that the other person's emotions are a waste of time ("Who needs to hear this? If she [or he] weren't so angry, we wouldn't have any problems"); a view of the relationship is a power struggle, which "necessarily" implies that one person is weak and the other is powerful; the reliance on rationality or facts to the exclusion of understanding and caring; and a view of an interaction's goal as "get to the truth." Whatever the underlying view(s) may be, the nature of communication and interaction becomes adversarial, based on truth-seeking, power, control, and winning arguments.

For example, a husband and wife discussed how he had told her he would meet her at 3:00 P.M. at the entrance to the park, but he showed up at 3:30 P.M. They debated for 10 minutes in session about what she had "really said": "You told me 3:30. I got there on time." Many of their other interactions were also about who was right or wrong, with each dredging up evidence of past mistakes, the "facts," or the illogical nature of the other person's position. Structuring their relationship as an adversarial contest about facts was associated with a wide range of negative emotional schemas, such as a rejection of the other person's right to express an opinion, the rejection of validation, refusal to see that others might have the same feelings, recognition of the wide range of other positive emotions, blaming the other, and overemphasis on rationality to the exclusion of emotions. Their typical maladaptive assumptions about the primacy of rationality and the adversarial contest included the following:

"It's absolutely essential to establish the facts."
"Emotions distract us from facts, logic, and getting things done."
"If I agree with my partner's interpretation, then it means I'm wrong."
"If I'm wrong, then I will be criticized and blamed for everything."
"It's important to win these arguments to prove that I'm right."

Refocusing on the importance of emotion, closeness, mutual respect, compassion, and nonjudgmental understanding will be difficult if partners such as this husband and wife are locked in a winner–loser script. The emotional schema therapist can address these impasses with a series of questions and techniques.

## Costs and Benefits of Winner–Lose Scripts

After identifying the pattern of adversarial dialogue, the therapist can help the partners identify what they see as the costs and benefits of viewing the relationship in terms of winning and losing. For example, the married man described in Chapter 4 and above indicated that the advantages of viewing the relationship in terms of "establishing the facts" and "logic" (which he believed represented his positions) were that things would get done; they could rely on reality rather than feelings; there would be less chaos in the family; and there was a moral obligation to focus on the truth and logic rather than his wife's emotions. He also described that the costs of focusing on winning and losing as follows: There were frequent arguments; both partners were resentful; they focused on past wrongs that they never seemed to escape; they had less emotional and sexual intimacy; both of them felt angry, sad, and discouraged; and they both felt as if they were walking on eggshells. Weighing out the costs and benefits suggested to him that his emphasis on facts was leading to more conflict—that it was not solving the problem.

## Establishing What "Winning" Would Look Like

As in any conflict, it is first important to establish what "winning" will look like, so that the partners can evaluate whether the goals have been achieved. In military conflict, the absence of defining winning is "mission creep," or a never-ending extension of hostilities to new targets and goals. Not knowing what the goal is may lead to endless escalation of conflict, as each party in the dyad attempts to "one-up" the other in a continual cycle of provocation and retaliation. In the case of the husband and wife who disagreed about their meeting time at the park, the therapist broached this question with the husband as follows:

> THERAPIST: Well, you seem to think that there is a way of winning these arguments. I wonder if you've ever thought about what "winning an argument" would look like. What do you see your wife saying or doing?
>
> PATIENT: (*Laughs*) It's hard to imagine. I guess she would just agree with me. But that's not going to happen.

THERAPIST: OK, so let's imagine if she agreed with you that she had the time wrong—that she had really said 3:30, not 3:00—then what would happen next?

PATIENT: I guess we would stop arguing.

THERAPIST: And then what would happen?

PATIENT: She would probably resent me and withdraw.

The therapist and patient can examine whether the attempt to dominate, control, or suppress the partner is a practical strategy to build the kind of relationship either party wants. As with many attempts to "control emotion," the solution (winning) may become the problem that simply perpetuates ongoing conflict and resentment. There may not be a winner or loser—or, more accurately, both partners may be losers if they play this game. Winning and losing can be replaced with understanding, caring, accepting, getting closer, and reaching a middle ground.

### Establishing the Meaning of Disagreement

Some individuals treat any disagreement as a negative occurrence that needs to be rectified—in other words, as a problem that needs an immediate solution. Disagreements are often interpreted as lack of respect, as manipulation, as attempts to gain power, as signs that the other partner is not reliable because he or she is not relying on "the truth," or as the beginnings of the unraveling of a relationship into tantrums and dramatic displays.

THERAPIST: I can see that it really bothers you when your wife disagrees with you. What does it mean to you when she doesn't see things your way?

PATIENT: It means she is patronizing me and treating me like I am a child.

THERAPIST: OK, that sounds like that must be unpleasant for you. Let's imagine that this might be true—that she is patronizing. What will happen if she does patronize you?

PATIENT: I couldn't respect myself if that happened. I need to be respected.

THERAPIST: So if she thinks that her facts are the right ones, it means that she doesn't respect you, and that you can't respect yourself. But why would you lose respect for yourself if your wife momentarily did not respect your facts or opinion?

PATIENT: I never thought about it. I guess I need her approval.

THERAPIST: So if you were less concerned about her approval, then you might be less angry and just let her have her opinion, even if you thought it wasn't right?

PATIENT: I guess that's true. I could just let it go.

### Evidence for and against "Happiness = Rationality"

An adversarial script is often based on the belief that establishing "the truth"—basing things on rationality and logic—will lead to a better relationship. But an overemphasis on rationality and logic can be dismissive and even contemptuous of the other person's emotional needs.

THERAPIST: It sounds like you think that if you can establish the truth and make sure that discussions are really rational and logical and based on facts, things will be better. I wonder if there is any evidence for that.

PATIENT: Well, if we aren't arguing, then we aren't upset with each other.

THERAPIST: OK, so if your wife agreed with you and you both had the facts on your side, then there wouldn't be arguments. But is it reasonable to expect that two people will always see things the same way? Don't you have disagreements with friends and colleagues?

PATIENT: Of course, but it doesn't seem to bother me as much.

THERAPIST: Maybe you take it less personally if it's just a friend or a colleague. But do you think that satisfying relationships are based on logic, or on closeness and warmth and caring?

PATIENT: I know, I know. But the facts are important.

THERAPIST: Can you imagine someone saying, "My wife and I have a great relationship, we have wonderful sex, because we both agree on the facts"?

PATIENT: (*Laughs*) No, no. I know that sounds crazy.

THERAPIST: So when you have both felt really close and warm toward each other what is going on?

PATIENT: I guess we both appreciate the other person and feel warm toward each other and trust each other.

THERAPIST: Is that based on rationality and facts, or on care and compassion?

PATIENT: Care and compassion.

## Listening to and Respecting a Problem versus Solving a Problem

A winner–loser script is often overly focused on solving problems, getting things done, and getting to the "bottom line." The "logical" married man often said to his wife, "Give me the net–net"; in other words, he wanted to get to the "bottom line" to find out what the problem was, so that he could suggest a solution. This made her feel that he had no time to listen—no time to respect her feelings and the pace of her sorting through her thoughts.

THERAPIST: I noticed that you said, "Get to the net–net." It sounds like you want to hurry to the bottom line in a business discussion. When you say that to your wife, how does she feel?

PATIENT: I guess she feels like I don't want to hear about her feelings. Maybe she thinks I'm controlling. She's told me that I am too controlling.

THERAPIST: I see. So I wonder what her feelings are. Do you think she feels hurt, sad, angry, frustrated?

PATIENT: Yeah. All those things. I know. But I just want to get to the bottom line and figure out what needs to be done. She just wants to dwell on these negative things, which only makes her feel worse.

THERAPIST: So you really want her to feel better, and you think that getting to the bottom line will work. Is it working?

PATIENT: No, it just makes her feel worse.

THERAPIST: What if you were to look at this as a series of steps? The first step might be setting aside some time to listen and maybe validate her feelings. Just *be* a great listener for a while. And then, after you have listened and validated her and told her you can understand that she is upset, you can ask her if there is anything that you can do to help solve the problem. Maybe she wants problem solving; maybe she just wants you to listen. You might need to find out by letting her express herself and ask her what she needs from you at this moment in time.

PATIENT: It's frustrating just to listen.

THERAPIST: Yes, it might be hard for you. But you have done difficult things before—especially in your work. And look at it this way: It might be harder to solve problems when all she wants you to do is listen to the problem.

PATIENT: You have a point. Yeah. She sometimes just wants to get things out there and talk about the way she feels.

THERAPIST: What if you were to reframe this in terms of problem solving? Maybe, from her point of view at that moment in time, the problem that she wants solved is your listening. So if you listen, you have solved her problem.

## Accepting Two (or More) Truths

People locked in a winner–loser script, focusing on "the truth," believe that there is *one* truth that needs to be discovered (and, in fact, imposed). But interpersonal systems consist of many perspectives, different needs, different past histories, and different personalities. One partner may be especially sensitive to requests being made of her, because of a past history of a controlling mother; she may interpret her partner's requests as domination and coercion. Another partner may view affection as an intrusion on his "space" and may rebuff his partner when she attempts to get physically closer. In discussions about what has transpired at a party, one individual may focus on the nonverbal expressions of another guest and find this person to be "phony," while the other partner may focus on whether the guest agrees with him or her and will find the guest a pleasure to be around. The emotional schema approach shares with DBT a recognition that there are two (or more) truths, and that understanding how both partners see something and what is important to them may be more important than establishing a definitive truth.

> THERAPIST: It seems that you think at times that there is one way to see things—that there is one truth, and that the two of you need to agree on that. But I wonder if what feels true to her may be different to what feels true to you.
>
> PATIENT: I don't understand. Truth is truth.
>
> THERAPIST: Yes, that is how we are taught in school. But another way of looking at it is that each person sees the world in a different way. We have our own histories, our own vulnerabilities, our own needs, and our own preferences—and we may only be focusing on one thing at the moment, and that seems true to us at that time.
>
> PATIENT: But if you look at things that way, aren't you just saying that there are no facts?
>
> THERAPIST: Facts are understood in terms of what we see as important to us at the moment. For example, if you look around the room right now, what do you notice at first?
>
> PATIENT: There's a blue painting on the wall and your computer screen.
>
> THERAPIST: Yes, that seems true, of course. But there are thousands of other things that you and I might notice—the books, the papers, the diplomas on the wall, the lamps, the windows, the light, and the shades of gray. So what if you accepted that your wife might

be focusing on one thing rather than another, and for the moment that thing seems important to her?

PATIENT: But how do we ever get to any agreement?

THERAPIST: Maybe you don't need to agree on a fact. Maybe you need to agree that you have different experiences, perspectives, and needs at the moment, and that you can accept that. For example, when you both see a movie, do you agree on everything?

Patient: No. There are times that we agree, but she might focus on something that I didn't notice.

THERAPIST: The same is true in everyday life. Many perspectives, many experiences, many truths. What feels true for you may not feel true for her.

## Understanding That Differences Are Not Devastation

Unrealistic models of close relationships often involve the idea that there will be perfect agreement, complete meeting of minds, and absolute soulmate congruence, rather than a realistic recognition that two adults have different histories, values, information, perspectives, and styles of thinking and speaking. Similar to the illusion of "total validation" discussed earlier, partners can become increasingly conflicted simply because they cannot accept that differences between them exist and will continue to exist, regardless of attempts to persuade or intimidate. For example, a man with more conservative beliefs was intolerant of his wife, who held more liberal beliefs; he often castigated her in contemptuous language for her "unrealistic" ideas.

THERAPIST: When your wife tells you about her political beliefs about a candidate, it seems to anger you. Why is that?

PATIENT: I can't stand it when she is so unrealistic. I mean, how many times do I have to go over this with her?

THERAPIST: OK, so it seems to frustrate you that you can't persuade her, but I am wondering why it is so problematic that these differences exist. Why does it bother you so much?

PATIENT: I know this sounds a little crazy, but it makes me think that we are two different people—completely different people.

THERAPIST: Well, you are two different people, but you view these political differences as a sign that you have nothing in common?

PATIENT: Yeah, I know, I know. That's all-or-nothing thinking.

THERAPIST: OK, if you had nothing in common, then what would that mean?

PATIENT: I guess it means to me that we don't belong together.

THERAPIST: So that would be really devastating, I guess—to not have a single thing in common, and to be completely different from one another and not belong together. I can see why this bothers you. But do you really believe that you have nothing in common?

PATIENT: No, no, we have a lot in common. Our values are very much the same on almost everything, and we love our two daughters, and we really like a lot of the same things.

THERAPIST: I wonder if these disagreements remind you a little of how your father always had to have his way and dismissed any disagreement, and how he made you feel that you were less than him. Is there a parallel here?

PATIENT: It feels like the same issue. And my wife, you know, is so completely different from him.

## Rephrasing, Validating, and Asking for More

An emphasis on winning or establishing dominance may lead to ridiculing, dismissing, or attacking what the other partner is saying, and thus may result in further escalation of conflict and more counterattacks on both sides. By contrast, practicing active listening, empathizing, validating, and asking for more from the partner communicates that one is interested in hearing the perspective and feelings of the other in a respectful manner; this communication typically helps the couple to move away from the roles of prosecutor and defendant. As indicated earlier, individuals focused on winning may be reluctant to take an active listening role: They may fear that their partners will overwhelm them, humiliate them, go on forever, never give them a chance to speak, and ultimately win. Changing the dynamic from winning to understanding can temporarily short-circuit these fears. When both partners in a relationship believe that they have a monopoly on the truth, allowing "competition" by listening to the other threatens the winning strategy. Shifting to an understanding strategy may subvert the adversarial pattern. In the case of the couple with political disagreements, the therapist introduced this approach as follows:

THERAPIST: So far, you have been thinking that the goal is to win these arguments by showing your partner that you are right—that the logic, facts, and your experience show that she is wrong, and that this means you are right. So the goal here is winning by defeating, which seems to escalate the conflicts. Let's try something different, if you are willing, and that is to redefine "winning" as "understanding your partner." I am going to give you a notebook here, and you are going to listen very carefully to what she says, and your goal—your assignment—is to be able to state her position and her feelings as accurately as possible. And the only way that you succeed is if she agrees that you understand her message. You don't have to agree with anything she says; you just have to understand it.

PATIENT: OK, I'll try. I just have to understand.

THERAPIST: Right.

[Wife describes her views on a political issue that they disagree on.]

PATIENT: So you think that he's going to be a good mayor because he is going to do more for the poor? But how about the taxes? Won't that make everything worse?

THERAPIST: OK, it sounds like you rephrased her on the mayor's goals for the poor, but then you began editorializing for yourself. Your assignment is to allow your opinions to disappear for a few minutes, put them up on the shelf, and only try to understand exactly what she thinks and feels. You are recording and reflecting her, not yourself.

PATIENT: Won't I get a chance to speak?

THERAPIST: Yes, later, and you are speaking now by telling her what you hear her saying. The first step is being the best listener that you can be.

## Practicing Agreeing

Because the adversarial pattern places such emphasis on proving that the other person is wrong, it can also lead to selective filtering of what is being heard, and to discounting any possible points of agreement between the two parties. Using the technique of practicing agreeing—and temporarily refraining from disagreeing—allows each individual to experience giving up the winning role and taking on an accepting, collaborative, understanding, and reflecting role. When partners take turns in practicing agreement, this helps them both to feel understood, to step away from adversarial dynamics, and to experience more acceptance of differences. In the following example, a couple with an 8-month-old baby argued often that the husband was often disengaged when he returned home and did not interact with the wife or child.

THERAPIST: So it sounds like the two of you have had some difficulties since the baby has come along, and I know that can be stressful for both of you. I wonder if each of you could simply practice saying what you see to be the case, and, for the time being, just focus and reflect on the few points that you might agree on.

HUSBAND: (*To wife*) I guess that you are saying that I come home and

I am not really interacting with you and Rachel, and this really bothers you. I guess there's some truth in that. I am so burned out by the end of the day that I can't give my full attention.

THERAPIST: Well, you started by pointing out your agreement with her, but then you defended yourself, and I am wondering if the arguments jut begin again when you defend yourself. Let's try to stay in the role of just agreeing for a moment.

HUSBAND: (*To wife*) You're right that I am still preoccupied with things at work, and I am not fully focused on you and Rachel. And, I agree, this is frustrating to you.

WIFE: Yeah, you are just in another world at times.

HUSBAND: You're right. Sometimes I am.

THERAPIST: Now, Susan [wife], I wonder if you can allow Marv to speak about his experience, and if you could find some points of agreement with him.

HUSBAND: (*To wife*) I am working all day, taking calls; I have a difficult boss; and you know I'm always worried about losing my job, and then how would I support you and Rachel? I know that you took a break from work to take care of Rachel, and I appreciate that, but I am so anxious about losing my job that it's hard for me to concentrate sometimes.

WIFE: (*To husband*) I agree that your job is demanding and that you are working long hours. And you have been worried about losing your job for so long, but you are really good at what you do . . .

THERAPIST: (*Interrupting*) That started off with some good rephrasing and agreeing, but then you began giving advice, which sounds like you are trying to change his mind. Right now we are just trying to see what it feels like to agree. The goal is to understand his mind, not to change his mind.

WIFE: (*To husband*) I guess you are saying that you are bringing that stress home from work, and that it makes it hard for you to shift gears when you are with me and Rachel.

HUSBAND: Yeah. It's not like I don't love both of you. I'm just anxious.

THERAPIST: How did this feel to both of you?

WIFE: Much better.

HUSBAND: I guess I am just worried a lot.

## Structuring Sharing Emotions

Although most couples will agree that it is important for partners to share their respect for each other's feelings is important, the logistics, style, and extent of this communication can become problematic. Effective communication entails structuring what is being said; how, when, and why it is being said; and what is expected in response. As our research indicates, blaming, invalidation, and acting in a dismissive, condescending, and adversarial style lead to greater relationship conflict and dysfunction, and perpetuate conflict or withdrawal. To guide couples in communicating more effectively, the therapist can go over the "ten secrets to getting heard" outlined in Figure 12.1. (These guidelines are intended for therapist use only and do not constitute a reproducible handout.)

## Resistance to Allowing the Partner to Share Feelings: Reasons Not to Listen

As with many cognitive-behavioral techniques, suggesting how thoughts, behaviors, and communication can change may sound much easier than it is in the real world of therapy with individuals who have been battling each other for months or years. I have reviewed one of the styles of structuring communication—the winner–loser dynamic—and discussed how it might be changed. But for each technique for improvement, there are a wide variety of reasons why individuals will resist using these techniques. Noncompliance or resistance is usually based on an underlying belief system that makes sense to these individuals and that is believed to protect them from further loss. It is often helpful to troubleshoot with patients all the reasons why they would choose not to use these techniques, in order to clarify their rationale for noncompliance.

### "It's a Power Struggle"

As emphasized above, many couples are locked in a power struggle about winning and losing. If one partner is venting feelings, then he or she is "winning" by taking the floor, dominating discussion, and making his or her feelings the most important topic. One man viewed the idea of active listening as "feminizing" him in the power struggle game, saying that he would not be a "wuss": "You want me to be a doormat?" (See also "Gendered Thinking," below.) As a result of his belief that he had to exercise power and control, he utilized marginalization, humiliation, and criticism ("You are never logical—just all emotion"). Examining the pros and cons of viewing an intimate relationship as a power struggle can sometimes lead to uncovering core beliefs or schemas. In the case of the man who was afraid of being a "wuss," he described his childhood experience with his dominating and humiliating father:

> "He would just tell us to shut up and that we didn't really know anything, and if you disagreed he'd slap us. I was so afraid. And I just kept

1. **Pick the right time.** Sometimes you think you need to be heard the minute you have a thought or feeling. But your partner may be wrapped up in something else at the moment—watching a game, fixing dinner, trying to go to sleep, working on something—or just may not be in the right mood right now. Use your experience to tell you what is definitely not the right time. For example, "big-process discussions" are seldom helpful right before bed, or the minute your partner walks in the door from work. If you start talking—and he or she isn't listening—then ask, "Is there a better time to talk?" And, if you are the listener, play fair; give your partner a reasonable alternative. Don't use sarcasm or stonewalling.

2. **Edit it down.** Many times you may start talking and just get carried away. Your partner is losing interest and drifting off. Nothing is getting through. OK, maybe you need to edit what you say. Try to limit your comments to relatively clear and short sentences. Pause, ask for feedback, and wait for your partner. Don't try to get on a soapbox and hold the floor. Make the discussion more give-and-take. Think about what is essential, and try to focus on that. One way of editing it down is to agree with your partner that there might be a reasonable period of time to spend on the topic—for example, "Can we spend about 10 minutes talking about this?" This helps you focus on the essentials and gives your listener a reasonable time frame.

3. **Pause and ask for feedback.** Sometimes as a speaker you will go on and on, without pausing. Perhaps you think that you need to stay on your topic so that everything is heard—or you fear that your partner will jump in and take the floor, and you won't ever get a chance to speak again. Again, slow it down, edit it down, and stop and ask for feedback. Make the communication two-way. If you feel your partner hasn't really heard what you are saying, then try asking, "Can you rephrase what I said?" Or, if you want your partner to help you think of things differently, you might say, "I wonder if I'm seeing things the right way here." Or, if you want problem solving, you might say, "I wonder what I can do to make it work."

4. **Don't catastrophize.** Sometimes you may think that the only way to get heard is to make everything sound awful. Sometimes that's a legitimate point of view, but if you make too many things sound awful, you will lose your credibility. Try to keep things in perspective, try to stay with the facts, and try to keep things from escalating. Keep your voice calm; don't get carried away. Slow it down, and quiet it down. You will be heard more clearly with a softer tone. In fact, if you stand back and think it through, some of the things that you are talking about may be unpleasant, inconvenient, or simply matters of opinion. But "awful" might be a bit extreme. Think it through, and decide whether it is really as awful as you think and feel it to be.

5. **Don't attack.** Your listener is not likely to be a good audience if your discussion is a series of attacks and criticisms. Labeling your partner ("idiot," "moron," "big baby") or overgeneralizing ("You always do that") is going to be a turnoff. This doesn't mean that you can't get your point across and assert yourself. It simply means that you need to communicate in a way that is not as hostile. Making suggestions for change ("It would be helpful if you cleaned up a bit more"), while giving credit for some positives ("I do appreciate your helping with the shopping"), can get you more attention and cooperation than outright attacks ("You are the most selfish person I have ever known").

*(continued)*

**FIGURE 12.1.** Ten secrets to getting heard. From Leahy (2010). Adapted with permission. (Do not reproduce.)

6. **Tell your partner whether you want to solve problems or share feelings.** Sometimes you may just want to vent your feelings and have a sympathetic ear from your partner. That's OK, but your partner needs to know where you are going with this. For example, it may be that you might want to divide it up: After a few minutes of venting and sharing, you either drop the topic or go on to problem solving. A lot of people just want to be heard and cared for.

7. **Listening is not agreeing.** Sometimes we have the belief that a listener should agree with everything we say and be just as upset as we are. We may think that this is the only way for the other person to show that he or she is really listening. However, it's wrong. Listening is hearing, understanding, reflecting, and processing information. I can listen to your thoughts and feelings without agreeing with your point of view. You and I are different people. It doesn't mean that I don't care for you if I don't agree with you. It means I am hearing you. But sometimes a speaker can attack a listener for not agreeing 100%. That seems unrealistic and unfair. We all need to accept the differences that make us unique. In fact, the differences can be opportunities for growth. When you talk to someone who understands you and cares about your feelings—but doesn't agree with your interpretation of events—it opens your mind to the fact that there is more than one way to think about things.

8. **Respect advice.** If you are turning to your partner for support and advice, you are likely to get feedback—and probably some advice. Now you might be unfortunate and get sarcasm and contempt. However, let's assume that your partner is trying to do what he or she can to be supportive—but it's not exactly what you want. Maybe the advice is not helpful; maybe it's irrational. But if you want to be heard, you have to be willing to respect the advice giver. You don't have to take the advice or like the advice. But if you are playing to an audience that you then attack, you won't have an audience the next time around. Think of advice or feedback as information: Take it or leave it, but don't hit the other person over the head with it.

9. **If you describe a problem, describe a solution.** As I said earlier, you might just want to vent, share feelings, and explore your thoughts. But I think it also makes sense—some of the time—to describe potential solutions if you describe potential problems. Some of us actually love to jump to problem solving, but it may be premature with other people. However, if you are a speaker, you might consider this as an option: Describe a solution if you describe a problem. Your solution doesn't have to be an *order* to do something. It can be tentative, reasonable, one of several possibilities. In fact, if you begin thinking of the problem as something to solve, you might begin feeling more empowered. But it's your call if you want to go there—now, later, or never.

10. **Validate the validator.** One of the most helpful things that you can do as a speaker is to support the person who is supporting you. You don't want to be a "downer," and you don't want to act entitled to every minute of the other person's time. Think about it from the listener's point of view: He or she is listening to you go on about something that is bothering you. Well, this may not be the most fun for the listener—but he or she is with you on this. Why not turn around and thank the listener for spending the time? Thank him or her for caring enough to listen and support you. Validate the validator.

**FIGURE 12.1.** *(continued)*

it in for a while until he pushed my mother. I was 16 and bigger than he was, and I grabbed him and slammed him against the wall."

The power struggle about emotion for this individual was a replay of the power struggle with his abusive father.

## Contempt for the Partner or the Partner's Views

Some people believe that the way to get their partners to stop "complaining" is to use contempt or sarcasm as a form of punishment. For example, one man would respond to his partner's perceived "complaints" with "It must be that time of the month," "Get me a beer," or other problematic and self-defeating comments. He indicated that he thought that by "joking," he would make her see how ridiculous she was being. The therapist asked him how he thought she felt and what she thought of him when he was contemptuous: "I guess she thinks I'm a jerk—because, to tell you the truth, I know I am. I just don't know what to say, though, when she gets emotional." He also indicated that he viewed her complaints as criticisms of him—and that, to some extent, he was correct—but he feared that if he acknowledged she was correct, then he would be humiliated and would have to criticize himself, and she would use this against him. The therapist suggested that an alternative to sarcasm or self-criticism might be apologizing and changing his behavior. He reluctantly agreed to experiment with apologizing to his wife and telling her that he was going to work on his contempt and sarcasm.

## Gendered Thinking

Some men, like the man described above who was afraid of being a "wuss," comment that to validate or to use emotional language to support a woman is unmanly. They believe that a man's role is to be strong, "above it," and domineering. In their view, validating and allowing emotional ventilation are for feminized men—men who have lost their dignity as "real men." The therapist can help such a patient examine the consequences of gendered thinking: Does it lead to more happiness? Does he feel like a "real man"? Is he becoming the kind of man that he would admire? Would he like these behaviors if he saw a man directing them at his mother or daughter? Replacing "gendered thinking" with "universal thinking" can help.

For example, a divorced man would describe women in objectified sexual terms—"good-old-boy" comments that sounded like fraternity banter with the male therapist. He would describe sarcastic and domineering behavior toward the woman he was currently involved with. The therapist asked him how his macho, sexualized thinking affected his ability to love and get emotionally close to a woman, and how it made his current partner feel. As he reflected on these issues, he described how he had been dev-astated in his previous marriage when he learned that his wife had been cheating on him—which he had discovered while they were in marital therapy. Humiliated, fearing that he was getting older and less attractive to women, and worrying that his current partner (who was younger than he was) might leave him, he tried to bolster his ego by playing the role of "the macho man with confidence." The therapist suggested that he try another role—that of "a real human being" or a "Mensch" (a compassionate, car-ing person), who treated his partner with love and respect, as an end in herself, a person with human dignity. The patient was encouraged to treat his partner the way he would want to be treated himself, or the way he would want a man to treat his 23-year-old daughter. This "mensch ther-apy" appealed to this patient because he did see himself as someone who valued human dignity and wanted to be loved for what was good about him, rather than the bravado-laced act that he was putting on. He replaced the goal of "being a macho man" with "being a mensch"—someone who was compassionate and caring, someone he would be proud of being.

## Emotion Dysregulation

Some people find it so upsetting or emotionally arousing to listen to their partners that they feel they have to ventilate their anger or withdraw. In fact, this is supported by research, which shows that such persons' pulse rates escalate during conflict, and they find this unbearable; this escalation of arousal is more common in men than in women (Gottman & Krokoff, 1989). As a result of their own escalating emotion—which they cannot tolerate—such persons either try to suppress their partners' communi-cation or leave the room. An emotionally overwhelmed individual feels trapped by emotional discussions and often fears that these will be never-ending, while the other partner feels controlled, marginalized, and aban-doned. In such a case, the therapist can identify the emotion dysregulation problem as the key issue to solve, and can suggest a number of techniques to help the overwhelmed individual manage his or her own emotion. These can include anticipating the situations that will elicit these feelings; iden-tifying the automatic thoughts (e.g., "They're going to go on and on for-ever"); practicing mindful detachment and observing rather than judging and controlling; practicing active listening and validating; experimenting with allowing time and space for feelings; taking the role of understand-ing and reflecting rather than winning and persuading; and trying mutual problem solving as a way of coping with disagreements. Because feeling overwhelmed is often another way for such individuals to say that they feel helpless and trapped, providing a wide range of techniques often helps these individuals feel empowered rather than overwhelmed. Other tech-niques for emotion regulation can include distraction, leaving the room for a few minutes ("time out"), rational restructuring, self-soothing, opposite action, improving the moment, acceptance, and pursuing other rewarding behaviors and goals.

## "I Don't Want to Reinforce Whining"

A common belief—even among some therapists—is that actively listening to and validating others when they are expressing their emotions will only reinforce continued complaining or "whining." This model of emotion views complaining as opening the floodgates to an inevitable deluge of overwhelming emotional expression from which there will be no escape. As a consequence, the individual attempts to stop it immediately by using sarcasm, trying to exert control, or stonewalling. The therapist can indicate that a baby will continue to cry until it is picked up and comforted, and that a partner will continue to complain until he or she is heard and validated. Of course, many people believe in the law of effect (i.e., the principle that behavior that is reinforced will increase in frequency), but emotional expression is like other attachment behaviors: It will continue to be expressed until the "system" is completed. This can be put to the test by engaging in role plays of escalated validation in session, with the patient taking the role of the "complainer" while the therapist actively takes the role of validating and asking for more. Typically, the "complainer" runs out of things to complain about and finally acknowledges that the listener "understands." This confirms the model that complaining will continue until it reaches an understanding: "Once I think you understand me, I stop complaining." Alternatively, the therapist can take the role of "invalidator," asking the patient to complain while the therapist argues against and rejects everything that the patient says. This reversed role play can illustrate that complaining will escalate in the face of invalidation, thereby demonstrating that the patient's strategy of invalidating because of "fear of whining" will prove to be a self-defeating strategy. The therapist can indicate that complaining is a journey in search of validation and understanding. Once it reaches its goal, it is finished.

## "Problems Have to Be Solved"

A common belief that interferes with the communication of emotion and its validation is an overinvestment in problem solving as the only strategy that makes sense. This belief is predicated on a model of communication as sharing facts in a concise manner, identifying a goal, and solving a problem. The individual believes that venting and sharing feelings are pointless, and that if the partner is not willing to initiate problem solving, then he or she is being self-indulgent and wasting everyone's time and energy. However, if the speaker's goal is to be understood and feel cared for, an overly rapid focus on problem solving may lead him or her to believe that the partner does not care about the speaker's feelings and is, at best, being patronizing. Ironically, the "problem solver" will claim, "I do care about my partner's feelings, and that is precisely why I want to begin problem solving." The therapist can suggest that both goals are valuable—being heard and solving problems—but that the speaker can have the privilege of deciding which goal is the one for the moment. If the speaker notices that the listener is jumping to solving problems too quickly, he or she can indicate, "I just want to share with you what my experience is, and I am not sure if I want to problem-solve right now." Both partners can acknowledge that problem solving *could* be an option now, later, or never, but that the speaker is the one to determine this. In some cases, the problem can be rephrased to "hearing what your partner is saying" so that the solution can be "understanding your partner."

## SUMMARY

Emotional schemas are core factors in relationship conflict. Partners either escalate and ruminate about their own emotions in order to be heard, or attempt to regulate each other's emotions by unwanted problem solving, sarcasm, stonewalling, withdrawal, or contempt. Underlying these dysfunctional patterns of communication and listening are problematic schemas about the duration, normality, control, and validity of the partner's emotions, with beliefs that listening, encouraging expression, or validating will only perpetuate further unraveling of these emotions. The emotional schema model helps highlight how these beliefs about emotion in close relationships can be addressed, and how specific behavioral and cognitive techniques can enhance relationship harmony.

# CHAPTER 13

# Emotional Schemas and the Therapeutic Relationship

We may define therapy as a search for value.
—ABRAHAM MASLOW

When I began learning cognitive-behavioral therapy, I became enamored of its powerful techniques and rational basis. My personality was focused on achieving goals, solving problems, thinking rationally, and staying on task. I thought I was particularly skilled in winning arguments, and I often enjoyed the repartee that I could experience in a good discussion with an energetic and intelligent opponent. In my own life, I would use the traditional cognitive and behavioral techniques to reverse rumination, overcome procrastination, address my worries, cope with loneliness, and further my career. It was working for me—why not for everyone else?

But my patients taught me that I was too narrow, too egocentric, and too rational. And, I must say, I owe a lot to them. They helped me rediscover who I really was. And who was that? In fact, when I was in college my dream was to be a playwright and occasional poet. I went looking for the wisdom in tragedy, moved by the insights of Nietzsche, Kierkegaard, and Sartre. When I look back on my earlier years and my education, I see that there was always this dialectic going on: I was moved by the emotional and existential, but also entranced with the rigors of British analytic philosophy and the challenges of deconstructing meaning in a rational manner. I think that the therapeutic relationship also reflects this dialectic. On the one hand, we therapists are trying to utilize the powerful behavioral and cognitive techniques available to us, while, on the other hand, opening the therapeutic relationship to the intensity, depths, and richness of each patient's emotional experiences. Both approaches are of value, and neither is sufficient for a deeper, more meaningful therapy. We are only in some ways like Plato's charioteer: although we may need to rein in the wild horse that is dragging us away, we may also need to pay attention to where that horse wants to lead us. Our emotions tell us what we may need to hear. And our emotions also tell us when we have heard it.

We can think of this dialectic in another way: Patients are looking for two things in therapy—usually not at the same time. Some patients come to therapy to be "put back together," while others come to therapy to "fall apart." In either case, it is our job as therapists to catch them, help them feel safe, and help them feel cared about. In particular, if patients are going to fall apart, we want it to be in safe, caring hands.

Therapists may differ in their beliefs about emotions in therapy. I ask you, my therapist readers, to consider the questions in Figure 13.1, and consider how you are approaching therapy. Try to be honest. Don't respond the way you *think* you should feel; just be as honest as you can. Do you notice any pattern? Are you often feeling critical of patients because they are "irrational"? Do you think they are wasting time in therapy when they are talking about their emotions? Do you focus a lot on "diagnosing their pathology" rather than humanizing their suffering? Do you think they need to change the way they think and feel—the sooner the better? How do you feel when patients are crying? Does it make you feel uncomfortable? Do you think you should not feel uncomfortable? Do you want to get them to feel better as soon as possible? Is it hard to tolerate their pain? Do you jump in and try to get them to feel better? Do you ever think to yourself, "They shouldn't feel this way"?

Now let's imagine that some of your patients are filling out the form in Figure 13.2. (Note, by the way, that both this and Figure 13.1 are for private use and are not intended to be reproducible.) How do your patients think you respond to their emotions? Do they think you give them time and space to express their feelings? Do they think you are too ready to "dispute" the way they are thinking or feeling? Do they feel labeled by you, criticized, afraid to reveal their most "shameful" thoughts and feelings? Do they think you want them to be rational and effective, even though they are feeling distraught and chaotic? Do they think you want them to "think rationally," "move on," "get over it," "not be so emotional," or "feel good"? Now ask yourself how you would want them to think about how you respond to their emotions. What is missing?

**Instructions**: Rate yourself as a therapist on each emotional schema dimension, using the following scale:

| | | |
|---|---|---|
| 1 = Very untrue | 2 = Somewhat untrue | 3 = Slightly untrue |
| 4 = Slightly true | 5 = Somewhat true | 6 = Very true |

1. Comprehensibility — I help my patients make sense of their emotions. _____

2. Validation — I help my patients feel understood and cared for when they talk about their emotions. _____

3. Guilt/Shame — I make my patients feel guilty and ashamed about the way they feel. _____

4. Simplistic View of Emotion — I help my patients understand that it is OK to have mixed feelings. _____

5. Values — I help my patients relate their feelings to important values. _____

6. Control — I often think that my patients' feelings are out of control. _____

7. Numbness — I often feel numb and indifferent when my patients talk about their feelings. _____

8. Rationality — I think that my patients are irrational a lot of the time. _____

9. Duration — I think that my patients' negative feelings just go on and on. _____

10. Consensus — I help my patients understand that others have the same feelings. _____

11. Acceptance — I accept and tolerate my patients' painful feelings, and don't try to force them to change. _____

12. Rumination — I often think over and over about, and seem to dwell on, why my patients feel the way they do. _____

13. Expression — I encourage my patients to express their feelings and talk about the way they feel. _____

14. Blame — I am critical of my patients for feeling so upset. _____

**FIGURE 13.1.** Therapist Emotional Schema Scale. (Do not reproduce.)

**Instructions**: Rate your therapist as you see him or her in responding to your emotions, using the following scale:

| 1 = Very untrue | 2 = Somewhat untrue | 3 = Slightly untrue |
| 4 = Slightly true | 5 = Somewhat true | 6 = Very true |

1. Comprehensibility   My therapist helps me make sense of my emotions.              _____

2. Validation          My therapist helps me feel understood and cared for          _____
                       when I talk about my feelings.

3. Guilt/Shame         My therapist criticizes me and tries to make me feel         _____
                       guilty and ashamed about the way I feel.

4. Simplistic View     My therapist helps me understand that it is OK to have        _____
   of Emotion          mixed feelings.

5. Values              My therapist relates my feelings to important values.        _____

6. Control             My therapist thinks that my feelings are out of control.     _____

7. Numbness            My therapist seems to be numb and indifferent when I         _____
                       talk about my feelings.

8. Rationality         My therapist thinks that I am irrational a lot of the time.   _____

9. Duration            My therapist thinks that my painful feelings just go on      _____
                       and on.

10. Consensus          My therapist helps me realize that many people also          _____
                       feel the way I feel.

11. Acceptance         My therapist accepts and tolerates my painful feelings,      _____
                       and doesn't try to force me to change.

12. Rumination         My therapist seems to think over and over about, and         _____
                       seems to dwell on, why I feel the way I feel.

13. Expression         My therapist encourages me to express my feelings and        _____
                       talk about the way I feel.

14. Blame              My therapist blames me for feeling upset.                    _____

**FIGURE 13.2.** How I think my therapist views my emotions. (Do not reproduce.)

## HOW PATIENTS' NEGATIVE EMOTIONAL SCHEMAS
## CAN AFFECT THERAPY

Imagine what it is like for a patient coming to see you for the first time. Let's say that this is a woman who has been ridiculed by her parents for her feelings, whose husband has labeled her as "crazy," and whose depression has gone unabated for several years. She feels ashamed of her feelings, afraid of being humiliated again, worried that she will never "get better," and convinced that no one can really understand her or help her. Imagine that she is coming to talk to you—a total stranger, a person of "authority," someone who reminds her of a parent or spouse, and someone who she has only a thread of hope will be able to help her. What are her fears about how you will respond to her emotions? She does not know you, but she is now going to consider exposing her secrets and sharing her vulnerability with you. How can she trust you?

This woman may believe that her emotions do not make sense; that others do not have the same feelings as she does; that her painful feelings are out of control and will go on and on; that she must keep her feelings in check; and that she will eventually be humiliated for being too emotional, out of control, selfish, childish, irrational, or even repulsive. How is she going to learn to trust you—a therapist, a stranger—with these beliefs that sustain her sense of defectiveness and leave her feeling alone with the demons that haunt her? How can she put herself in *your* hands—the hands of a stranger?

Consider the following examples of the effects of patients' negative emotional schemas on therapists and therapy:

- Shame in sharing feelings
- Fear of allowing themselves to "let my feelings happen"
- Shame and fear of crying
- Fear of arousing painful emotion when trying new behavior
- Feeling defective for feeling emotional
- Thinking that there are "good" versus "bad" emotions
- Equating emotion with the self (e.g., "If I feel angry, then I am a hateful person")
- Wanting therapists to "control" or "soothe" their emotions
- Viewing "soothing" as a sign that they are pathetic and weak

These negative emotional schemas may make therapy difficult—unless therapists are able to recognize that patients' beliefs about emotions will almost necessarily affect how the patients view sharing or experiencing emotions in therapy. The fear of emotion may make it difficult to engage patients in exposure to feared stimuli, or may make it difficult for the patients to utilize behavioral activation if this involves activities that are anticipated to be unpleasant. The patients may avoid difficult topics, be reluctant to access painful memories, or hesitate to describe traumatic and humiliating experiences, since these would activate intense emotion. If the patients fear experiencing or sharing intense emotion, they will avoid these topics, inhibit these emotions when they arise, catch themselves before they start to cry, and eventually terminate therapy if it becomes too threatening.

And patients may have beliefs about their therapists and how the therapists will relate to the patients' emotions. For example, the patients may believe that the therapists will be critical and dismissive of these emotions—or, alternatively, they may believe that the therapists need to hear about every feeling, every thought, every memory so as to understand the patients. Patients may believe that they themselves cannot regulate their emotions, and that their therapists are the only ones who can soothe these emotions. Or, in some cases, the patients may think that turning to others for compassion and comfort is a sign of weakness and should be avoided at all costs.

## HOW PROBLEMATIC THERAPIST STYLES
## CAN AFFECT THERAPY

As indicated above, therapists may have their own negative schemas about emotion in therapy. Some may view therapy as a set of techniques to be applied mechanically to the symptoms or behaviors that are presented. This "mechanical therapy" often appears to observers as robotic, superficial, and overly technique-driven, and it can be a turnoff for students new to cognitive-behavioral treatment. Overconcern with techniques, agendas, and protocols may lead the patients to think of their therapists as technicians who do not "get" the patients' experience or care about the patients' individuality, and do not really want to hear about the emotions with which the patients are struggling.

Let's consider some problematic approaches to therapy:

- Not eliciting emotion
- Overemphasizing rationality and problem solving
- Labeling patients as "irrational"
- Not allowing time for emotional expression
- Not exploring the variety of emotions underlying an experience
- Suggesting that the goal of therapy is to feel better
- Implying that painful feelings are problematic
- Suggesting that there is a solution to every problem

Some therapists are reluctant to elicit emotion, preferring to focus on agenda setting, problem solving, rational disputation, and accomplishing tasks. Eliciting emotion is not limited to asking, "How do you feel?" Rather, it can include having a patient describe the bodily sensations that accompany the feeling; the memories associated with the feeling; and images that come to mind that evoke more emotions. It can also involve observing the nonverbal expressions in the patient's face and body; the intonation of the voice; the hesitations in speech; and moments when emotion seems to be blocked, or when an emotion inconsistent with the topic seems to emerge. Eliciting emotion is really the reason why the patient came to therapy. No one comes to therapy because of an irrational thought or even a behavioral deficit. People come to therapy because they are having difficulty with their emotions, and learning about them is the first order of business.

Therapists who are overly focused on rationality and problem solving may believe that they are doing empirically validated therapy and may feel proud of following the protocols. But I remember learning from Aaron T. Beck, the founder of cognitive therapy, that helping the patient feel cared for, respected, and encouraged—and thus helping the patient access emotions—are all part of cognitive therapy. In videos of Beck doing therapy, his gentle, compassionate, quiet, caring manner is striking. The techniques are seamless, often not apparent to the observer, as he gently guides the patient and listens to the voice of the emotion. Beck is not only a great cognitive therapist; he is what some might call a "real therapist." Real therapists elicit, care for, and have time for emotion. And I have noticed that there are "real therapists" in all the camps, all the approaches to therapy.

Labeling a patient as "irrational" is criticizing the patient. I recall that, years ago, a rather inexperienced therapist contacted me to do a consultation. He wanted to talk about a patient who was self-critical. I asked him to do a role play where I would play the role of the patient. The trainee then launched into me with an intense, disputatious attack on my self-critical thinking—hammering me with one technique after another. I then asked him, "How do you think this patient would feel if you said these things?" He replied, "I don't know. I haven't thought about that." I replied, "I would have thought, if I were the patient, that you thought I was stupid. I would have felt sad and angry, and I would have thought all I could expect would be more criticism. And my problem is self-criticism." We always need to think about how it feels, what it sounds like, from where a patient is sitting.

Another problematic style is not to allow time for the experience or expression of emotions. For example, pacing a session may mean allowing the patient to be silent at times, since this may be a time when the patient is reflecting, trying to access feelings and thoughts, considering whether it is a good idea to disclose what is being felt at the moment. Therapists often feel uncomfortable with silence—especially if they think that something needs to be happening every second. Silence may also trigger therapists' feelings of frustration or anxiety: "Nothing is happening. I need to move this forward." In fact, cognitive-behavioral therapists may be especially vulnerable to frustration with silence, since the emphasis in this type of therapy is very much on techniques and interventions. Silence may also be a "test" by a patient: "Let's see if you can allow me to be myself," or "Let's see if you jump in and try to find out what is going on." Therapists need to be aware that they often "talk over the silence"; that is, they may feel so uncomfortable with the silence that they feel a need to "fill the void." Of course, they would be unwise to allow silence to go on indefinitely, since little is exchanged with silence. After some time has elapsed (a few minutes), a therapist might inquire, "I noticed that you became quiet, and I was wondering what you were feeling while you were quiet." The therapist might also consider a paradoxical observation: "I noticed that you were trusting me with your silence—as if you might understand that it is OK for us to just sit here and reflect quietly." Or the therapist might inquire, "Silence is often part of relationships—allowing each person some private moments, some feeling of reflection. I wonder what you thought I might do or say when you were silent."

Silence may also be a behavior reflecting a patient's thought that "If I said something, you might be critical. Or you might not understand." The therapist might inquire, "Sometimes we remain silent because we are not sure if the other person will hear us—will understand us—if we speak. I wonder if that is a feeling that you have had in the past." Silence may simply be the most efficient way of saying, "No one hears me anyway." Silence may be speaking to both the therapist and the patient.

Another problematic style is not exploring the *variety* of emotions underlying an experience. A therapist who is too quick to jump into a patient's automatic thoughts may overlook other emotions underlying the first emotion described. For example, one man complained that coworkers at meetings were not listening to him, and that they were coming up with ideas that he thought were not useful. Ostensibly, his emotion was anger, and he expressed his anger by being critical of them. However, further inquiry indicated that the more important emotion was anxiety: "I am afraid that if I don't get the job done right, then I will get fired. If I listen to them, we won't be productive, and then they'll blame me." Exploring a range of emotions means giving time to that inquiry, as well as suggesting that the patient may be having a lot of different feelings. One emotion may be the door that opens into other emotions—but the patient may struggle to keep the door shut.

Although therapy ultimately should help in relieving suffering, there is a risk that therapy can appear glib and superficial, especially if the therapist conveys the idea that the goal of therapy is to "feel better." Although "feeling good" may be pleasurable (and may even be a goal that the patient clearly states), the fear of negative feelings may make it difficult for the patient to confront necessary losses and dilemmas. For example, a patient of mine who was going through a separation from her husband said to me, "I don't understand why I am so emotional." Her previous therapist had been focused primarily on behavioral activation, while dismissing the value of the marital relationship that she had lost. This made her wonder what was wrong with her that she was not feeling good. Indeed, she was self-invalidating while discussing her experience, alternating between a polite smile and tears. I suggested that it made sense that she felt badly now, since things mattered to her, she valued the idea of family, and she was going through a difficult time:

"Sometimes we just don't feel good because things are going really badly. Right now, for you, although you love your daughter, you have plenty of friends, and your parents are immensely supportive, you are having a hard time because family and marriage matter to you. So I imagine that you will have a lot of feelings—some of which will be unpleasant—until you come out the other side and find yourself again."

This validation that "bad feelings" can come from meaning and caring was very helpful to her, since she had viewed herself as someone who should be happy and content. I added, "You don't want to feel bad about feeling bad. After all, you are human."

Another approach that some therapists take is to view painful feelings as problematic. For example, the "problem" becomes a patient's anger, anxiety, fear, sadness, lethargy, distrust, or other emotions. This may help confirm for some patients that "I can't get on with my life as long as I have these feelings." In contrast, the emotional schema approach proposes that patients can do almost everything that is important even if they have these feelings. For example, they can engage in public speaking even if they are anxious; they can treat their partners with kindness even if they are angry; and they can work together with other people even if they don't completely trust them. Indeed, they can "act as if" they feel better—as George Kelly (1955) recommended 60 years ago. Kelly described a "fixed role" therapy technique in which patients acted as if they were confident (for example) to collect information that disconfirmed their "construct." For example, if I believed that I could not give a good talk, I would adapt the role of a confident speaker—"acting as if"—and give the talk to find out if the audience would ridicule me. This is similar to the "opposite action" recommended in DBT (Linehan, 1993, 2015). Opposite action helps patients move from behavior determined by feelings to behavior determined by the intention to obtain valued goals. Thus, in the emotional schema model, emotions are not the real problem; the real problem is the impairment in functioning that often results from maladaptive coping, such as avoidance, escape, self-injury, or substance misuse.

Finally, a therapist may unfortunately suggest to a patient that every problem has a solution, and that the goal of therapy is to find the solution. I recall that, years ago, a very experienced cognitive-behavioral therapist offered this rather glib suggestion: "If the problem doesn't have a solution, then it is not a real problem." This kind of glib, dismissive comment gives cognitive-behavioral treatment a reputation for being superficial and dismissive of the real tragedies of life. For example, imagine saying to someone whose child has died, "If it doesn't have a solution it's not a real problem." Of course, it is a real problem that the child has died—but it is not a solvable problem. In fact, its inability to be solved makes it ever more real. Sometimes we all have to learn to live with real problems rather than solve them. Sometimes our patients will need to recognize that difficulties, unfairness, emotional ups and downs, loneliness, and histories of mistakes and rejections are realities that they will need to accept, to tolerate, and (if they are lucky) to learn from. But these are not problems that will be solved. They are problems that require endurance—and courage.

## HOW CONSTRUCTIVE THERAPIST BEHAVIORS CAN ENHANCE THERAPY

Therapists can focus on the importance of emotion in therapy, while simultaneously working toward growth and change. The following are useful and constructive approaches to working with emotions in therapy, reminding patients and therapists alike that the reason the patients came to therapy is that they are having difficulty living with their emotions:

- Indicating that emotions are the key in therapy
- Pointing out that respect for patients' feelings is paramount
- Asking more about a range and variety of feelings
- Acknowledging that cognitive-behavioral therapy can seem invalidating
- Linking painful emotions to higher values
- Making emotions universal
- Acknowledging that sometimes life "feels awful"
- Recognizing that an emotion may "feel like it's going to last forever," but can also pass with time
- Validating that people can have apparently contradictory emotions, and there is "space" for many feelings
- Suggesting that other emotions can also be legitimate goals
- Acknowledging that the foregoing statements may not be helpful right now

A patient's first session is an ideal time to focus on both emotions and thoughts while noting to the patient that "The goal of therapy is to help you with your emotions." Learning how to live with emotions; how to develop the capacity for a wide range of emotions; how to include emotions in everyday life; and how to relinquish problematic strategies such as avoidance, in order to achieve goals and live according to values, are all important aspects of therapy—but, more importantly, of a complete life. The therapist can convey to the patient: "I am particularly interested in how these things feel to you and what they mean, and I hope that you will be able to tell me about the feelings that you have while we work together. The most important thing is how you are feeling and how you can make your life fuller, more meaningful, and more rewarding."

Unfortunately, some patients may have chosen cognitive-behavioral therapy because they thought that feelings would not be discussed. Some people view this form of therapy as an escape from emotions. For example, one man said, "I thought that CBT focused on your thoughts and your behavior. Why are we talking about my feelings? Why are we talking about how my mother and father responded to my feelings? I don't want to talk about feelings." This was a patient who needed to talk about and gain access to his feelings. He needed to learn that he could trust the therapist; that having feelings would not lead to humiliation and decompensation; and that being able to go through feelings and live with them would help him form closer relationships, make decisions that "felt right," and tell him what he valued. This was a patient who needed to learn to cry—and did.

It is important to make room for feelings from the first session onward, while conveying the idea that respecting these feelings helps create a safe emotional environment in which the patient can "open up." The therapist can focus on astute awareness of feelings that are being discussed, feelings that underlie what is being said, and feelings that are shown nonverbally. For example, the therapist can empathize, "That must have been hard for you, making you very sad," while at the same time reflecting the nonverbal expression of feeling that the patient is displaying: "I can see sadness in your eyes and hear the sadness in your voice as you tell me this. Your sadness is completely here, with you and me."

In her first session, a woman indicated that in the past 2 months her father had died, her boyfriend had broken up with her, and she had lost her job. As she told her story, she wept, and her voice was sometimes barely audible as she choked her words through her tears. She said, "What's wrong with me? I sometimes cry for no reason. I don't know why I can't control myself." She described her boyfriend as cold, overly rational, and ultimately dismissive. Toward the end of the session, the following exchange occurred:

THERAPIST: You seem to think there is something terribly wrong with you that you are crying. But it may be that you have things to cry about. You have lost your relationship, your father, and your job. Things matter to you. You are upset because you are not superficial. You describe your boyfriend as aloof and out of touch, and you sound like you are criticizing yourself from that perspective. But everything about you today is real. Your feelings come through in every way: Your voice quivers, you cry, your eyes show your feelings, you move your hands around. You are completely here in the present moment, completely alive.

PATIENT: Well, that sounds atypically sensitive to me. Thank you, though.

THERAPIST: Imagine if you were to talk like that to yourself about the reality of your feelings?

PATIENT: Yeah. But what can I do when I am feeling this way?

THERAPIST: You can say, "At this moment I am feeling this way because I am real and I am alive."

The therapist can ask about a range of feelings: "It sounds like you were feeling sad after [a negative event occurred], and that makes a lot of sense. And I am wondering if you had other feelings as well." As Greenberg and his colleagues suggest in emotion-focused therapy, a patient may be experiencing a wide range of feelings, and the initial emotion that is described may not be the most important for the patient (see, e.g., Greenberg, 2002). For example, a patient may describe sadness as the first emotion, but may reveal on further discussion that other emotions, such as anxiety and hopelessness, are more troubling. If so, the therapist might ask, "If you were more confident that you would be happier in the future, what would you think about the sadness you are having now?" In many such cases, the current sadness might be more tolerable if the patients believed that the future would be less bleak.

I have found it quite helpful to tell patients with intense emotions that cognitive-behavioral therapy can seem invalidating at times. Even if I intend to do the best I can to validate each patient, this acknowledgment of limitations and its sincerity can go a long way to establish trust in the relationship. Ironically, we might trust a doctor more who tells us that an injection will be painful than one who just jabs us in the arm. Acknowledging that the rational challenges and behavioral recommendations can seem invalidating, and suggesting that this may sometimes constitute a dilemma ("I want to help you with your feelings and help build a meaningful life, but sometimes I will say things that move us away from discussing your feelings"), set the stage for the possibility of future invalidation—while suggesting that "We can talk about it when this happens and work on it together" helps prepare the patient for ruptures that might occur.

Moreover, it is helpful to link emotions to higher values. This is very different from the idea that the goal of therapy is to get rid of emotions or to medicate a patient so that the emotions disappear. For example, a young mother described how she worried about her child going off to preschool: "I know I shouldn't be worried, but I am." The therapist responded, "Even though worries are troublesome, it may simply be part of being a mother at times to worry about your child. Perhaps the goal is not to eliminate your worries, but rather to put them in perspective in your life." A patient who experiences difficulties with loneliness after a breakup can be told, "Loneliness means that you care about intimacy and love—because you are a loving person." The desire to connect with others can sometimes feel painful when it is not available. This is similar to the idea that our emotions may be telling us something that we need to listen to. Another helpful approach is to make emotions universal: "This is how many of us feel when we are lonely." Normalizing emotions by helping the patient realize that others feel this way under similar circumstances helps the patient feel less alone, less pathologized.

The therapist can also suggest to the patient that sometimes life "feels awful." Rather than trying to reduce the impact of a negative life event by immediately "putting things in perspective" with cognitive-behavioral techniques, the therapist can acknowledge that life often involves experiences that just feel terrible. This initial approach to the intensity of the emotion that the patient is experiencing helps establish trust in what the therapist will say later. Unlike some therapists, who will dispute that there is anything that is "awful," the emotional schema therapist may initially join in reflecting and empathizing with the awfulness of the experience for the patient. "Life sometimes feels awful" is a universal truth for many people who are suffering, and acknowledging this will help the patient feel heard, respected, and cared for. This can then be followed by an observation that the patient's emotion may "feel like it's going to last forever," but can also pass with time. The therapist can convey respect for the moment: "Right now is a moment in time when things feel awful, and we must both respect this moment. This is where you are right now. We can listen together and hear what it feels like for you. Although these feelings may pass, there is no question that this where you are at now." This observation and appreciation of the present moment of emotion are similar to mindful awareness and nonjudgmental acceptance. The patient can reflect on what the emotion is telling him or her, what it feels like—while recognizing the possibility that, like all moments, this moment will pass. The emotion is here for the present moment.

The goal of emotional schema therapy is not to eliminate emotions; it is to expand the range of emotions available to the patient. The therapist can validate that it is possible to have apparently contradictory emotions, and that there is "space" for many feelings. For example, a man who is feeling lonely on a Saturday night can examine whether he has other emotions—and can do so not only on this night, but throughout the week and month ahead. The therapist can say:

> "We often think that the emotion we are having at this one moment is the only emotion that we will have—because we get so focused on a painful emotion. But I wonder if there are a lot of other emotions that you could have right now—or over the next week or month. Think about emotions as all the notes available to a musician or all the colors available to a painter, and think about all the emotions that you have known. What could they be?"

While expanding on the awareness of the complexity and richness of emotion, the therapist can also expand on the possibility of experiencing other emotions. For example, a therapist suggested to a man who was angry over an incident at work that other emotions can also be a legitimate goal:

> "Right now you are feeling angry because your boss treated you unfairly, and anger is a feeling that we often have when this happens. It's perfectly human to feel angry about unfairness. What if you were to set aside that anger for a few minutes and consider other emotions in your life—perhaps unrelated to work or to your boss or the current incident? Certainly what happened to you is important, but we can also examine if there are other things that are important. For example, let's take 'appreciation' as an emotion—that is, the awareness that certain things in life are important to you and that you value them. Close your eyes for a moment, and try to focus on something or someone that you appreciate, and tell me what you value in them."

The patient reflected that he appreciated his parents, who were loving and kind; his sister and her husband; his partner; his education and his ability to learn; many things about his job (including even his boss at times); and living in the city where he lived. The therapist commented:

> "Sometimes we focus on an emotion or an experience that is important at the moment and we get stuck on it—almost like we get hijacked by it—and we lose sight of so many other emotions, experiences, and possibilities. It's like going to a great museum and standing in front of a painting all day—*one that you don't like.* There are other great works of art to be seen. You can think, 'What else is there to experience? Where else can I turn?' Each experience is an opportunity for a different emotion, and each emotion opens new opportunities."

Early in therapy—and, often, throughout future sessions when difficult experiences arise—I find it helpful to reiterate the limitations of what we are doing. For example, even after describing many of the foregoing validating, respectful, hopeful, flexible, and empowering possibilities, I find it helpful to acknowledge that what I am saying may not be helpful right now. Although therapy offers a "promise," it is also helpful to reflect that the promise may take quite some time to be fulfilled. Indeed, like many promises, it may never be completely fulfilled. From the perspective of the distraught patient, a facile claim that "Changing your behaviors and thoughts will change the way you feel" may be true in the long run, but it may fall on its face in the short run. Just as the patient can hear the suggestions for changing behavior and thinking, the patient also hears the promise that is implied. Ironically, suggesting that the immediate feelings may not change for a while is helpful both if the feelings persist (since the therapist is sug-gesting it will take a while) and if the feelings change (since that is what the patient wants). Either way, it is validating and encouraging.

The constructive therapist behaviors described in this section con-vey that the therapist cares, validates, allows for feelings, makes emotion "safe," understands, and is not controlling. The therapist also shares a view of "suffering"—that it makes sense for now, is not a flaw, reflects impor-tant values, does not need to be controlled, will not necessarily harm the patient, and is part of being human. The manner in which the therapist talks about emotions is related to many of the emotional schema dimensions. For example, expression is encouraged, and validation is a continuing part of the relationship. The patient is not blamed or shamed; the therapist is not telling the patient, "Control your feelings," or "Get a handle on yourself." Emotions are accepted; they are linked to human nature and higher val-ues; and they are considered a source of rich information about needs. The therapist is expanding on emotions, viewing other emotions as possibilities, encouraging emotional flexibility, and reframing conflicting feelings as the richness of experience and possibility. Since emotions are accessed in the session—and since they will abate during the session—the patient directly experiences evidence that emotions are not durable and dangerous. The manner in which the therapist relates to the emotions that are presented is a continuing experiential test of the patient's negative beliefs about emotion.

## THE NATURE OF TRANSFERENCE
## IN EMOTIONAL SCHEMA THERAPY

Cognitive-behavioral therapists have consistently recognized the thera-peutic relationship as an important component of the process of change (Gilbert, 1992, 2007; Gilbert & Irons, 2005; Greenberg, 2001; Katzow & Safran, 2007; Leahy, 2001, 2005b, 2007b, 2009b; Safran, 1998; Saf-ran & Muran, 2000; Strauss et al., 2006). Although cognitive-behavioral therapists seldom refer to the patient's predispositions as "transference," we can conceptualize the schemas, assumptions, and coping strategies that are activated in therapy as representing prior experiences from other relationships, particularly the family of origin. We can think of "trans-ference" or "countertransference" in an emotional schema perspective as representing stimulus and response generalization from prior relationships; this view was first advanced by Dollard and Miller (1950). Indeed, Dol-lard and Miller attempted to view the therapeutic relationship in terms of stimulus and response generalization—concepts familiar to learning theorists. Similar to the transference concept in psychoanalytic theory (Menninger & Holzman, 1973), the strategies, schemas, and scripts in the emotional schema therapy relationship may reflect personal schemas about the self (inadequate, special, helpless); interpersonal schemas about others (superior, judgmental, nurturing); intrapsychic processes (repression, denial, displacement); interpersonal strategies (provoking, stonewalling, clinging); and past and present relationships that affect how the current therapeutic relationship is experienced (Leahy, 2001, 2007b, 2009b). There is no reason why the transference concept needs to be limited to psychodynamic theory. However, emotional schema therapy, unlike psychodynamic models, entails implicit expectations about the patient's role in actively engaging with current thoughts, feelings, relationships, and behavior. As a consequence of these expectations and therapeutic procedures, noncompliance or resistance may take specific forms (Leahy, 2001, 2003b). Since emotional schema therapy (like other forms of cognitive-behavioral therapy) establishes an expectation of following an agenda, staying in the here and now, conducting rational evaluations, encouraging behavioral activation, and engaging self-help, patients will have many "opportunities" to bring personal schemas of defectiveness, unlovability, and helplessness to the experience of therapy, as well as their beliefs about their own emotions and how others respond to them.

Patients with specific personality disorders function differently in the transference relationship (Leahy, 2005b). For example, dependent patients, fearing abandonment and isolated helplessness, may seek considerable reassurance from the therapist, relying on the therapist to comfort and reassure them. In contrast, narcissistic patients, viewing therapy as a potential humiliation and feeling entitled to their emotions, may devalue and provoke the therapist in order to test their "power." These role enactments in therapy also reflect the social relational systems described by Gilbert (1989, 2000a, 2005, 2007), as well as the interpersonal schemas elaborated by Safran and his colleagues (Muran & Safran, 1993, 1998; Safran, 1998; Safran & Greenberg, 1988, 1989, 1991) and the relational schemas identified by Baldwin and Dandeneau (2005). These schemas can be seen as dimensions that are not mutually exclusive, and different therapists may "pull on" them in different ways (Leahy, 2007b). For example, one therapist may stimulate hostility or dependency in patients in a way that another therapist may not. Another therapist may find a particular patient very hard to work with, while another therapist may not. The therapeutic relationship is a co-construction between therapist and patient; both parties bring to the experience their own personal and emotional schema predispositions.

## AN EMOTIONAL SCHEMA MODEL OF COUNTERTRANSFERENCE

Although we therapists would ideally like to believe that we can work effectively with a wide range of people, clinical experience suggests that each of us has our own difficulties with specific groups of patients. As therapists, we are similar to our patients in holding certain personal and interpersonal schemas. I have listed a number of patients' personal schemas in Table 13.1.

We can ask ourselves, "What issues concern me most? Which patients are most troubling to me? Are there certain patients I feel too comfortable with? How do I feel about telling patients things that might disturb them?" For example, some therapists are more concerned about the nature of the relationship, others about the expression of emotion, and still others about encouraging patients to become more active. While some therapists are intimidated by narcissistic patients, others prefer patients who are self-effacing, and yet others have difficulty with intense emotional experiences. We can note which patients and issues "push our buttons," and what automatic thoughts and personal schemas are activated (e.g., "If the patient is disappointed in me, it must be because I am an inadequate therapist").

When I have asked therapists which patients they find most difficult to work with, the general agreement is that they have problems with narcissistic patients. Typical responses by therapists are the following: "They are egocentric and selfish," "They devalue me," "They act entitled," and "They treat people unfairly." Of course they do; these are defining characteristics

**TABLE 13.1. Patients' Personal Schemas in Therapy**

| Schema | Example |
|---|---|
| Incompetent (avoidant) | Avoids difficult topics and emotions. Appears vague. Looks for signs that therapist will reject him or her. Believes that therapist will criticize him or her for not doing homework well enough. Reluctant to do behavioral exposure homework assignments. |
| Helpless (dependent) | Seeks reassurance. Does not have an agenda of problems to solve. Frequently complains about "feelings." Calls frequently between sessions. Wants to prolong sessions. Does not think he or she can do the homework, or believes that homework will not work. Upset when therapist takes vacations. |
| Vulnerable to control (passive–aggressive) | Comes late to or misses sessions. Views cognitive "challenges" as controlling. Reluctant to express dissatisfaction directly. Vague about goals, feelings, and thoughts—especially as related to therapist and therapy. "Forgets" to do homework or pay bills. |
| Responsible (obsessive–compulsive) | Feels emotions are "messy" and "irrational." Criticizes self for being irrational and disorganized. Wants to see immediate results and expresses skepticism about therapy. Views homework as a test to be done perfectly or not at all. |
| Superior (narcissistic) | Comes late or misses sessions. "Forgets" to pay for sessions. Devalues therapy and the therapist. Expects special arrangements. Feels humiliated to have to talk about problems. Believes that therapy will not work, since the problem resides in other people. |
| Glamorous (histrionic) | Focuses on expressing emotions, alternating rapidly from crying, laughing to anger. Tries to impress therapist with appearance, feelings, or problems. Rejects the rational approach and demands validation. |

*Note.* From Leahy (2001). Copyright 2001 by Robert L. Leahy. Adapted by permission.

of narcissism. A therapist's negative response to such a patient can be viewed in several ways. First, the therapist's response may be a "normal" response to narcissism—and may simply be information about how this individual elicits similar feelings in others. Second, the therapist can ask, "How would I respond in normal social interactions with someone like this?" The answer might be that the therapist might avoid them or, in some cases, criticize them. This may also be informative about how others respond. Third, these countertransference responses may motivate the therapist to distance him- or herself from or criticize the patient. It may be difficult to show empathy or even curiosity. This may confirm the patient's view that people cannot be trusted, that the therapist is not competent, and that the therapist "should be punished." Fourth, the patient's narcissism and tendency to devalue the therapist may activate the therapist's schemas and conditional assumptions about inadequacy ("Maybe I'm not competent"), fear of conflict ("It's terrible when people are angry with me"), need for approval ("I need my patients to like me"), or emphasis on fairness ("My patients should be fair and ethical all the time").

As a result of these negative responses by the therapist—which are often judgments of character and emphasis on traits (e.g., "selfishness")—the therapist may have difficulty focusing on the patient's emotions. For example, many narcissistic patients experience anxiety, emptiness, anger, helplessness, and sadness, but may avoid focusing on these inner experiences by provoking these emotions in others. Thus, if a narcissistic patient provokes anger in a therapist, the therapist may pay little attention to the feelings of anxiety, humiliation, and defeat that the patient is experiencing. Moreover, if the therapist experiences the patient as attempting to attack or humiliate the therapist, it may be especially difficult to use compassion and validation. Yet those might be the best strategies. For example, a divorced narcissistic man was describing how his girlfriend did not make him feel appreciated and how she seemed "selfish." When the therapist made a comment, he responded, "Shut up and listen." Now, in daily life, such a comment would lead to rejection or counterattack. However, the therapist commented, "I can see you are angry with me, but tell me what it felt like when she didn't show appreciation." This led to a discussion of his feelings of being criticized and humiliated by her, as well as his fears that he was becoming old and unattractive and that he would end up a sick old man with no one to take care of him. Thus his underlying profound vulnerabilities were masked by his bravado, condescension, and attack. In the next session, the therapist focused on how the patient structured relationships in terms of power and judgment: He tried to have all the power, and he bolstered his ego by judging other people. The therapist described this power assertion strategy as a way in which the patient thought he could avoid being "one-down" in a relationship. The patient observed, "My mother never made me feel like I was good enough." His compensating strategy was to make others feel that they were inadequate (e.g., berating the therapist).

Problems in the relationship can arise even when things seem to be going well. Feeling especially "comfortable" with a patient may make it difficult to identify and address problematic behavior such as substance misuse, lack of financial responsibility, or self-defeating patterns (Leahy, 2001). The therapist can ask him- or herself, "If I didn't like this patient so much, what would I be noticing and talking about?" and "If I did bring up some less 'desirable' issues, what do I fear would happen?" In fact, the therapist positive regard for the patient—if the patient perceives it as authentic—can often be a significant facilitating factor in bringing up problems.

Some therapists are reluctant to confront patients with "disturbing" information, fearing that the patients may get angry, become sad, or leave therapy. A threat to terminate therapy may activate a therapist's schemas about abandonment, loss of reputation, or being controlled by the patient. These perceptions of relationships are reflected in the countertransference schemas held by the therapist. These include demanding standards, fears of abandonment, need for approval, viewing the self as rescuer, or self-sacrifice (see Table 13.2). For example, a therapist may be reluctant to bring up uncomfortable material because she fears that the patient will become upset and leave therapy. This then can trigger the thoughts that "other patients will drop out," "My reputation will be ruined," and "I will become a failure."

In addition, as suggested above, therapists have different emotional philosophies: They may believe either that painful and difficult emotions can provide opportunities to deepen the therapeutic relationship, or that such emotions should be eliminated or avoided. Gottman's model of emotional philosophies, described in earlier chapters, provides a valuable taxonomy for identifying the shared emotional style within the therapeutic relationship (see Gottman et al., 1996; Katz et al., 1996); this taxonomy includes dismissive, critical, overwhelmed, and facilitative styles. Of particular interest is the "emotion-coaching" style, which reflects the therapist's authentic and nonjudgmental interest in all emotions, while encouraging the patient to differentiate and explore these emotions, and to consider ways in which self-soothing can be facilitated. This style is similar to the empathic and supportive style advocated by Rogers (1955) and Greenberg (2002, 2007), and by Gilbert (2005, 2007) in his discussion of compassion as a complex set of abilities that can help the therapeutic relationship. Some therapists, who view painful emotions as distracting or self-indulgent, may communicate a dismissive attitude ("We need to get back to the agenda"), or they may take a critical approach, such as that reflected in Ellis's (1994) sarcastic comments about patients who whine. Sometimes patients need to "be with" their feelings, become familiar with them, and learn to tolerate them. However, therapists who are uncomfortable "being with" a feeling may constantly ask patients about their thoughts, or may intrude and inadvertently model emotional avoidance. In psychodynamic approaches, the idea is for patients to feel that their emotions can be "contained," and

**TABLE 13.2. Therapist Schemas in the Therapeutic Relationship**

| Schema | Assumptions |
|---|---|
| Demanding standards | "I have to cure all my patients. I must always meet the highest standards. My patients should do an excellent job. We should never waste time." |
| Special, superior person | "I am entitled to be successful. My patients should appreciate all that I do for them. I shouldn't feel bored when doing therapy. Patients try to humiliate me." |
| Rejection sensitivity | "Conflicts are upsetting. I shouldn't raise issues that will bother the patient." |
| Abandonment | "If my patients are bothered with therapy, they might leave. It's upsetting when patients terminate. I might end up with no patients." |
| Autonomy | "I feel controlled by the patient. My movements, feelings, or what I say are limited. I should be able to do or say what I wish. Sometimes I wonder if I will lose myself in the relationship." |
| Control | "I have to control my surroundings or the people around me." |
| Judgmental | "Some people are basically bad people. People should be punished if they do wrong things." |
| Persecution | "I often feel provoked. The patient is trying to get to me. I have to guard against being taken advantage of or hurt. You usually can't trust people." |
| Need for approval | "I want to be liked by the patient. If the patient isn't happy with me, then it means I'm doing something wrong." |
| Need to like others | "It's important that I like the patient. It bothers me if I don't like a patient. We should get along—almost like friends." |
| Withholding | "I want to withhold thoughts and feelings from the patient. I don't want to give patients what they want. I feel I am withdrawing emotionally during the session." |
| Helplessness | "I feel I don't know what to do. I fear I'll make mistakes. I wonder if I'm really competent. Sometimes I feel like giving up." |
| Goal inhibition | "The patient is blocking me from achieving my goals. I feel like I'm wasting time. I should be able to achieve my goals in sessions without the patient's interference." |
| Self-sacrifice | "I should meet the patient's needs. I should make patients feel better. The patient's needs often take precedence over my needs. I sometimes believe that I would do almost anything to meet patients' needs." |
| Emotional inhibition | "I feel frustrated when I'm with this patient because I can't express the way I really feel. I find it hard to suppress my feelings. I can't be myself." |

*Note.* From Leahy (2001). Copyright 2001 by Robert L. Leahy. Adapted by permission.

that they do not threaten the therapists or the therapy. In this way, the patients learn that their emotions are understandable, acceptable, tolerable and meaningful—but also can change.

A therapist's emotional philosophy—and the strategies that are implemented—will have a significant impact on a patient's own emotional schemas (Leahy, 2005a, 2007a, 2009a). For example, the therapist who takes the dismissive approach ("Let's get back to the agenda") conveys the unsympathetic messages that "Your emotions are not interesting to me," "Emotions are a waste of time," and "You are indulging yourself." As a consequence of a dismissive or critical stand by the therapist, the patient may conclude, "My emotions don't make sense," "No one cares about them," "I should feel ashamed or guilty for having these feelings," and "Focusing on my emotions won't help me." As the patient dutifully follows the lead of the agenda-setting therapist, emotions become secondary to compliance with an agenda that may never really address the very reason the patient sought therapy—that is, for help with feelings.

Crucially, interpersonal styles differ among therapists—some are distancing, overly attached, engage in rigid boundary setting, appear deferent, or are dominating, soothing, or reassuring. Therapists who view emotions as a waste of time may appear somewhat distancing (aloof and condescending), deferential (intellectualized), relentlessly boundary-setting ("That's not on our agenda" or "We don't have time for that today"), or dominating ("This is cognitive-behavioral therapy, and we try to focus only on your thoughts and on getting things done"). Other therapists—also viewing painful emotions as intolerable—may be quick to rescue patients from their feelings ("Oh, you'll be OK. Don't worry, it will work out"), may directly tell patients to stop crying ("Don't cry. Things will be OK"), or may be quick to soothe ("You'll be fine in a while"). The implicit message of these well-meaning interactions is that "Your painful emotions need to be eliminated as soon as possible." Thus, rather than sharing, differentiating, exploring, and clarifying these emotional experiences (as in emotion coaching or in emotion-focused therapy), these therapists may communicate through rescue and support that painful emotions do not have a place in a therapeutic relationship and that the patients are too vulnerable to deal with their own emotions. Rescuing someone from painful emotions confirms the belief that experiential avoidance is a desirable coping strategy.

## PATIENT–THERAPIST SCHEMA MISMATCH

Some therapists are more likely to "explain" behavior by reference to diagnostic labels (e.g., "She's saying that because she is a borderline") than to specific thoughts (e.g., "She thinks I don't understand her") or to specific emotions (e.g., "She is hurt, afraid, and angry"). A therapist who harbors a negative view of specific emotions (e.g., anger) may be likely to attribute these emotions to fixed personality traits than to situational factors or specific interpretations held for the moment by the patient. For example, "She's angry because she is a borderline" actually explains nothing, is not helpful, and ultimately is dismissive. The individual becomes a category, a case, a diagnosis—someone different from the rest of us. Is it possible to imagine a patient saying, "I really felt understood and cared for today because my therapist labeled me a 'borderline' and said my behavior was typical of borderlines"? Labeling and diagnosing a patient may be helpful in enabling a therapist to use information about psychopathology, but focusing on the idiographic rather than the nomothetic is considerably more helpful (Meehl, 1954/1996). The emotional schema approach recognizes the value of diagnosis, but treats each patient as a unique individual, with a unique case conceptualization and a focus on the patient's unique emotions and thoughts.

Moreover, it is often difficult for us (as both therapists and human beings) to understand how our own behavior may elicit behavior in other persons, partly because the behavior of the others "engulfs the field" of our experience, since we are observing the others' behavior at this moment in time (Heider, 1958; Jones & Davis, 1965). We seldom have access to the variability of the others' behavior across time and situations, and we have difficulty taking the perspective of ourselves interacting with others. Once a trait concept is activated, it leads to confirmation bias; that is, we tend to selectively attend to and remember information consistent with the trait concept. The therapeutic relationship is both interactive and iterative, characterized by a series of interactions over time with a bias toward self-fulfilling prophecies by both therapist and patient (Leahy, 2007b). As a result, patient and therapist may both have difficulty seeing the "larger picture"; the other person's behavior may be attributed to unchangeable traits; the other person's behavior may be personalized; it is hard for each party to get information that runs counter to his or her expectations; and the roles enacted lead to further confirmation bias and further self-fulfilling prophecies.

## Types of Patient–Therapist Mismatches

What happens when a patient's schemas about self, others, and emotions are in conflict with the therapist's schemas or core beliefs? Imagine the following: A man has an avoidant personality; his goal is to keep people from knowing him so he cannot get rejected. He is cautious, since he does not want to take any chances of getting rejected or failing. Consequently, he is reluctant to carry out self-help assignments, he seldom has an agenda (since he either does not have direct access to his emotions—since he has avoided emotions—or does not want to "make a stand" in therapy). In contrast to this man's avoidant personality, consider the possibility that the therapist has demanding standards; she expects patients to conform to her agenda and treatment plans. In this interaction, the therapist has little tolerance for "vague complaints," "procrastination" or lack of clear goals. The patient with the avoidant personality may believe that he cannot express his emotions, they will not be validated, and his emotions are different from those of others, and he may feel ashamed and guilty about his emotions. In concert with these negative beliefs, the therapist with demanding standards believes that emotions are a waste of time, the patient's reluctance to share openly thoughts and feelings is an impediment to the "success of the therapy," and the patient is blocking the therapist from achieving her goals.

Both parties in the dyad collect information to confirm their beliefs. For example, the patient is trying to find out whether the therapist can be trusted; thus the patient hesitates, remains vague, and waits to see how the therapist reacts. The therapist's behavior is attributed either to dispositions or traits that the therapist has ("She is critical") or to defects in the self ("I am a loser"). (The patient does not recognize the situational game-like quality: "When I hesitate, some people will either probe or withdraw from me.") Similarly, the therapist with demanding standards will activate probes, controls, criticisms, and exhortations if the patient is "noncompliant." The therapist will attribute her own behavior to the patient's "noncompliance," not recognizing that this kind of controlling and demanding behavior creates a self-fulfilling prophecy: When the therapist demands, the patient withdraws. This confirms the schematic perception of the patient as noncompliant.

Other types of schematic mismatches can occur, in which therapists inadvertently confirm the negative beliefs held by their patients by utilizing either avoidant or compensatory strategies. For example, a dependent patient (with fears of abandonment and beliefs about personal helplessness) and a therapist who also is dependent and fears abandonment by patients are locked in a self-fulfilling prophecy. The dependent therapist, fearing the "loss" of the patient, may use avoidant strategies. She does not bring up difficult topics, avoids discussing the patient's dependent behavior, does not set limits on the patient, and avoids using exposure techniques. As a result, the patient may interpret this hesitancy or avoidance as confirming the following beliefs: "My emotions must be overwhelming to other people. Doing new things will be risky and terrifying. My therapist must think I am incapable of doing things on my own. I should avoid independent behavior." Or the therapist may try to compensate for the patient's dependency by constantly reassuring the patient, prolonging sessions, or apologizing for absences. The patient may then interpret these behaviors as confirming his beliefs: "I need to rely on others to solve my problems, I must be incompetent, I can't get better on my own, the only way to get better is to find someone to take care of me and protect me."

Or consider the schematic mismatch that arises for the dependent patient whose therapist has demanding standards. The dependent patient seeks reassurance, does not have an agenda of problems to solve, frequently complains about "feelings," calls frequently between sessions, wants to prolong sessions, does not think he can do the homework or believes that homework will not work, and is upset when the therapist takes vacations. The therapist with demanding standards may believe, "I have to cure all my patients; I must always meet the highest standards; my patients should do an excellent job; and we should never waste time." This therapist may view this patient's lack of progress as "personal" resistance and may impose a more demanding agenda, insist on task compliance, become critical of lack of progress, and label the patient as "dependent." The patient may then conclude, "I can't count on my therapist. I will be abandoned if I don't improve. My emotions are not important to my therapist. I am a failure in therapy. I can't solve any problems." Alternatively, the therapist may avoid the patient's emotions and dependency by losing interest in the patient, not exploring the patient's need for validation and emotional expression, and terminating the patient for "noncompliance" ("You are not ready for therapy"), thereby leading the patient to conclude, "I must be boring. My therapist has no interest in me. Therefore, my therapist will leave me." These two versions of this type of patient–therapist mismatch are illustrated in Figure 13.3.

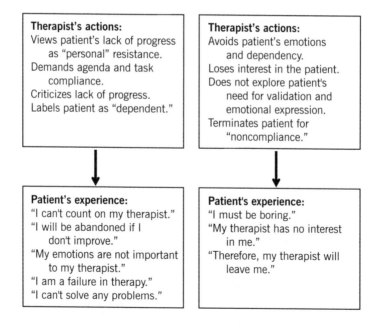

**FIGURE 13.3.** Two versions of a schematic mismatch between a dependent patient and a therapist with demanding standards.

## Using the Countertransference

The therapist is not a neutral object onto which internal dynamics are projected. Rather, the therapist is a dynamic part of the patient's interpersonal world. In the examples just given, the therapist with demanding standards can recognize *her own resistance to the patient*—in her tendency to impose her agenda onto the patient, coerce him into changing, or withdraw from the patient with indifference (Leahy, 2001, 2009b). Indeed, if the therapist acts and feels this way, then the patient may be eliciting these responses from other "demanding" people. Three questions can be posed: (1) How does the patient respond when other demanding people interact with him? (2) What are the typical personality characteristics of the people in the patient's life? and (3) What is the patient's developmental history of relationships and dysfunctional strategies?

Consider another example. A patient of mine was a married woman with long-standing relationship problems, characterized by feeling she was not heard, not feeling emotionally or physically in touch with her husband, and feeling guilty. She responded to the homework "demands" in therapy with statements of her own helplessness and inadequacy, complaining that her problem resided in her controlling and narcissistic husband. In this context, I recognized my own demanding standards coming up. These would have led me to set strict agendas, "challenge" her automatic thoughts, suggest alternatives, and help lay out some problem-solving strategies. Unfortunately, as I quickly realized, this would replicate the domineering, dismissive, and emotionally empty experiences that she had had with other people in her life—from her parents to her husband. I thus decided to back away from imposing homework on the patient, in order to examine the patient's pattern of deferring to other people in intimate relationships. In fact, her deference to others—based on her view that she did not know her own needs and that she did not have a right to have needs—resulted in others' taking charge or taking the lead. This reinforced her view that she was secondary in relationships, although she hoped that a strong, determined man "who knew what he wanted" would be able to satisfy her and take care of her. Just as she deferred in her relationship to me in therapy, she also deferred in her family and intimate relationships.

Prior to seeing me, this patient had seen an argumentative, "rational" therapist who lectured her. The earlier therapist was highly focused on rational disputation, going on at great length about cognitive distortions and irrational "shoulds." The patient indicated that this prior therapy reminded her of her father and mother, who would tell her how to feel and how to act, but who never appeared to validate her individuality. She experienced the prior therapist as dismissive, critical, and condescending—experiences that she also complained of with her husband. While recognizing the importance of change, we focused on her emotional schemas. I indicated that "the most important thing in our relationship is for both of us to understand and respect your emotions—it's what you feel that counts the most." As she began to focus on her emotions and attempt to discuss them, she noticed that she had difficulty labeling her emotions, and also would often suddenly start crying "for no reason" (as she would say). She believed that her emotions made no sense; that no one could understand her emotions; and that she had no right to feel upset, since she had a lucrative job and a husband who loved her. She believed she needed to keep a tight hold on her emotions in order to prevent them from going out of control. The emotional philosophies of her mother and father were that her emotions were self-indulgent, manipulative, and unwarranted. In fact, she observed that much of her life around her father was focused on trying to "put out" *his* emotional tirades. There was no room for her emotions in their lives—or in the life of her husband.

We decided to view her pain and suffering as a window into her needs and values, and as a signal that her painful emotions needed to be heard and respected. Her new emotional schemas included the following: "It's important to recognize a wide range of my emotions," "My emotions come from human needs for love, closeness, and sensuality," "I have a human need for validation, warmth, and acceptance," and "I want to seek this out in a new relationship." Although she had come for "cognitive therapy" (with an emphasis on "rationality"), she acknowledged that focusing on her rights to have emotions and needs—and to develop relationships where that is possible—would be worth pursuing.

Let's review the different therapeutic styles that this patient experienced. With the demanding and antiemotional didactic therapist, the "coercive" and "intellectual" style reflected the belief that she was whining, had too many "shoulds," and had low frustration tolerance. Indeed, these were the very terms he used with her. The messages were "Get over it" and "It shouldn't matter that much." The therapist appeared to her to be condescending, out of touch, and critical of her feelings. This confirmed her belief that her feelings didn't make sense, that she was self-indulgent, and that "I must be too needy." In contrast, in taking an emotional schema approach in treatment with me, she was able to recognize and differentiate her various emotions; experiment with expressing emotions and getting validation; explore how her emotions were linked to important needs that were going unmet; and recognize that although she was good at supporting and validating others, she would need to direct this nurturing and compassionate mind toward herself. The contrast between a didactic and overly rational approach therapist's and an emotional schema therapist's approach is shown in Figure 13.4.

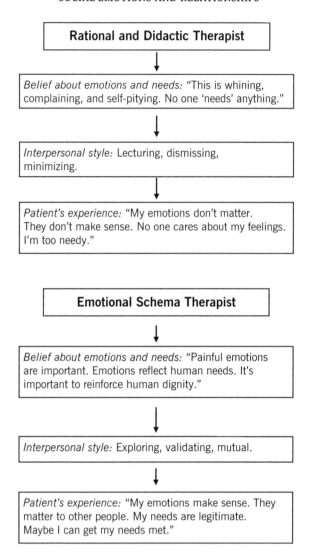

**FIGURE 13.4.** Contrasting an overly rational therapist with an emotional schema therapist.

## Responding to Schematic Mismatch

A therapist can take several productive steps to address a schematic mismatch with a patient. The first three steps have been illustrated above, and I briefly describe them here for you, my readers.

First, as indicated above, it is helpful to recognize your own vulnerabilities. Do you have negative beliefs about specific emotions in therapy—for example, about expression and validation of these emotions? Are there certain emotions (like anger or extreme sadness) that make you uncomfortable in general? Is your approach characterized by demanding standards, fears of being abandoned, concerns about helplessness, or other personal schemas? All of us have our vulnerabilities; the most serious one is not recognizing what yours are.

Second, do certain kinds of patients or problems make you more uncomfortable? What automatic thoughts and assumptions are triggered for you? How would you use cognitive therapy to address these beliefs? What avoidant or compensatory strategies do you use and with which patients? Third, given a specific patient's personal and emotional schemas, how can your behavior as a therapist inadvertently lead to confirmation of the patient's negative beliefs? What would be the consequence for the patient if you confirm these beliefs? How have others in the patient's life confirmed these beliefs?

A fourth step you can take is this: Rather than compensating for or avoiding the patient's emotional schemas, focus on the specific beliefs about emotional regulation that the patient may hold. This is particularly important, because patients who have negative beliefs about their emotions may have seen other therapists who have been overly rational, demanding, and controlling (as in many earlier examples). This approach may have reinforced their negative emotional schemas. The emotional schema approach can help reverse this.

As an emotional schema therapist, you can directly address an avoidant patient's beliefs about emotions by asking the following questions:

"Are there topics or feelings that you find it hard to talk about? What are they?"

"What would you fear would happen if you did talk about these things?"

"You seem vague. Is there an advantage in not specifying what you think or feel?"

"Is it hard for you to identify or label your emotions?"

For instance, avoidant patients might comment that angry and sexual feelings are difficult to discuss, since they fear that they will be criticized and humiliated. In one case, this led to a discussion of how sexual feelings and angry feelings were not discussed in the family during the patient's childhood and adolescence, and that there was a rigid formality in the home, with the parents eating separately and seldom showing affection. Thus sexual feelings became secretive and shameful—and, in the patient's own experience, had been directed toward clandestine phone sex. The patient indicated that he still feared being humiliated and viewed as "less than a man" for his sexual "preoccupations." He also feared that he would lose control over these feelings and that his fantasies would easily lead to sexual acting out, even though this had never happened. His belief that he had to keep a tight control on his fantasies led him to worry about these thoughts and images, which only intensified them. He feared that talking about them would only make them more real. The emotional message from childhood was that he needed to control sexual and aggressive thoughts, images, and feelings, lest they escalate and destroy everything. The therapist suggested that he reframe his fantasies as an indication that he was alive and well, that he enjoyed sexy images about sexy women, and that he could use these fantasies to enrich his sexual relationship with his wife. Rather than try to distract himself from these fantasies, the therapist suggested that he "welcome them in as energy and enrichment" and "note that 'I am alive at this moment.'" His fears were significantly reduced, and he reported less guilt and more sexual desire with his wife.

Another patient characterized by an avoidant personality indicated that remaining vague in his discussion of his thoughts and feelings allowed him to disown them: "If I am vague, then you and I will not really know what I am thinking and feeling. And if we don't know, then I can't be responsible." His fear was that being "clear" would commit him to certain responsibilities for his inner life, and that he would have them to change in ways that would be threatening. Indeed, he also observed that he often "spaced out," seldom mindful of what was present, and that he had a "rich fantasy life" of escape and even heroism. He also commented that it was difficult to label his emotions, and he recalled that emotions were seldom discussed in his family of origin: "The emphasis was on being polite and doing the right thing. In fact, I was an excellent athlete as a kid, but I remember not trying so hard because I didn't want to make the other kids feel that they weren't good enough." In his family, holding up the image of respectability and not threatening others with one's abilities was valued. It is no surprise that anger was an emotion he had difficulty recognizing and tolerating in himself. The therapist suggested that one of the most misleading ideas that people tend to have is that they need to be good in every way at all times. "This idea of being good, pure, and nice goes against human nature. There are so many feelings, urges, thoughts, desires, and resentments that brew in each and every one of us. Owning them as part of human nature can be a great relief." The therapist suggested, "Perhaps you are too good for your own good."

Many avoidant patients also believe that a therapist will criticize them for not doing homework correctly, and as a result the patient is reluctant to do behavioral exposure homework assignments. The therapist might ask such a patient the following questions:

> "What do you fear I might think if you did your homework and it was not perfect?"
> "Is this fear of being evaluated in therapy the same as your fear with other people?"
> "Are you afraid that doing exposure or homework will make you feel uncomfortable?"
> "What will happen if you are uncomfortable?"

These patients will often think that the therapist will be like other people (e.g., their parents) and will criticize them, humiliate them, and compare them unfavorably with others who do better. The therapist can then inquire about the history of being criticized for not doing well enough and how this made the patients feel. One such patient described his mother's continual demands for academic excellence, with frequent criticisms that the patient, as a child, did not get all A's. This led him to resent his mother, but still feel the need for her attention and approval. In his current job, he often personalized the behavior of other people as reflecting their lack of respect for him, derogation of his achievement, or marginalization within the group. On further examination, however, the behavior of others was not actually directed toward him, but was part of the company culture. The "marginalization" that he did experience was primarily due to his own withdrawing, ruminating, and pouting over his imagined exclusion.

A therapist can also directly inquire as to a patient's beliefs about the desirability (or necessity) of avoiding all discomfort. For example, behavioral activation assignments and exposure assignments will often elicit discomfort—and much of the discomfort may stem from the anticipation of discomfort. Rather than label such a patient as noncompliant or not ready for therapy, the therapist can inquire into the patient's predictions about what discomfort will lead to. These predictions can then be tested, as described in earlier chapters. For example, the prediction "I will fall apart if I do the exposure" can be examined for the costs and benefits of the belief and the evidence for and against it. In-session exposure that arouses discomfort can help disconfirm these beliefs. Moreover, the therapist can encourage the patient to refocus from "comfort" to "effectiveness," and to realize that short-term discomfort may be a small price to pay for longer-term self-efficacy. Other possible inquiries regarding avoidance and dependency include the following:

> "What would it mean if you did not get reassurance?"
> "Do you need to know for sure that things will be OK? What if it is uncertain? Does uncertainty mean it will be bad?"

"What is the advantage of not having an agenda?"

"Is the lack of an agenda similar to your lack of goals and plans in life?"

"Do you let other people set the agenda for you?"

"Do you believe that you cannot handle your feelings on your own?"

"What do you typically do when you have unpleasant feelings? Do you get other people to take care of them?"

"Do your feelings make sense to you? Do other people have these feelings? Will your painful feelings go away on their own?"

"If you were not able to get in touch with me, could you use some techniques to handle your thoughts and feelings?"

"What does it mean to you when the session ends before you are ready to end it? Do you feel abandoned? Do you feel angry? Does it make you think I don't care?"

"If I prolong the session, does it mean I care about you?"

"Which part of the homework do you think you can't do?"

"When you start to do something to help yourself, do you give up because you are not sure if you can do it?"

"What would be the worst thing about not doing it correctly?"

"When I go away, what thoughts and feelings are triggered? Do you feel abandoned? Do you think I don't care?"

"Do you think that you are helpless, unable to take care of your feelings?"

"What are some self-help plans that you can use?"

Such inquiries as these open the door to sharing thoughts and feelings, tolerating discomfort, and focusing on effectiveness and personal growth rather than the suppression and elimination of emotion. Therapists who simply impose a set of rules in therapy, or who engage in formulaic therapy—such as imposing an agenda, labeling patients as noncompliant, overdiagnosing rather than empathizing, or attempting to get patients to be rational and happy—will find that patients will drop out, make less progress, or even resent the therapy. In contrast, developing an inquisitive and validating approach to a patient's difficulties can strengthen the collaborative set.

## SUMMARY

The therapeutic relationship may be as important as the therapeutic model. There are effective and ineffective approaches to therapy, and there are productive and unproductive therapeutic relationships. In this chapter, I have reviewed some of the personal and interpersonal schemas that a patient and therapist bring to the therapeutic relationship. "Resistance" or "noncompliance" may be viewed as an opportunity to learn more about the patient's tolerance of frustration, emotional intensity, beliefs about the danger and durability of emotion, and ability to trust the therapist. Therapists who continue to ask themselves about what is going on within themselves (e.g., "Why am I so bothered by this?") are more likely to overcome their own roadblocks in dealing with certain patients. I advise my readers: knowing your own vulnerabilities as a therapist, and working on modifying them—especially on recognizing how your own responses may mirror the responses of others—may help you transcend the limits of your own personal and emotional schemas to help patients enrich their experience in therapy.

# CHAPTER 14

# Conclusions

Similar to other cognitive-behavioral models, the emotional schema model proposes that emotion may arise from situational factors, loss of rewards, aversive factors, cognitive biases, or physiological processes. In other words, the activation of emotion in the first instance may be due to factors that a variety of cognitive and behavioral models might suggest. However, once emotion is aroused, an individual then activates a theory about emotion and a strategy of emotion regulation. These appraisals and strategies constitute "emotional schemas." Depending on the particular appraisals, either problematic strategies (e.g., worry, rumination, blaming, avoidance, bingeing) or adaptive strategies (e.g., reappraisal, problem solving, behavioral activation, acceptance) are utilized. Theories of emotion have implications for strategies of regulation. In the emotional schema model, emotion itself is an object of cognition, and the interpretations, evaluations, and strategies that follow once emotion arises will have significant implications for psychopathology.

The emotional schema model posits that emotions have arisen partly as modular responses to threats that have evolutionary significance, partly as physiological responses, and partly as cognitive biases. Although it acknowledges the significance of each of the major cognitive-behavioral models in developing a case conceptualization of emotion, the emotional schema model adds to these models by suggesting that appraisals of emotions are singularly important in the maintenance, escalation, and recurrent fear of emotional experience. Experiential avoidance is viewed as the result of these problematic appraisals; metacognitive strategies of worry and rumination are also viewed as problematic approaches to emotion regulation; and passivity and isolation are viewed as partly the consequences of beliefs that behavioral activation will result in intolerable emotional experiences. In each of these instances, the emotional schema model advances other models and expands what a therapist may be able to accomplish—that is, changing a patient's theory of emotion and strategies of engagement and regulation.

As indicated in Chapter 1, emotion and rationality have alternately assumed a privileged position throughout the history of Western philosophy and society. Cultural differences in beliefs about emotion—and regulation of emotion—also attest to the social construction of emotional experience. And certain specific emotions, such as jealousy, have also risen and fallen in their desirability in human society; in its earlier history, jealousy had a higher value because it was associated with honor. The emotional schema model does not privilege rationality or emotion; both are viewed as essential, depending on the context and the purpose that one strives for. Moreover, all emotions are viewed as having legitimacy in the human experience, and there is no distinction between "higher" and "lower" mind. Emotions are part of being human.

The emotional schema model does not view the goal of therapy as ridding the patient of sadness, anger, anxiety, or fear, but rather as incorporating these emotions into the full complexity of existence. As Martha Nussbaum (2001) eloquently observed after the death of her mother, not to feel sadness—not to experience the depths of grief—would be inconsistent with affirming her love for her mother. Where there is love, there is grief. One suffers because things matter. The goal that is advocated here is to live a life worth suffering for. Rather than "feeling good," the goal is the capacity to feel *everything* within the context of a meaningful life—one that is filled with sorrow, joy, confusion, doubt, envy, jealousy, courage, and awe. Although some might argue that nothing can be truly "awful" if there is still the possibility of some rewarding experience, we are reminded that the original meaning of the word "awful" is "filled with awe." This is what Herman Melville meant when he wrote to Nathaniel Hawthorne that he had written an "awful" story: It was *Moby Dick*, the story of a symbolic Leviathan in the form of a great white whale. Melville's novel included all the emotions of rage, courage, love, and revenge—and depicted man as challenging and being conquered by nature. It was a book about awe.

The emotional schema model stresses the importance of the ability to do what patients do not want to do, so that they can accomplish what they really need to accomplish. Emotions—and the ability to tolerate discomfort—are placed in the context of a purposeful means–ends relationship: The goal is to learn the ability to endure, to embrace resilience, to take pride in discomfort where it is linked to valued goals. Accordingly, the therapist will emphasize constructive discomfort; pride in enduring and tolerating discomfort; the value of overcoming obstacles, rather than making life easy and pleasant at all times; and the recognition that although life may be a struggle, it is worth the fight. Rather than lowering a patient's expectations so that anything becomes an "achievement," and rather than setting impossible standards that will only demoralize, the emotional schema therapist will emphasize successful imperfection in all areas of life. Moving forward imperfectly, accepting setbacks, and recognizing that no one ever gets things exactly right are all part of the journey and part of the challenge. Perfectionism underlies a great deal of confusion about emotion, including the intolerance of uncertainty and ambivalence, "pure mind," "pure emotion," and "existential perfectionism" (in which the individual seeks out some unattainable ideal of thinking, feeling, and being). In contrast, the emotional schema model assists the patient in recognizing that all experiences in life are temporary, filled with noise and contradiction at times, and part of the changing landscape that one travels on and lives in. The patient who is seeking complete fulfillment or happiness will need to recognize that unpleasant emotions, such as boredom, frustration, anger, jealousy, and envy, are all part of the landscape. This "normalization of the abnormal" is often a great relief for individuals who have come to recognize that life is more complex than they had bargained for. It may be more complex, even disappointing at times, but it may be worth it.

An individual who fears painful emotion may say, "I do not want to fall in love again, since I might get hurt." The consequence is a life without love, without commitment—a life robbed of meaning. The real question should be "Was it worth it to have experienced the pain?" Great commitments involve great pain; there is no way to get out of life without facing disappointment, disillusionment, and ultimately death. The emotional schema model helps patients realize that unpleasant emotions can either be means to an end (as with exposure treatment) or can lead to a long, steady, dull experience, such as isolation or passivity. The therapist can help patients relinquish emotional and existential perfectionism, challenge the idea of "pure mind," and recognize that life contains a lot of noise that people need to push through and move past. By helping patients clarify what they value and how these values affect their relationships, work, and identity, the therapist can assist them in determining what they can find worth working toward. By helping the patients clarify purpose, the therapist can help them endure what is difficult and learn to say, "I am a person who does hard things." The goal is not to make life easy or always to have happy experiences. The goal is to enrich life and make it worth the fight.

Emotional schema therapy does not view emotions as good or bad, but simply as experiences that humans have. These emotions are linked to evolutionary adaptiveness (as in the case of jealousy) and to the values that matter to a patient. Allowing the patient to acknowledge unwanted emotions, such as anger, resentment, jealousy, envy, the desire for revenge, humiliation, and hopelessness, brings these emotions "into the light." They can then be examined as valid and sensible responses at the moment—the "fluttering of the soul" that Plato described. But they can also be viewed as a starting point from which a patient can decide recognizing if these emotions are "human" and "universal," whether they are linked to important values, whether they are temporary, and whether they need to dictate the patient's choices. The ultimate question is always "Now that I feel this way, what is the best choice for me, given what my values are?" The classic view of virtue can help individuals decide. In particular, it can help them break away from the entrapment of a negative emotion and choose self-control, kindness, forgiveness, or prudence over the emotion of the present moment. Indeed, these choices can change the emotion that is experienced, once again demonstrating that emotions come and go, but one's values may endure.

Emotional schema therapy is not a model of catharsis or expression. It suggests that simply ventilating an emotion may be insufficient if this is not linked to validation and purposeful action. Moreover, unskilled ventilation, marked by blaming, rumination, and escalating affect, may serve to alienate valued support. The emotional schema model recognizes that validation can address a wide range of emotional schemas. It can also help patients universalize and make sense of emotion, experience an emotion and observe it subsiding, and realize that having an emotion need not lead to loss of control. Thus validation has a number of cognitive implications, making it a central process in developing more adaptive beliefs and responses to the experience of emotion.

Emotions are often the core element in intimate relationships. Not to recognize the importance of one's partner's emotions is to live a life in parallel, never truly touching. Thinking about the partner's emotions as a "goal" ("How do I want my partner to feel?") allows individuals to step outside fruitless struggles for the facts, for power, or for being heard above all else. It can connect partners in a mutual exercise in "mentalization," where both partners understand that the mind (thoughts and feelings) of each partner is important and can be affected by how the other partner responds. In some cases, even the nature of simple conversation reflects this lack of understanding: Some people think that conversation is an exchange of information, but what most conversation entails is taking turns being heard. Changing the metaphor for conversation from "pointing to the facts as if they are a landscape of information" to "passing the ball back and forth" can help modify endless struggles about getting the facts "right." It may be less important what the facts are and more important that the partners are taking turns. We have seen that one partner can put up considerable resistance to validating the other partner, marked by beliefs that "facts" need to be established, that relationships are about seeking the "truth," that the resistant partner has a monopoly on the truth, and that validation will only lead to endless complaining. An alternative is to view communication as an attempt to connect, and until the connection is made (and felt to be secure), the complaining will continue—and escalate. Thus the emotional schema model views communication and emotion as part of an ongoing interactive behavioral system that seeks completion—sometimes at high cost.

Similarly, patients and therapists may find themselves locked in struggles about the meaning and regulation of emotion. Therapists come to therapy with their own schemas about relationships and about emotions. If they view emotional expression as a waste of time and view their patients' role as requiring compliance to agendas, the patients may interpret these responses as dismissive, condescending, and critical, further verifying their negative beliefs about their emotions and how others see these. Even well-intentioned, experienced, and well-trained therapists will have specific beliefs about emotions that may affect the willingness to validate, encourage "unpleasant" exposure, or raise topics that may be troubling to patients. The concept of "schematic mismatch" allows therapists to evaluate the emotional and personal schemas that both patients and therapists may have, and can prevent the therapists from getting "carried away" by predetermined biases. Indeed, a mismatch experience may be a unique opportunity to inquire, "When has this happened before?" This model allows cognitive-behavioral therapists to address the issues of "transference" and "countertransference" in new ways, while recognizing that therapy can still find the balance between focusing on the current experience while recognizing the importance of all that has happened before. Moreover, a therapist who often feels caught up in a patient's emotions—especially the patient's anger or intense anxiety—may recognize that the boundaries that can exist between patient and therapist may be necessary for effective treatment to proceed, but do not preclude empathy and compassion. It may be difficult to have empathy and compassion when one is being criticized, but it may be the first time that the patient's anger has been confronted with acceptance. Knowing that the emotion exists in the other person may help the patient avoid "contagion." Standing back with detached, mindful acceptance may assist the patient in taking the next steps toward inquiry, validation, and acceptance.

Certainly you, my readers, will realize the debt that the emotional schema model owes to a wide range of cognitive-behavioral models. You can see the influence of Beckian cognitive therapy, metacognitive therapy, emotion-focused therapy, ACT, DBT, and behavioral activation therapy. You can choose to approach your patients with any of these models and consider integrating the emotional schema model with the chosen model(s), or you can approach your patients with the emotional schema model while using any or all of the other approaches. This is not a model that replaces what has already been accomplished by others. It is one that seeks to enrich, inform, broaden, and empower.

# References

Abramson, L. Y., Metalsky, G. I., & Alloy, L. B. (1989). Hopelessness depression: A theory-based subtype of depression. *Psychological Review, 96*, 358–372.

Ahrens, A. H., & Alloy, L. B. (1997). Social comparison processes in depression. In B. Buunk & R. Gibbons (Eds.), *Health, coping, and well-being: Perspectives from social comparison theory* (pp. 389–410). Mahwah, NJ: Erlbaum.

Ainsworth, M. S., Blehar, M. C., Waters, E., & Wall, S. (1978). *Patterns of attachment: A psychological study of the Strange Situation.* Hillsdale, NJ: Erlbaum.

Aldao, A., & Nolen-Hoeksema, S. (2010). Specificity of cognitive emotion regulation strategies: A transdiagnostic examination. *Behaviour Research and Therapy, 48*(10), 974–983.

Aldao, A., & Nolen-Hoeksema, S. (2012a). The influence of context on the implementation of adaptive emotion regulation strategies. *Behaviour Research and Therapy, 50*, 493–501.

Aldao, A., & Nolen-Hoeksema, S. (2012b). When are adaptive strategies most predictive of psychopathology? *Journal of Abnormal Psychology, 121*(1), 276–281.

Alloy, L. B., Abramson, L. Y., Metalsky, G. I., & Hartledge, S. (1988). The hopelessness theory of depression. *British Journal of Clinical Psychology, 27*, 5–12.

Ameli, R. (2014). *25 lessons in mindfulness: Now time for healthy living.* Washington, DC: American Psychological Association.

Arend, R. A., Gove, F. L., & Sroufe, L. A. (1979). Continuity of individual adaptation from infancy to kindergarten: A predictive study of ego-resiliency and curiosity in preschoolers. *Child Development, 50*, 950–959.

Ariès, P. (1962). *Centuries of childhood: A social history of family life.* New York: Random House.

Aristotle. (1984). *The rhetoric and poetics of Aristotle.* New York: Random House.

Aristotle. (1995). *Aristotle: Selections* (T. Irwin & G. Fine, Eds.). Indianapolis, IN: Hackett.

Arntz, A., & Haaf, J. (2012). Social cognition in borderline personality disorder: Evidence for dichotomous thinking but no evidence for less complex attributions. *Behaviour Research and Therapy, 50*(11), 707–718.

Austin, J. L. (1975). *How to do things with words* (2nd ed.). Cambridge, MA: Harvard University Press.

Ayer, A. J. (1946). *Language, truth, and logic* (2nd ed.). London: Gollancz.

Baldwin, M. W., & Dandeneau, S. D. (2005). Understanding and modifying the relational schemas underlying insecurity. In M. W. Baldwin (Ed.), *Interpersonal cognition* (pp. 33–61). New York: Guilford Press.

Bar-Anan, Y., Wilson, T. D., & Gilbert, D. T. (2009). The feeling of uncertainty intensifies affective reactions. *Emotion, 9*(1), 123–127.

Bargh, J. A., & Morsella, E. (2008). The unconscious mind. *Perspectives on Psychological Science, 3*(1), 73–79.

Barlow, D. H. (2002). *Anxiety and its disorders: The nature and treatment of anxiety and panic* (2nd ed.). New York: Guilford Press.

Bateman, A., & Fonagy, P. (2004). *Psychotherapy for borderline personality disorder: Mentalization-based treatment.* Oxford, UK: Oxford University Press.

Bateman, A., & Fonagy, P. (2006). *Mentalization-based treatment for borderline personality disorder: A practical guide.* Oxford, UK: Oxford University Press.

Beck, A. T., Emery, G., & Greenberg, R. L. (1985). *Anxiety disorders and phobias: A cognitive perspective.* New York: Basic Books.

Beck, A. T., Freeman, A., & Davis, D. D. (2004). *Cognitive therapy of personality disorders* (2nd ed.). New York: Guilford Press.

Beck, A. T., Rush, A. J., Shaw, B. F., & Emery, G. (1979). *Cognitive therapy of depression.* New York: Guilford Press.

Beck, A. T., & Steer, R. A. (1993). *Beck Anxiety Inventory manual.* San Antonio, TX: Psychological Corporation.

Beck, A. T., Steer, R. A., & Brown, G. K. (1996). *Manual for the Beck Depression Inventory–II.* San Antonio, TX: Psychological Corporation.

Beck, J. S. (2011). *Cognitive therapy: Basics and beyond* (2nd ed.). New York: Guilford Press.

Becker, G. S. (1976). *The economic approach to human behavior.* Chicago: University of Chicago Press.

Becker, G. S. (1991). *A treatise on the family.* Cambridge, MA: Harvard University Press.

Bishay, N. R., Tarrier, N., Dolan, M., Beckett, R., & Harwood, S. (1996). Morbid jealousy: A cognitive outlook. *Journal of Cognitive Psychotherapy, 10,* 9–22.

Blackledge, J. T., & Hayes, S. C. (2001). Emotion regulation in acceptance and commitment therapy. *Journal of Clinical Psychology, 57*(2), 243–255.

Blanchard, D. C., & Blanchard, R. J. (1990). Behavioral correlates of chronic dominance-subordination relationships of male rats in a seminatural situation. *Neuroscience and Biobehavioral Reviews, 14,* 455–462.

Boehm, C. (2001). *Hierarchy in the forest: The evolution of egalitarian behavior.* Cambridge, MA: Harvard University Press.

Bonanno, G. A., & Burton, C. L. (2013). Regulatory flexibility: An individual differences perspective on coping and emotion regulation. *Perspectives on Psychological Science, 8*(6), 591–612.

Bonanno, G. A., & Gupta, S. (2009). Resilience after disaster. In Y. Neria, S. Galea, & F. Norris (Eds.), *Mental health consequences of disasters* (pp. 145–160). New York: Cambridge University Press.

Bond, F. W., Hayes, S. C., Baer, R. A., Carpenter, K. C., Guenole, N., Orcutt, H. K., et al. (2011). Preliminary psychometric properties of the Acceptance and Action Questionnaire–II: A revised measure of psychological flexibility and acceptance. *Behavior Therapy, 42*, 676–688.

Borkovec, T. D. (1994). The nature, functions, and origins of worry. In G. C. L. Davey & F. Tallis (Eds.), *Worrying: Perspectives on theory, assessment, and treatment* (pp. 5–33). Chichester, UK: Wiley.

Borkovec, T. D., Alcaine, O. M., & Behar, E. (2004). Avoidance theory of worry and generalized anxiety disorder. In R. G. Heimberg, C. L. Turk, & D. S. Mennin (Eds.), *Generalized anxiety disorder: Advances in research and practice* (pp. 77–108). New York: Guilford Press.

Borkovec, T. D., Lyonfields, J. D., Wiser, S. L., & Deihl, L. (1993). The role of worrisome thinking in the suppression of cardiovascular response to phobic imagery. *Behaviour Research and Therapy, 31*, 321–324.

Borkovec, T. D., Newman, M. G., & Castonguay, L. G. (2003). Cognitive-behavioral therapy for generalized anxiety disorder with integrations from interpersonal and experiential therapies. *CNS Spectrums, 8*(5), 382–389.

Borkovec, T. D., Ray, W. J., & Stoeber, J. (1998). Worry: A cognitive phenomenon intimately linked to affective, physiological, and interpersonal behavioral processes. *Cognitive Therapy and Research, 22*, 561–576.

Bowlby, J. (1969). *Attachment and loss: Vol. 1. Attachment.* London: Hogarth Press.

Bowlby, J. (1973). *Attachment and loss: Vol. 2. Separation.* London: Hogarth Press.

Bowlby, J. (1980). *Attachment and loss: Vol. 3. Sadness and depression.* London: Hogarth Press.

Brickman, P., & Campbell, D. T. (1971). Hedonic relativism and planning the good society. In M. H. Apley (Ed.), *Adaptation-level theory: A symposium* (pp. 287–302). New York: Academic Press.

Brigham, N. L., Kelso, K. A., Jackson, M. A., & Smith, R. H. (1997). The roles of invidious comparisons and deservingness in sympathy and *Schadenfreude. Basic and Applied Social Psychology, 19*, 363–380.

Brown, L. (Ed.). (2009). *Aristotle: The Nicomachean ethics* (D. Ross, Trans.). New York: Oxford University Press.

Buss, D. M. (1989). Conflict between the sexes: Strategic interference and the evocation of anger and upset. *Journal of Personality and Social Psychology, 56*, 735–747.

Buss, D. M. (2000). *Dangerous passion: Why jealousy is as necessary as love and sex.* New York: Free Press.

Buss, D. M., Larsen, R., Westen, D., & Semmelroth, J. (1992). Sex differences in jealousy: Evolution, physiology, and psychology. *Psychological Science, 3*, 251–255.

Buss, D. M., & Schmitt, D. P. (1993). Sexual strategies theory: An evolutionary perspective on human mating. *Psychological Review, 100*(2), 204–232.

Butler, R. (1963). The life review: An interpretation of reminiscence in the aged. *Psychiatry, 26*, 65–76.

Buunk, B. (1981). Jealousy in sexually open marriages. *Alternative Lifestyles, 4*, 357–372.

Carnap, R. (1967). *The logical structure of the world.* Berkeley: University of California Press.

Cassidy, J. (1995). Attachment and generalized anxiety disorder. In D. Cicchetti & S. L. Toth (Eds.), *Rochester Symposium on Developmental Psychopathology: Vol. 6. Emotion, cognition, and representation* (pp. 343–370). Rochester, NY: University of Rochester Press.

Castella, K. D., Goldin, P., Jazaieri, H., Ziv, M., Dweck, C. S., & Gross, J. J. (2013). Beliefs about emotion: Links to emotion regulation, well-being, and psychological distress. *Basic and Applied Social Psychology, 35*(6), 497–505.

Chesterfield, P. D. S. (2008). *Lord Chesterfield's letters.* Oxford, UK: Oxford University Press. (Original work published 1776)

Chiu, C.-Y., Hong, Y.-Y., & Dweck, C. S. (1997). Lay dispositionism and implicit theories of personality. *Journal of Personality and Social Psychology, 73*(1), 19–30.

Clark, D. A., & Beck, A. T. (2010). *Cognitive therapy of anxiety disorders: Science and practice.* New York: Guilford Press.

Clark, D. M. (1996). Panic disorder: From theory to therapy. In P. M. Salkovskis (Ed.), *Frontiers of cognitive therapy* (pp. 318–344). New York: Guilford Press.

Clark, D. M. (1999). Anxiety disorders: Why they persist and how to treat them. *Behaviour Research and Therapy, 37*, S5–S27.

Clark, D. M., Salkovskis, P. M., & Chalkley, A. (1985). Respiratory control as a treatment for panic attacks. *Journal of Behavior Therapy and Experimental Psychiatry, 16*(1), 23–30.

Clark, D. M., Salkovskis, P. M., Hackmann, A., Wells, A., Ludgate, J., & Gelder, M. (1999). Brief cognitive therapy for panic disorder: A randomized controlled trial. *Journal of Consulting and Clinical Psychology, 67*(4), 583–589.

Cosmides, L., & Tooby, J. (2002). Unraveling the enigma of human intelligence: Evolutionary psychology and the multimodular mind. In R. J. Sternberg & J. C. Kaufman (Eds.), *The evolution of intelligence* (pp. 145–198). Mahwah, NJ: Erlbaum.

Crusius, J., & Mussweiler, T. (2012). When people want what others have: The impulsive side of envious desire. *Emotion, 12*(1), 142–153.

Daly, M., & Wilson, M. (1988). *Homicide.* New York: Aldine de Gruyter.

Darwin, C. (1965). *The expression of the emotions in man and animals.* Chicago: University of Chicago Press. (Original work published 1872)

Davidson, R. J., & McEwen, B. S. (2012). Social influences on neuroplasticity: Stress and interventions to promote well-being. *Nature Neuroscience, 15*(5), 689–695.

De Botton, A. (2004). *Status anxiety.* New York: Vintage.

de Unamuno, M. (1954). *Tragic sense of life* (J. E. Crawford Fitch, Trans.). Mineola, NY: Dover. (Original work published 1921)

De Wolff, M. S., & van IJzendoorn, M. H. (1997). Sensitivity and attachment: A meta-analysis on parental antecedents of infant attachment. *Child Development, 68*(4), 571–591.

Deutsch, H. (1944–1945). *The psychology of women: A psychoanalytic interpretation* (Vols. 1–2). New York: Grune & Stratton.

Dolan, M., & Bishay, N. (1996). The effectiveness of cognitive therapy in the treatment of non-psychotic morbid jealousy. *British Journal of Psychiatry, 168*(5), 588–593.

Dollard, J., & Miller, N. E. (1950). *Personality and psychotherapy: An analysis in terms of learning, thinking, and culture.* New York: McGraw-Hill.

Donnellan, M. B., Burt, S. A., Levendosky, A. A., & Klump, K. L. (2008). Genes, personality, and attachment in adults: A multivariate behavioral genetic analysis. *Personality and Social Psychology Bulletin, 34*(1), 3–16.

Dugas, M. J., Buhr, K., & Ladouceur, R. (2004). The role of intolerance of uncertainty in the etiology and maintenance of generalized anxiety disorder. In R. G. Heimberg, C. L. Turk, & D. S. Mennin (Eds.), *Generalized anxiety disorder: Advances in research and practice* (pp. 143–163). New York: Guilford Press.

Dugas, M. J., Freeston, M. H., & Ladouceur, R. (1997). Intolerance of uncertainty and problem orientation in worry. *Cognitive Therapy and Research, 21*(6), 593–606.

Dugas, M. J., Gosselin, P., & Ladouceur, R. (2001). Intolerance of uncertainty and worry: Investigating specificity in a nonclinical sample. *Cognitive Therapy and Research, 25,* 13–22.

Dunbar, R. I. M. (1998). *Grooming, gossip, and the evolution of language.* Cambridge, MA: Harvard University Press.

Dunbar, R. I. M. (2012). *The science of love and betrayal.* London: Faber & Faber.

Dunsmore, J. C., & Halberstadt, A. G. (1997). How does family emotional expressiveness affect children's schemas? In K. C. Barrett (Ed.), *New directions for child development: No. 77. The communication of emotion: Current research from diverse perspectives* (pp. 45–68). San Francisco: Jossey-Bass.

Dutton, D. G., van Ginkel, C., & Landolt, M. A. (1996). Jealousy, intimate abusiveness, and intrusiveness. *Journal of Family Violence, 11*(4), 411–423.

Dweck, C. S. (2000). *Self-theories: Their role in motivation, personality and development.* Philadelphia: Psychology Press.

Dweck, C. S. (2006). *Mindset: The new psychology of success.* New York: Random House.

Eibl-Eibesfeldt, I. (1972). *Love and hate: The natural history of behavior patterns.* New York: Holt.

Eisenberg, N., Cumberland, A., & Spinrad, T. L. (1998). Parental socialization of emotion. *Psychological Inquiry, 9*(4), 241–273.

Eisenberg, N., & Fabes, R. A. (1994). Mothers' reactions to children's negative emotions: Relations to children's temperament and anger behavior. *Merrill–Palmer Quarterly, 40*(1), 138–156.

Eisenberg, N., & Spinrad, T. L. (2004). Emotion-related regulation: Sharpening the definition. *Child Development, 75*(2), 334–339.

Elias, N. (2000). *The civilizing process: Sociogenetic and psychogenetic investigations* (rev. ed.). Oxford: Blackwell. (Original work published 1939)

Elicker, J., Englund, M., & Sroufe, L. A. (1992). Predicting peer competence and peer relationships in childhood from early parent–child relationships. In R. Parke & G. Ladd (Eds.), *Family–peer relationships: Modes of linkage* (pp. 77–106). Hillsdale, NJ: Erlbaum.

Ellis, A. (1994). *Reason and emotion in psychotherapy* (2nd ed.). Secaucus, NJ: Carol.

Ellis, A. (1996). The treatment of morbid jealousy: A rational emotive behavior therapy approach. *Journal of Cognitive Psychotherapy, 10*(1), 23–33.

Ellis, A., & Harper, R. A. (1975). *A new guide to rational living.* Englewood Cliffs, NJ: Prentice-Hall.

Emmons, R. A., & Mishra, A. (2011). Why gratitude enhances well-being: What we know, what we need to know. In K. Sheldon, T. B. Kashdan, & M. F. Steger (Eds.), *Designing positive psychology: Taking stock and moving forward* (pp. 248–262). New York: Oxford University Press.

Englund, M. M., Kuo, S. I., Puig, J., & Collins, W. A. (2012). Early roots of adult competence: The significance of close relationships from infancy to early adulthood. *International Journal of Behavioral Development, 35,* 490–496.

Epstein, S., & O'Brien, E. J. (1985). The person–situation debate in historical and current perspective. *Psychological Bulletin, 98*(3), 513–537.

Erickson, T. M., & Newman, M. G. (2007). Interpersonal and emotional processes in generalized anxiety disorder analogues during social interaction tasks. *Behavior Therapy, 38*(4), 364–377.

Ermer, E., Guerin, S. A., Cosmides, L., Tooby, J., & Miller, M. B. (2006). Theory of mind broad and narrow: Reasoning about social exchange engages ToM areas, precautionary reasoning does not. *Social Neuroscience, 1*(3–4), 196–219.

Euripides. (1920). *The Bacchae of Euripides.* New York: Longmans, Green.

Feeney, B. C., & Thrush, R. L. (2010). Relationship influences on exploration in adulthood: The characteristics and function of a secure base. *Journal of Personality and Social Psychology, 98*(1), 57–76.

Festinger, L. (1957). *A theory of cognitive dissonance.* Palo Alto, CA: Stanford University Press.

Field, T., Sandberg, D., Garcia, R., Vega-Lahr, N., Goldstein, S., & Guy, L. (1985). Pregnancy problems, postpartum depression, and early mother–infant interactions. *Developmental Psychology, 21*(6), 1152–1156.

Finucane, M., Alhakami, A., Slovic, P., & Johnson, S. (2000). The affect heuristic in judgments of risks and benefits. *Journal of Behavioral Decision Making, 13,* 1–13.

Fiske, S. T. (2010). Envy up, scorn down: How comparison divides us. *American Psychologist, 65*(8), 698–706.

Fleeson, W., & Noftle, E. E. (2009). The end of the person–situation debate: An emerging synthesis in the answer to the consistency question. *Social and Personality Psychology Compass, 2*(4), 1667–1684.

Foa, E. B., & Kozak, M. J. (1986). Emotional processing of fear: Exposure to corrective information. *Psychological Bulletin, 99,* 20–35.

Fonagy, P. (1989). On tolerating mental states: Theory of mind in borderline patients. *Bulletin of the Anna Freud Centre, 12,* 91–115.

Fonagy, P. (2002). *Affect regulation, mentalization, and the development of the self.* New York: Other Press.

Fonagy, P., & Target, M. (2006). The mentalization-focused approach to self pathology. *Journal of Personality Disorders, 20*(6), 544–576.

Forgas, J. P. (1995). Mood and judgment: The affect infusion model (AIM). *Psychological Bulletin, 117*(1), 39–66.

Fraley, R. C., Waller, N. G., & Brennan, K. A. (2000). An item-response theory analysis of self-report measures of adult attachment. *Journal of Personality and Social Psychology, 78,* 350–365.

Frankl, V. E. (1959). The spiritual dimension in existential analysis and logotherapy. *Journal of Individual Psychology, 15,* 157–165.

Frankl, V. E. (1963). *Man's search for meaning: An introduction to logotherapy.* Boston: Beacon Press.

Franklin, B. (1914). *Poor Richard's almanac.* Waterloo, IA: U.S.C. Publishing. (Original work published 1759)

Frederick, S., Loewenstein, G., & O'Donoghue, T. (2002). Time discounting and time preference: A critical review. *Journal of Economic Literature, 40,* 351–401.

Fredrickson, B. L. (1998). What good are positive emotions? *Review of General Psychology, 2,* 300–319.

Fredrickson, B. L. (2004). Gratitude (like other positive emotions) broadens and builds. In R. A. Emmons & M. E. McCullough (Eds.), *The psychology of gratitude* (pp. 145–166). New York: Oxford University Press.

Fredrickson, B. L. (2013). Positive emotions broaden and build. In P. G. Devine & E. A. Plant (Eds.), *Advances in experimental social psychology* (Vol. 47, pp. 1–53). Burlington, MA: Academic Press.

Fredrickson, B. L., Cohn, M. A., Coffey, K. A., Pek, J., & Finkel, S. M. (2008). Open hearts build lives: Positive emotions, induced through loving-kindness meditation, build consequential personal resources. *Journal of Personality and Social Psychology, 95,* 1045–1062.

Froh, J. J., Emmons, R. A., Card, N. A., Bono, G., & Wilson, J. A. (2011). Gratitude and the reduced costs of materialism in adolescents. *Journal of Happiness Studies, 12*(2), 289–302.

Fromm, E. (1976). *To have or to be?* New York: Harper & Row.

Funder, D. C., & Colvin, C. R. (1991). Explorations in behavioral consistency: Properties of persons, situations, and behaviors. *Journal of Personality and Social Psychology, 60,* 773–794.

Gay, P. (2013). *The Enlightenment: The science of freedom* (Vol. 2. Enlightenment: An interpretation). New York: Norton.

Gigerenzer, G., & Selten, R. (2001). *Bounded rationality: The adaptive toolbox.* Cambridge, MA: MIT Press.

Gilbert, D. T., Driver-Linn, E., & Wilson, T. D. (2002). The trouble with Vronsky: Impact bias in the forecasting of future affective states. In L. F. Barrett & P. Salovey (Eds.), *The wisdom in feeling: Psychological processes in emotional intelligence* (pp. 114–143). New York: Guilford Press.

Gilbert, D. T., Pinel, E. C., Wilson, T. D., Blumberg, S. J., & Wheatley, T. P. (1998). Immune neglect: A source of durability bias in affective forecasting. *Journal of Personality and Social Psychology, 75*(3), 617–638.

Gilbert, P. (1989). *Human nature and suffering.* Hove, UK: Erlbaum.

Gilbert, P. (1990). Changes: Rank, status and mood. In S. Fischer & C. L. Cooper (Eds.), *On the move: The psychology of change and transition* (pp. 33–52). New York: Wiley.

Gilbert, P. (1992). *Counselling for depression.* London: Sage.

Gilbert, P. (1992). *Depression: The evolution of powerlessness.* Hove, UK: Erlbaum.

Gilbert, P. (2000a). Social mentalities: Internal "social" conflict and the role of inner warmth and compassion in cognitive therapy. In P. Gilbert & K. G. Kent (Eds.), *Genes on the couch: Explorations in evolutionary psychotherapy* (pp. 118–150). Hove, UK: Brunner-Routledge.

Gilbert, P. (2000b). Varieties of submissive behavior as forms of social defense: Their evolution and role in depression. In L. Sloman & P. Gilbert (Eds.), *Subordination and defeat: An evolutionary approach to mood disorders and their therapy* (pp. 3–46). Mahwah, NJ: Erlbaum.

Gilbert, P. (2003). Evolution, social roles and the differences in shame and guilt. *Social Research, 70,* 401–426.

Gilbert, P. (Ed.). (2005). *Compassion: Conceptualisations, research and use in psychotherapy.* Hove, UK: Routledge.

Gilbert, P. (2007). Evolved minds and compassion in the therapeutic relationship. In P. Gilbert & R. L. Leahy (Eds.), *The therapeutic relationship in the cognitive behavioural psychotherapies* (pp. 106–142). Hove, UK: Routledge.

Gilbert, P. (2009). *The compassionate mind.* London: Constable.

Gilbert, P., & Allen, S. (1998). The role of defeat and entrapment (arrested flight) in depression: An exploration of an evolutionary view. *Psychological Medicine, 28,* 585–598.

Gilbert, P., & Irons, C. (2005). Focused therapies and compassionate mind training for shame and self-attacking. In P. Gilbert (Ed.), *Compassion: Conceptualisations, research and use in psychotherapy* (pp. 263–326). Hove, UK: Routledge.

Gottman, J. M., Katz, L. F., & Hooven, C. (1996). Parental meta-emotion philosophy and the emotional life of families: Theoretical models and preliminary data. *Journal of Family Psychology, 10*(3), 243–268.

Gottman, J. M., Katz, L. F., & Hooven, C. (1997). *Meta-emotion: How families communicate emotionally.* Mahwah, NJ: Erlbaum.

Gottman, J. M., & Krokoff, L. J. (1989). Marital interaction and satisfaction: A longitudinal view. *Journal of Consulting and Clinical Psychology, 57*(1), 47–52.

Greenberg, L. S. (2001). *Toward an integrated affective, behavioral, cognitive psychotherapy for the new millennium.* Paper presented at the meeting of the Society for the Exploration of Psychotherapy Integration, Washington, DC.

Greenberg, L. S. (2002). *Emotion-focused therapy: Coaching clients to work through their feelings.* Washington, DC: American Psychological Association.

Greenberg, L. S. (2007). Emotion in the therapeutic relationship in emotion-focused therapy. In P. L. Gilbert & R. L. Leahy (Eds.), *The therapeutic relationship in the cognitive behavioural psychotherapies* (pp. 43–62). Hove, UK: Routledge.

Greenberg, L. S., & Paivio, S. C. (1997). *Working with emotions in psychotherapy.* New York: Guilford Press.

Greenberg, L. S., & Safran, J. D. (1987). *Emotion in psychotherapy: Affect, cognition, and the process of change.* New York: Guilford Press.

Greenberg, L. S., & Safran, J. D. (1989). Emotion in psychotherapy. *American Psychologist, 44*(1), 19–29.

Greenberg, L. S., & Safran, J. D. (1990). Emotional-change processes in psychotherapy. In R. Plutchik & H. Kellerman (Eds.), *Emotion: Theory, research, and experience: Vol. 5. Emotion, psychopathology, and psychotherapy* (pp. 59–85). San Diego, CA: Academic Press.

Greenberg, L. S., & Watson, J. C. (2005). *Emotion-focused therapy for depression.* Washington, DC: American Psychological Association.

Gross, J. J. (1998). Antecedent- and response-focused emotion regulation: Divergent consequences for experience, expression, and physiology. *Journal of Personality and Social Psychology, 74*(1), 224–237.

Gross, J. J. (2002). Emotion regulation: Affective, cognitive, and social consequences. *Psychophysiology, 39*(3), 281–291.

Gross, J. J., & John, O. P. (1997). Revealing feelings: Facets of emotional expressivity in self-reports, peer ratings, and behavior. *Journal of Personality and Social Psychology, 72*(2), 435–448.

Gross, J. J., & John, O. P. (2003). Individual differences in two emotion regulation processes: Implications for affect, relationships, and well-being. *Journal of Personality and Social Psychology, 85*, 348–362.

Grossman, M., Chaloupka, F. J., & Sirtalan, I. (1998). An empirical analysis of alcohol addiction: Results from the Monitoring the Future panels. *Economic Inquiry, 36*(1), 39–48.

Guerrero, L. K., & Afifi, W. A. (1999). Toward a goal-oriented approach for understanding communicative responses to jealousy. *Western Journal of Communication, 63*(2), 216–249.

Hackmann, A. (2005). Compassionate imagery in the treatment of early memories in Axis I anxiety disorders. In P. Gilbert (Ed.), *Compassion: Conceptualisations, research and use in psychotherapy* (pp. 352–368). Hove, UK: Routledge.

Halberstadt, A. G., Dunsmore, J. C., Bryant, A., Jr., Parker, A. E., Beale, K. S., & Thompson, J. A. (2013). Development and validation of the Parents' Beliefs About Children's Emotions questionnaire. *Psychological Assessment, 25*(4), 1195–1210.

Hanish, L. D., Eisenberg, N., Fabes, R. A., Spinrad, T. L., Ryan, P., & Schmidt, S. (2004). The expression and regulation of negative emotions: Risk factors for young children's peer victimization. *Development and Psychopathology, 16*(2), 335–353.

Hansen, G. L. (1982). Reactions to hypothetical, jealousy producing events. *Family Relations, 31*, 513–518.

Hassin, R. R., Uleman, J. S., & Bargh, J. A. (2005). *The new unconscious.* New York: Oxford University Press.

Hawkley, L. C., & Cacioppo, J. T. (2010). Loneliness matters: A theoretical and empirical review of consequences and mechanisms. *Annals of Behavioral Medicine, 40*(2), 218–227.

Hayes, S. C. (2002). Acceptance, mindfulness, and science. *Clinical Psychology: Science and Practice, 9*(1), 101–106.

Hayes, S. C. (2004). Acceptance and commitment therapy, relational frame theory, and the third wave of behavioral and cognitive therapies. *Behavior Therapy, 35*, 639–665.

Hayes, S. C., Jacobson, N. S., & Follette, V. M. (Eds.). (1994). *Acceptance and change: Content and context in psychotherapy.* Reno, NV: Context Press.

Hayes, S. C., Levin, M., Plumb-Vilardaga, J., Villatte, J., & Pistorello, J. (2013). Acceptance and commitment therapy and contextual behavioral science: Examining the progress of a distinctive model of behavioral and cognitive therapy. *Behavior Therapy, 44*(2), 180–198.

Hayes, S. C., Luoma, J. B., Bond, F. W., Masuda, A., & Lillis, J. (2006). Acceptance and commitment therapy: Model, processes and outcomes. *Behaviour Research and Therapy, 44*(1), 1–25.

Hayes, S. C., Strosahl, K. D., & Wilson, K. G. (2003). *Acceptance and commitment therapy: An experiential approach to behavior change.* New York: Guilford Press.

Hayes, S. C., Strosahl, K. D., & Wilson, K. G. (2012). *Acceptance and commitment therapy: The process and practice of mindful change* (2nd ed.). New York: Guilford Press.

Hayes, S. C., Strosahl, K. D., Wilson, K. G., Bissett, R. T., Pistorello, J., Toarmino, D., et al. (2004). Measuring experiential avoidance: A preliminary test of a working model. *Psychological Record, 54*, 553–578.

Hayes, S. C., Wilson, K. G., Gifford, E. V., Follette, V. M., & Strosahl, K. (1996). Experiential avoidance and behavioral disorders: A functional approach to diagnosis and treatment. *Journal of Consulting and Clinical Psychology, 64*, 1152–1168.

Hazan, C., & Shaver, P. (1987). Romantic love conceptualized as an attachment process. *Journal of Personality and Social Psychology, 52*(3), 511–524.

Heidegger, M. (1962). *Being and time.* New York: Harper & Row.

Heider, F. (1958). *The psychology of interpersonal relations.* New York: Wiley.

Heimberg, R. G., Turk, C. L., & Mennin, D. S. (Eds.). (2004). *Generalized anxiety disorder: Advances in research and practice.* New York: Guilford Press.

Hernandez-Reif, M., Field, T., Ironson, G., Beutler, J., Vera, Y., Hurley, J., et al. (2005). Natural killer cells and lymphocytes increase in women with breast cancer following massage therapy. *International Journal of Neuroscience, 115*(4), 495–510.

Hernandez-Reif, M., Field, T., Largie, S., Diego, M., Manigat, N., Seoanes, J., et al. (2005). Cerebral palsy symptoms in children decreased following massage therapy. *Early Child Development and Care, 175*(5), 445–456.

Hertenstein, M. J., Keltner, D., App, B., Bulleit, B. A., & Jaskolka, A. R. (2006). Touch communicates distinct emotions. *Emotion, 6*(3), 528–533.

Hill, S. E., & Buss, D. M. (2006). Envy and positional bias in the evolutionary psychology of management. *Managerial and Decision Economics, 27*, 131–143.

Hill, S. E., & Buss, D. M. (2008). The evolutionary psychology of envy. In R. H. Smith (Ed.), *Envy: Theory and research* (pp. 60–70). New York: Oxford University Press.

Hill, S. E., DelPriore, D. J., & Vaughan, P. W. (2011). The cognitive consequences of envy: Attention, memory, and self-regulatory depletion. *Journal of Personality and Social Psychology, 101*(4), 653–666.

Hofmann, S. G., Alpers, G. W., & Pauli, P. (2009). Phenomenology of panic and phobic disorders. In M. M. Antony & M. Stein (Eds.), *Oxford handbook of anxiety and related disorders* (pp. 34–46). New York: Oxford University Press.

Ingram, R. E., Atchley, R. A., & Segal, Z. V. (2011). *Vulnerability to depression: From cognitive neuroscience to prevention and treatment.* New York: Guilford Press.

Inwood, B. (Ed.). (2003). *The Cambridge companion to the Stoics.* Cambridge, UK: Cambridge University Press.

Ironson, G., Field, T., Scafidi, F., Hashimoto, M., Kumar, M., Kumar, A., et al. (1996). Massage therapy is associated with enhancement of the immune system's cytotoxic capacity. *International Journal of Neuroscience, 84*(1–4), 205–217.

Job, V., Dweck, C. S., & Walton, G. M. (2010). Ego depletion—is it all in your head?: Implicit theories about willpower affect self-regulation. *Psychological Science, 21*(11), 1686–1693.

Johnson, S. L., Leedom, L. J., & Muhtadie, L. (2012). The dominance behavioral system and psychopathology: Evidence from self-report, observational, and biological studies. *Psychological Bulletin, 138*(4), 692–743.

Joiner, T. E., Jr., Brown, J. S., & Kistner, J. (Eds.). (2006). *The interpersonal, cognitive, and social nature of depression.* Mahwah, NJ: Erlbaum.

Joiner, T. E., Jr., Van Orden, K. A., Witte, T. K., & Rudd, M. D. (2009). *The interpersonal theory of suicide: Guidance for working with suicidal clients.* Washington, DC: American Psychological Association.

Jones, E., & Davis, K. E. (1965). From acts to dispositions: The attribution process in person perception. In L. Berkowitz (Ed.), *Advances in experimental social psychology* (Vol. 2, pp. 219–266). New York: Academic Press.

Kahneman, D., Krueger, A. B., Schkade, D., Schwarz, N., & Stone, A. A. (2006). Would you be happier if you were richer?: A focusing illusion. *Science, 312,* 1908–1910.

Kahneman, D., & Tversky, A. (1984). Choices, values, and frames. *American Psychologist, 39*(4), 341–350.

Kar, H. L., & O'Leary, K. D. (2013). Patterns of psychological aggression, dominance, and jealousy within marriage. *Journal of Family Violence, 28,* 109–119.

Katz, L. F., Gottman, J. M., & Hooven, C. (1996). Meta-emotion philosophy and family functioning: Reply to Cowan (1996) and Eisenberg (1996). *Journal of Family Psychology, 10*(3), 284–291.

Katzow, A. W., & Safran, J. D. (2007). Recognizing and resolving ruptures in the therapeutic alliance. In P. Gilbert & R. L. Leahy (Eds.), *The therapeutic relationship in the cognitive-behavioural psychotherapies* (pp. 90–105). Hove, UK: Routledge.

Kelley, H. H. (1973). The processes of causal attribution. *American Psychologist, 28*(2), 107–128.

Kelly, G. A. (1955). *The psychology of personal constructs.* New York: Norton.

Kermer, D. A., Driver-Linn, E., Wilson, T. D., & Gilbert, D. T. (2006). Loss aversion is an affective forecasting error. *Psychological Science, 17*(8), 649–653.

Kerns, K. A. (1994). A longitudinal examination of links between mother–child attachment and children's friendships in early childhood. *Journal of Social and Personal Relationships, 11,* 379–381.

Kessen, W. (1965). *The child.* New York: Wiley.

Kierkegaard, S. (1941). *The sickness unto death.* Princeton, NJ: Princeton University Press.

Kierkegaard, S. (1992). *Either/or: A fragment of life* (A. Hannay, Trans.). New York: Penguin. (Original work published 1843)

Klerman, G., Weissman, M. M., Rounsaville, B. J., & Chevron, E. (1984). *Interpersonal psychotherapy of depression.* New York: Basic Books.

Knobloch, L. K., Solomon, D. H., & Cruz, M. G. (2001). The role of relationship development and attachment in the experience of romantic jealousy. *Personal Relationships, 8,* 205–224.

Kohut, H. (1977). *The restoration of the self.* New York: International Universities Press.

Kohut, H. (2009). *The analysis of the self: A systematic approach to the psychoanalytic treatment of narcissistic personality disorders.* Chicago: University of Chicago Press. (Original work published 1971)

Kuyken, W., Padesky, C. A., & Dudley, R. (2009). *Collaborative case conceptualization: Working effectively with clients in cognitive-behavioral therapy.* New York: Guilford Press.

Labott, S. M., & Teleha, M. K. (1996). Weeping propensity and the effects of laboratory expression or inhibition. *Motivation and Emotion, 20,* 273–284.

Ladouceur, R., Gosselin, P., & Dugas, M. J. (2000). Experimental manipulation of intolerance of uncertainty: A study of a theoretical model of worry. *Behaviour Research and Therapy, 38*(9), 933–941.

Lasch, C. (1977). *Haven in a heartless world.* New York: Basic Books.

Lazarus, R. S. (1999). *Stress and emotion: A new synthesis.* New York: Springer.

Lazarus, R. S., & Folkman, S. (1984). *Stress, appraisal, and coping.* New York: Springer.

Leahy, R. L. (2001). *Overcoming resistance in cognitive therapy.* New York: Guilford Press.

Leahy, R. L. (2002). A model of emotional schemas. *Cognitive and Behavioral Practice, 9*(3), 177–190.

Leahy, R. L. (2003a). *Cognitive therapy techniques: A practitioner's guide.* New York: Guilford Press.

Leahy, R. L. (2003b). Emotional schemas and resistance. In R. L. Leahy (Ed.), *Roadblocks in cognitive-behavioral therapy: Transforming challenges into opportunities for change* (pp. 91–115). New York: Guilford Press.

Leahy, R. L. (2005a, November). *Integrating the meta-cognitive and meta-emotional models of worry.* Paper presented at the Association for the Advancement of Cognitive and Behavioral Therapy, Washington, DC.

Leahy, R. L. (2005b, September). *Overcoming resistance in cognitive therapy.* Paper presented at the meeting of the European Association for Behavioral and Cognitive Therapy, Thessaloniki, Greece.

Leahy, R. L. (2005c). A social cognitive model of validation. In P. Gilbert (Ed.), *Compassion: Conceptualisations, research and use in psychotherapy* (pp. 195–217). Hove, UK: Routledge.

Leahy, R. L. (2005d). *The worry cure: Seven steps to stop worry from stopping you.* New York: Harmony/Random House.

Leahy, R. L. (2007a). Emotional schemas and resistance to change in anxiety disorders. *Cognitive and Behavioral Practice, 14*(1), 36–45.

Leahy, R. L. (2007b). Schematic mismatch in the therapeutic relationship: A social-cognitive model. In P. Gilbert & R. L. Leahy (Eds.), *The therapeutic relationship in the cognitive behavioural psychotherapies* (pp. 229–254). Hove, UK: Routledge.

Leahy, R. L. (2009a). *Anxiety free: Unravel your fears before they unravel you.* Carlsbad, CA: Hay House.

Leahy, R. L. (2009b). Resistance: An emotional schema therapy (EST) approach. In G. Simos (Ed.), *Cognitive behaviour therapy: A guide for the practising clinician* (Vol. 2, pp. 187–204). Hove, UK: Routledge.

Leahy, R. L. (2010b). *Beat the blues before they beat you: How to overcome depression.* Carlsbad, CA: Hay House.

Leahy, R. L. (2010a, October). *Keynote: Emotional schemas and cognitive therapy.* Paper presented at the meeting of the European Association for Behavioral and Cognitive Therapies, Milan, Italy.

Leahy, R. L. (2010b). *Relationship Emotional Schema Scale (RESS).* Unpublished manuscript, American Institute for Cognitive Therapy, New York.

Leahy, R. L. (2011a, June). *Keynote: Emotional intelligence and cognitive therapy: A bridge over troubled waters.* Paper presented at the International Congress of Cognitive Psychotherapy, Istanbul, Turkey.

Leahy, R. L. (2011b). *Keynote: Emotional schemas and implicit theory of emotion: Overcoming fear of feeling.* Paper presented at the International Conference of Metacognitive Therapy, Manchester, UK.

Leahy, R. L. (2012a). *Emotional schemas as predictors of relationship dissatisfaction.* Unpublished manuscript, American Institute for Cognitive Therapy, New York.

Leahy, R. L. (2012b). *Leahy Emotional Schema Scale II (LESS II).* Unpublished manuscript, American Institute for Cognitive Therapy, New York.

Leahy, R. L. (2013). *Keeping your head after losing your job: How to cope with unemployment.* London: Piatkus.

Leahy, R. L. (in press). Emotional schema therapy. In J. Livesley, G. Dimmagio, & J. Clarkin (Eds.), *Integrated treatment for personality disorders.* New York: Guilford Press.

Leahy, R. L., Beck, A. T., & Beck, J. S. (2005). Cognitive therapy of personality disorders. In S. Strack (Ed.), *Handbook of personology and psychopathology: Essays in honor of Theodore Millon* (pp. 442–461). New York: Wiley.

Leahy, R. L., Holland, S. J. F., & McGinn, L. K. (2012). *Treatment plans and interventions for depression and anxiety disorders* (2nd ed.). New York: Guilford Press.

Leahy, R. L., & Tirch, D. (2008). Cognitive behavioral therapy for jealousy. *International Journal of Cognitive Therapy, 1,* 18–32.

Leahy, R. L., Tirch, D. D., & Melwani, P. S. (2012). Processes underlying depression: Risk aversion, emotional schemas, and psychological flexibility. *International Journal of Cognitive Therapy, 5*(4), 362–379.

Leahy, R. L., Tirch, D., & Napolitano, L. A. (2011). *Emotion regulation in psychotherapy: A practitioner's guide.* New York: Guilford Press.

LeDoux, J. (2007). The amygdala. *Current Biology, 17*(20), R868–R874.

Linehan, M. M. (1993). *Cognitive-behavioral treatment of borderline personality disorder.* New York: Guilford Press.

Linehan, M. M. (2015). *DBT® skills training manual* (2nd ed.). New York: Guilford Press.

Linehan, M. M., Bohus, M., & Lynch, T. R. (2007). Dialectical behavior therapy for pervasive emotion dysregulation: Theoretical and practical underpinnings. In J. J. Gross (Ed.), *Handbook of emotion regulation* (pp. 581–605). New York: Guilford Press.

Loevinger, J. (1976). *Ego development.* San Francisco: Jossey-Bass.

Love, T. M. (2014). Oxytocin, motivation and the role of dopamine. *Pharmacology, Biochemistry and Behavior, 119,* 49–60.

Lundh, L.-G., Johnsson, A., Sundqvist, K., & Olsson, H. (2002). Alexithymia, memory of emotion, emotional awareness, and perfectionism. *Emotion, 2*(4), 361–379.

Mancini, A. D., Bonanno, G. A., & Clark, A. E. (2011). Stepping off the hedonic treadmill: Individual differences in response to major life events. *Journal of Individual Differences, 32*(3), 144–152.

Marazziti, D., Rucci, P., Nasso, E. D., Masala, I., Baroni, S., Rossi, A., et al. (2003). Jealousy and subthreshold psychopathology: A serotonergic link. *Neuropsychobiology, 47,* 12–16.

Marcus Aurelius. (2002). *Meditations.* New York: Modern Library.

Martell, C. R., Dimidjian, S., & Herman-Dunn, R. (2010). *Behavioral activation for depression: A clinician's guide.* New York: Guilford Press.

Mathes, E. W., & Severa, N. (1981). Jealousy, romantic love, and liking: Theoretical considerations and preliminary scale development. *Psychological Reports, 49*(1), 23–31.

Mayer, J. D., & Salovey, P. (1997). What is emotional intelligence? In P. Salovey & D. J. Sluyter (Eds.), *Emotional development and emotional intelligence: Educational implications* (pp. 3–34). New York: Basic Books.

McClure, S. M., Ericson, K. M., Laibson, D. I., Loewenstein, G., & Cohen, J. D. (2007). Time discounting for primary rewards. *Journal of Neuroscience, 27*(21), 5796–5804.

McFarland, C., & Miller, D. T. (1994). The framing of relative performance feedback: Seeing the glass as half empty or half full. *Journal of Personality and Social Psychology, 66,* 1061–1073.

McGillicuddy-De Lisi, A. V., & Sigel, I. E. (1995). Parental beliefs. In M. H. Bornstein (Ed.), *Handbook of parenting: Vol. 3. Status and social conditions of parenting* (pp. 333–358). Mahwah, NJ: Erlbaum.

McGregor, I. S., & Bowen, M. T. (2012). Breaking the loop: Oxytocin as a potential treatment for drug addiction. *Hormones and Behavior, 61*(3), 331–339.

McGuire, M. T., Raleigh, M. J., & Johnson, C. (1983). Social dominance in adult male vervet monkeys: Behavior–biochemical relationships. *Social Science Information, 22*(2), 311–328.

McIntosh, E. G. (1989). An investigation of romantic jealousy among black undergraduates. *Social Behavior and Personality, 17*(2), 135–141.

Meehl, P. E. (1996). *Clinical versus statistical prediction: A theoretical analysis and a review of the evidence.* Northvale, NJ: Jason Aronson. (Original work published 1954)

Mennin, D. S., Heimberg, R. G., Turk, C. L., & Fresco, D. M. (2002). Applying an emotion regulation framework to integrative approaches to generalized anxiety disorder. *Clinical Psychology: Science and Practice, 9*(1), 85–90.

Mennin, D. S., Heimberg, R. G., Turk, C. L., & Fresco, D. M. (2005). Preliminary evidence for an emotion dysregulation model of generalized anxiety disorder. *Behaviour Research and Therapy, 43*(10), 1281–1310.

Menninger, K. A., & Holzman, P. S. (1973). *Theory of psychoanalytic technique* (2nd ed.). New York: Basic Books.

Michalik, N. M., Eisenberg, N., Spinrad, T. L., Ladd, B., Thompson, M., & Valiente, C. (2007). Longitudinal relations among parental emotional expressivity and sympathy and prosocial behavior in adolescence. *Social Development, 16*(2), 286–309.

Mikulincer, M., Gillath, O., Halevy, V., Avihou, N., Avidan, S., & Eshkoli, N. (2001). Attachment theory and reactions to others' needs: Evidence that activation of the sense of attachment security promotes empathic responses. *Journal of Personality and Social Psychology, 81*(6), 1205–1224.

Millon, T., Millon, C., Davis, R., & Grossman, S. (1994). *Millon Clinical Multiaxial Inventory–III (MCMI-III).* Minneapolis, MN: Pearson Education.

Morrison, J. (2014). *The first interview* (4th ed.). New York: Guilford Press.

Muran, J. C., & Safran, J. D. (1993). Emotional and interpersonal considerations in cognitive therapy. In K. T. Kuehlwein & H. Rosen (Eds.), *Cognitive therapies in action: Evolving innovative practice* (pp. 185–212). San Francisco: Jossey-Bass.

Muran, J. C., & Safran, J. D. (1998). Negotiating the therapeutic alliance in brief psychotherapy: An introduction. In J. D. Safran & J. C. Muran (Eds.), *The therapeutic alliance in brief psychotherapy* (pp. 3–14). Washington, DC: American Psychological Association.

Needleman, L. D. (1999). *Cognitive case conceptualization: A guidebook for practitioners.* Mahwah, NJ: Erlbaum.

Neff, K. D. (2009). Self-compassion. In M. R. Leary & R. H. Hoyle (Eds.), *Handbook of individual differences in social behavior* (pp. 561–573). New York: Guilford Press.

Neff, K. D. (2012). The science of self-compassion. In C. Germer & R. D. Siegel (Eds.), *Wisdom and compassion in psychotherapy* (pp. 79–92). New York: Guilford Press.

Nesse, R. M. (1994). An evolutionary perspective on substance abuse. *Ethology and Sociobiology, 15,* 339–348.

Nesse, R. M., & Ellsworth, P. C. (2009). Evolution, emotions, and emotional disorders. *American Psychologist, 64*(2), 129–139.

Nietzsche, F. (1956). *The birth of tragedy* and *The genealogy of morals.* Garden City, NY: Doubleday.

Nolen-Hoeksema, S. (1991). Responses to depression and their effects on the duration of depressive episodes. *Journal of Abnormal Psychology, 100*(4), 569–582.

Nolen-Hoeksema, S. (2000). The role of rumination in depressive disorders and mixed anxiety/depressive symptoms. *Journal of Abnormal Psychology, 109,* 504–511.

Nussbaum, M. C. (2001). *Upheavals of thought: The intelligence of emotions.* Cambridge, UK: Cambridge University Press.

Nussbaum, M. C. (2005). *Frontiers of justice: Disability, nationality, species membership.* Cambridge, MA: Belknap Press.

O'Donoghue, T., & Rabin, M. (1999). Doing it now or later. *American Economic Review, 89*(1), 103–124.

O'Leary, K. D., Smith Slep, A. M., & O'Leary, S. G. (2007). Multivariate models of men's and women's partner aggression. *Journal of Consulting and Clinical Psychology, 75,* 752–764.

Olff, M., Frijling, J. L., Kubzansky, L. D., Bradley, B., Ellenbogen, M. A., Cardoso, C., et al. (2013). The role of oxytocin in social bonding, stress regulation and mental health: An update on the moderating effects of context and interindividual differences. *Psychoneuroendocrinology, 38,* 1883–1894.

Paivio, S. C., & McCulloch, C. R. (2004). Alexithymia as a mediator between childhood trauma and self-injurious behaviors. *Child Abuse and Neglect, 28*(3), 339–354.

Panzarella, C., Alloy, L. B., & Whitehouse, W. G. (2006). Expanded hopelessness theory of depression: On the mechanisms by which social support protects against depression. *Cognitive Therapy and Research, 30*(3), 307–333.

Papageorgiou, C. (2006). Worry and its psychological disorders: Theory, assessment, and treatment. In G. C. L. Davey & A. Wells (Eds.), *Worry and rumination: Styles of persistent negative thinking in anxiety and depression* (pp. 21–40). Hoboken, NJ: Wiley.

Papageorgiou, C., & Wells, A. (2001a). Metacognitive beliefs about rumination in major depression. *Cognitive and Behavioral Practice, 8,* 160–163.

Papageorgiou, C., & Wells, A. (2001b). Positive beliefs about depressive rumination: Development and preliminary validation of a self-report scale. *Behavior Therapy, 32*(1), 13–26.

Papageorgiou, C., & Wells, A. (2004). *Depressive rumination: Nature, theory, and treatment.* Chichester, UK: Wiley.

Papageorgiou, C., & Wells, A. (2009). A prospective test of the clinical metacognitive model of rumination and depression. *International Journal of Cognitive Therapy, 2,* 123–131.

Parker, G., Roussos, J., Hadzi-Pavlovic, D., Mitchell, P., Wilhelm, K., & Austin, M.-P. (1997). The development of a refined measure of dysfunctional parenting and assessment of its relevance in patients with affective disorders. *Psychological Medicine, 27,* 1193–1203.

Parsons, T. (1951). *The social system.* New York: Free Press.

Parsons, T. (1967). *Sociological theory and modern society.* New York: Free Press.

Parsons, T., & Bales, R. F. (1955). *Family, socialization and interaction process.* Glencoe, IL: Free Press.

Pennebaker, J. W., & Chung, C. K. (2011). Expressive writing: Connections to mental and physical health. In H. S. Friedman (Ed.), *The Oxford handbook of health psychology* (pp. 417–437). New York: Oxford University Press.

Persons, J. B. (1993). Case conceptualization in cognitive-behavior therapy. In K.

T. Kuehlwein & H. Rosen (Eds.), *Cognitive therapies in action: Evolving innovative practice* (pp. 33–53). San Francisco: Jossey-Bass.

Pinker, S. (2002). *The blank slate: The modern denial of human nature.* New York: Viking.

Pirie, D. (1994). *The Romantic period.* New York: Viking Penguin.

Plato. (1991). *The republic of Plato* (A. D. Bloom, Trans.). New York: Basic Books.

Price, J. (1967). The dominance hierarchy and the evolution of mental illness. *Lancet, 290,* 243–246.

Purdon, C., & Clark, D. A. (1994). Obsessive intrusive thoughts in nonclinical subjects: II. Cognitive appraisal, emotional response and thought control strategies. *Behaviour Research and Therapy, 32,* 403–410.

Purdon, C., Rowa, K., & Antony, M. M. (2005). Thought suppression and its effects on thought frequency, appraisal and mood state in individuals with obsessive–compulsive disorder. *Behaviour Research and Therapy, 43*(1), 93–108.

Rachman, S. J. (1997). A cognitive theory of obsessions. *Behaviour Research and Therapy, 35,* 793–802.

Raes, F., Pommier, E., Neff, K. D., & Van Gucht, D. (2011). Construction and factorial validation of a short form of the Self-Compassion Scale. *Clinical Psychology and Psychotherapy, 18,* 250–255.

Raleigh, M. J., McGuire, M. T., Brammer, G. L., Pollack, D. B., & Yuwiler, A. (1991). Serotonergic mechanisms promote dominance acquisition in adult male vervet monkeys. *Brain Research, 559*(2), 181–190.

Rapee, R. M., & Heimberg, R. G. (1997). A cognitive-behavioral model of anxiety in social phobia. *Behaviour Research and Therapy, 35*(8), 741–756.

Rawls, J. (1971). *A theory of justice.* Cambridge, MA: Belknap Press.

Read, D., & Read, N. L. (2004). Time discounting over the lifespan. *Organizational Behavior and Human Decision Processes, 94*(1), 22–32.

Ridley, C. R., Mollen, D., & Kelly, S. M. (2011a). Beyond microskills: Toward a model of counseling competence. *The Counseling Psychologist, 39*(6), 825–864.

Ridley, C. R., Mollen, D., & Kelly, S. M. (2011b). Counseling competence: Application and implications of a model. *The Counseling Psychologist, 39*(6), 865–886.

Riskind, J. H. (1997). Looming vulnerability to threat: A cognitive paradigm for anxiety. *Behaviour Research and Therapy, 35*(8), 685–702.

Riskind, J. H., & Kleiman, E. M. (2012). Looming cognitive style, emotion schemas, and fears of loss of emotional control: Two studies. *International Journal of Cognitive Therapy, 5*(4), 392–405.

Riskind, J. H., Tzur, D., Williams, N. L., Mann, B., & Shahar, G. (2007). Short-term predictive effects of the looming cognitive style on anxiety disorder symptoms under restrictive methodological conditions. *Behaviour Research and Therapy, 45*(8), 1765–1777.

Roemer, E., & Orsillo, S. M. (2002). Expanding our conceptualization of and treatment for generalized anxiety disorder: Integrating mindfulness/acceptance-based approaches with existing cognitive-behavioral models. *Clinical Psychology: Science and Practice, 9*(1), 54–68.

Roemer, L., & Orsillo, S. M. (2009). *Mindfulness- and acceptance-based behavioral therapies in practice.* New York: Guilford Press.

Rogers, C. R. (1951). *Client-centered therapy: Its current practice, implications, and theory.* Boston: Houghton Mifflin.

Rogers, C. R., & American Psychological Association. (1985). *Client-centered therapy* [Sound recording]. Washington, DC: American Psychological Association.

Ross, L., & Nisbett, R. E. (1991). *The person and the situation: Perspectives of social psychology.* New York: McGraw-Hill.

Rotenberg, K. J., & Eisenberg, N. (1997). Developmental differences in the understanding of and reaction to others' inhibition of emotional expression. *Developmental Psychology, 33*(3), 526–537.

Rumi, J. A.-D. (1997). *The illuminated Rumi* (C. Barks, Trans.). New York: Random House.

Ryle, G. (1949). *The concept of mind.* London: Hutchinson.

Saarni, C. (1999). *The development of emotional competence.* New York: Guilford Press.

Saarni, C. (2007). The development of emotional competence: Pathways for helping children to become emotionally intelligent. In R. Bar-On & M. J. Elias (Eds.), *Educating people to be emotionally intelligent* (pp. 15–35). Westport, CT: Praeger.

Safran, J. D. (1998). *Widening the scope of cognitive therapy: The therapeutic relationship, emotion and the process of change.* Northvale, NJ: Jason Aronson.

Safran, J. D., & Greenberg, L. S. (1988). Feeling, thinking, and acting: A cognitive framework for psychotherapy integration. *Journal of Cognitive Psychotherapy, 2*(2), 109–131.

Safran, J. D., & Greenberg, L. S. (Eds.). (1989). The treatment of anxiety and depression: The process of affective change. In P. C. Kendall & D. Watson (Eds.), *Anxiety and depression: Distinctive and overlapping features* (pp. 455–489). San Diego, CA: Academic Press.

Safran, J. D., & Greenberg, L. S. (Eds.). (1991). *Emotion, psychotherapy, and change.* New York: Guilford Press.

Safran, J. D., & Muran, J. C. (2000). Resolving therapeutic alliance ruptures: Diversity and integration. *Journal of Clinical Psychology, 56*(2), 233–243.

Sale, E., Sambrano, S., Springer, J. F., & Turner, C. W. (2003). Risk, protection, and substance use in adolescents: A multi-site model. *Journal of Drug Education, 33*(1), 91–105.

Salkovskis, P. M. (1989). Cognitive-behavioural factors and the persistence of intrusive thoughts in obsessional problems. *Behaviour Research and Therapy, 27*(6), 677–682.

Salkovskis, P. M., & Campbell, P. (1994). Thought suppression induces intrusion in naturally occurring negative intrusive thoughts. *Behaviour Research and Therapy, 32*(1), 1–8.

Salkovskis, P. M., Clark, D. M., & Gelder, M. G. (1996). Cognition–behaviour links in the persistence of panic. *Behaviour Research and Therapy, 34*, 453–458.

Salkovskis, P. M., & Kirk, J. (1997). Obsessive–compulsive disorder. In D. M. Clark & C. G. Fairburn (Eds.), *Science and practice of cognitive behaviour therapy* (pp. 179–208). New York: Oxford University Press.

Sallquist, J. V., Eisenberg, N., Spinrad, T. L., Reiser, M., Hofer, C., Zhou, Q., et al.

(2009). Positive and negative emotionality: Trajectories across six years and relations with social competence. *Emotion, 9*(1), 15–28.

Salovey, P., & Rodin, J. (1991). Provoking jealousy and envy: Domain relevance and self-esteem threat. *Journal of Social and Clinical Psychology, 10*(4), 395–413.

Sartre, J.-P. (1956). *Being and nothingness* (H. Barnes, Trans.). New York: Gallimard.

Scafidi, F., Field, T., Schanberg, S., Bauer, C., Tucci, K., Roberts, J., et al. (1990). Massage stimulates growth in preterm infants: A replication. *Infant Behavior and Development, 13*, 167–188.

Segal, Z. V., Williams, J. M. G., & Teasdale, J. D. (2002). *Mindfulness-based cognitive therapy for depression: A new approach to preventing relapse*. New York: Guilford Press.

Seligman, M. E. (2002). *Authentic happiness: Using the new positive psychology to realize your potential for lasting fulfillment*. New York: Free Press.

Sennett, R. (1996). *The fall of public man*. New York: Norton.

Sheets, V. L., Fredendall, L. L., & Claypool, H. M. (1997). Jealousy evocation, partner reassurance, and relationship stability: An exploration of the potential benefits of jealousy. *Evolution and Human Behavior, 18*(6), 387–402.

Simon, H. A. (1956). Rational choice and the structure of the environment. *Psychological Review, 63*(2), 129–138.

Simon, H. A. (1979). Rational decision making in business organizations. *American Economic Review, 69*, 493–513.

Simpson, C., & Papageorgiou, C. (2003). Metacognitive beliefs about rumination in anger. *Cognitive and Behavioral Practice, 10*(1), 91–94.

Sloman, L., Price, J., Gilbert, P., & Gardner, R. (1994). Adaptive function of depression: Psychotherapeutic implications. *American Journal of Psychotherapy, 48*, 401–414.

Slovic, P. (2000). Trust, emotion, sex, politics, and science: Surveying the risk-assessment battlefield. In P. Slovic (Ed.), *The perception of risk* (pp. 277–313). Sterling, VA: Earthscan.

Slovic, P., Finucane, M., Peters, E., & MacGregor, D. (2004). Risk as analysis and risk as feelings: Some thoughts about affect, reason, risk, and rationality. *Risk Analysis, 24*(2), 311–322.

Smith, R. H., & Kim, S. H. (2007). Comprehending envy. *Psychological Bulletin, 133*(1), 46–64.

Smith, R. H., Turner, T. J., Garonzik, R., Leach, C. W., Urch-Druskat, V., & Weston, C. M. (1996). Envy and *Schadenfreude*. *Personality and Social Psychology Bulletin, 22*, 158–168.

Smucker, M. R., & Dancu, C. V. (1999). *Cognitive-behavioral treatment for adult survivors of childhood trauma: Imagery rescripting and reprocessing*. Northvale, NJ: Jason Aronson.

Sookman, D., & Pinard, G. (2002). Overestimation of threat and intolerance of uncertainty in obsessive compulsive disorder. In R. O. Frost & G. Steketee (Eds.), *Cognitive approaches to obsessions and compulsions: Theory, assessment, and treatment* (pp. 63–89). Amsterdam: Pergamon/Elsevier.

Sorabji, R. (2000). *Emotion and peace of mind: From Stoic agitation to Christian temptation*. Oxford, UK: Oxford University Press.

Spanier, G. B. (1976). Measuring dyadic adjustment: New scales for assessing the quality of marriage and similar dyads. *Journal of Marriage and the Family, 38,* 15–28.

Spock, B. (1957). *Baby and child care* (2nd ed.). New York: Pocket Books.

Sroufe, L., & Waters, E. (1977). Heart rate as a convergent measure in clinical and developmental research. *Merrill–Palmer Quarterly, 23*(1), 3–27.

Stearns, P. N. (1994). *American cool: Constructing a twentieth-century emotional style.* New York: New York University Press.

Steinbeis, N., & Singer, T. (2013). The effects of social comparison on social emotions and behavior during childhood: The ontogeny of envy and *Schadenfreude* predicts developmental changes in equity-related decisions. *Journal of Experimental Child Psychology, 115*(1), 198–209.

Stevens, A., & Price, J. (1996). *Evolutionary psychiatry: A new beginning.* London: Routledge.

Strauss, J. L., Hayes, A. M., Johnson, S. L., Newman, C. F., Brown, G. K., Barber, J. P., et al. (2006). Early alliance, alliance ruptures, and symptom change in a nonrandomized trial of cognitive therapy for avoidant and obsessive-compulsive personality disorders. *Journal of Consulting and Clinical Psychology, 74*(2), 337–345.

Suls, J., & Wheeler, L. (2000). A selective history of classic and neo-social comparison theory. In J. Suls & L. Wheeler (Eds.), *Handbook of social comparison* (pp. 3–19). New York: Kluwer Academic/Plenum Press.

Tangney, J. P., Stuewig, J., & Mashek, D. J. (2007). Moral emotions and moral behavior. *Annual Review of Psychology, 58,* 345–372.

Tannen, D. (1986). *That's not what I meant!: How conversational style makes or breaks your relations with others.* New York: Morrow.

Tannen, D. (1990). *You just don't understand: Women and men in conversation.* New York: Morrow.

Tannen, D. (1993). *Gender and conversational interaction.* New York: Oxford University Press.

Taylor, G. J., Bagby, R. M., & Parker, J. D. (1991). The alexithymia construct: A potential paradigm for psychosomatic medicine. *Psychosomatics, 32,* 153–164.

Teasdale, J. D. (1999). Multi-level theories of cognition–emotion relations. In T. Dalgleish & M. J. Power (Eds.), *Handbook of cognition and emotion* (pp. 665–681). Chichester, UK: Wiley.

Thaler, R. H., & Shefrin, H. M. (1981). An economic theory of self-control. *Journal of Political Economy, 89*(2), 392–406.

Tirch, D. D., Leahy, R. L., Silberstein, L. R., & Melwani, P. S. (2012). Emotional schemas, psychological flexibility, and anxiety: The role of flexible response patterns to anxious arousal. *International Journal of Cognitive Therapy, 5*(4), 380–391.

Tolstoy, L. (1981). *The death of Ivan Ilyich.* New York: Bantam. (Original work published 1886)

Tooby, J., & Cosmides, L. (1992). The psychological foundations of culture. In J. H. Barkow & L. Cosmides (Eds.), *The adapted mind: Evolutionary psychology and the generation of culture* (pp. 19–136). New York: Oxford University Press.

Trivers, R. L. (1971). The evolution of reciprocal altruism. *Quarterly Review of Biology, 46*, 35–57.

Trivers, R. L. (1972). Parental investment and sexual selection. In B. Campbell (Ed.), *Sexual selection and the descent of man, 1871–1971* (pp. 136–179). Chicago: Aldine.

Troy, M., & Sroufe, L. (1987). Victimization among preschoolers: Role of attachment relationship history. *Journal of the American Academy of Child and Adolescent Psychiatry, 26*(2), 166–172.

Tse, W. S., & Bond, A. J. (2002). Serotonergic intervention affects both social dominance and affiliative behaviour. *Psychopharmacology, 161*, 324–330.

Tybur, J. M., Lieberman, D., Kurzban, R., & DeScioli, P. (2013). Disgust: Evolved function and structure. *Psychological Review, 120*(1), 65–84.

Urban, J., Carlson, E., Egeland, B., & Sroufe, L. (1991). Patterns of individual adaptation across childhood. *Development and Psychopathology, 3*(4), 445–460.

van de Ven, N., Zeelenberg, M., & Pieters, R. (2009). Leveling up and down: The experiences of benign and malicious envy. *Emotion, 9*, 419–429.

van de Ven, N., Zeelenberg, M., & Pieters, R. (2011). Why envy outperforms admiration. *Personality and Social Psychology Bulletin, 37*(6), 784–795.

van de Ven, N., Zeelenberg, M., & Pieters, R. (2012). Appraisal patterns of envy and related emotions. *Motivation and Emotion, 36*(2), 195–204.

van Dijk, W. W., Ouwerkerk, J. W., Goslinga, S., Nieweg, M., & Gallucci, M. (2006). When people fall from grace: Reconsidering the role of envy in *Schadenfreude. Emotion, 6*(1), 156–160.

Veen, G., & Arntz, A. (2000). Multidimensional dichotomous thinking characterizes borderline personality disorder. *Cognitive Therapy and Research, 24*(1), 23–45.

Watson, D., Clark, L. A., & Tellegen, A. (1988). Development and validation of brief measures of positive and negative affect: The PANAS scales. *Journal of Personality and Social Psychology, 54*(6), 1063–1070.

Watson, J. B. (1919). *Psychology from the standpoint of a behaviorist.* Philadelphia: Lippincott.

Weber, M. (1930). *The Protestant ethic and the spirit of capitalism.* London: Unwin Hyman.

Wegner, D. M. (1994). Ironic processes of mental control. *Psychological Review, 101*, 34–52.

Wegner, D. M., Schneider, D. J., Carter, S., & White, T. (1987). Paradoxical effects of thought suppression. *Journal of Personality and Social Psychology, 53*, 5–13.

Wegner, D. M., & Zanakos, S. (1994). Chronic thought suppression. *Journal of Personality, 62*, 615–640.

Weinberger, D. A. (1995). The construct validity of the repressive coping style. In J. L. Singer (Ed.), *Repression and dissociation: Implications for personality theory, psychopathology, and health* (pp. 337–386). Chicago: University of Chicago Press.

Weiner, B. (1974). *Achievement motivation and attribution theory.* Morristown, NJ: General Learning Press.

Weiner, B. (1986). *An attributional theory of motivation and emotion.* New York: Springer-Verlag.

Wells, A. (1995). An issue of intrusions [Editorial]. *Behavioural and Cognitive Psychotherapy, 23*(3), 202.

Wells, A. (2000). *Emotional disorders and metacognition: Innovative cognitive therapy.* New York: Wiley.

Wells, A. (2004). A cognitive model of GAD: Metacognitions and pathological worry. In R. G. Heimberg, C. L. Turk, & D. S. Mennin (Eds.), *Generalized anxiety disorder: Advances in research and practice* (pp. 164–186). New York: Guilford Press.

Wells, A. (2005a). Detached mindfulness in cognitive therapy: A metacognitive analysis and ten techniques. *Journal of Rational–Emotive and Cognitive-Behavior Therapy, 23,* 337–355.

Wells, A. (2005b). The metacognitive model of GAD: Assessment of meta-worry and relationship with DSM-IV generalized anxiety disorder. *Cognitive Therapy and Research, 29,* 107–121.

Wells, A. (2005c). Worry, intrusive thoughts, and generalized anxiety disorder: The metacognitive theory and treatment. In D. A. Clark (Ed.), *Intrusive thoughts in clinical disorders: Theory, research, and treatment* (pp. 119–144). New York: Guilford Press.

Wells, A. (2009). *Metacognitive therapy for anxiety and depression.* New York: Guilford Press.

Wells, A., & Carter, K. (2001). Further tests of a cognitive model of generalized anxiety disorder: Metacognitions and worry in GAD, panic disorder, social phobia, depression, and nonpatients. *Behavior Therapy, 32*(1), 85–102.

Wells, A., & Cartwright-Hatton, S. (2004). A short form of the Meta-Cognitions Questionnaire: Properties of the MCQ-30. *Behaviour Research and Therapy, 42,* 385–396.

Wells, A., & Papageorgiou, C. (1998). Relationships between worry, obsessive–compulsive symptoms and meta-cognitive beliefs. *Behaviour Research and Therapy, 36,* 899–913.

Wells, A., & Papageorgiou, C. (2001). Social phobic interoception: Effects of bodily information on anxiety, beliefs and self-processing. *Behaviour Research and Therapy, 39,* 1–11.

Wells, A., & Papageorgiou, C. (2004). Metacognitive therapy for depressive rumination. In C. Papageorgiou & A. Wells (Eds.), *Depressive rumination: Nature, theory, and treatment* (pp. 259–273). Chichester, UK: Wiley.

Wenzlaff, R. M., & Wegner, D. M. (2000). Thought suppression. *Annual Review of Psychology, 51,* 59–91.

White, G. L. (1980). Inducing jealousy: A power perspective. *Personality and Social Psychology Bulletin, 6,* 222–227.

White, G. L. (1981). A model of romantic jealousy. *Motivation and Emotion, 5,* 295–310.

White, G. L., & Mullen, P. E. (1989). *Jealousy: Theory, research, and clinical strategies.* New York: Guilford Press.

Whitman, W. (1959). Song of myself. In J. E. Miller, Jr. (Ed.), *Complete poetry and selected prose by Walt Whitman* (pp. 25–68). Boston: Houghton Mifflin.

Wilson, K. A., & Chambless, D. L. (1999). Inflated perceptions of responsibility and obsessive–compulsive symptoms. *Behaviour Research and Therapy, 37*(4), 325–335.

Wilson, K. G., & Murrell, A. R. (2004). Values work in acceptance and commitment therapy: Setting a course for behavioral treatment. In S. C. Hayes, V. M. Follette, & M. M. Linehan (Eds.), *Mindfulness and acceptance: Expanding the cognitive-behavioral tradition* (pp. 120–151). New York: Guilford Press.

Wilson, K. G., & Sandoz, E. K. (2008). Mindfulness, values, and the therapeutic relationship in acceptance and commitment therapy. In S. F. Hick & T. Bein (Eds.), *Mindfulness and the therapeutic relationship* (pp. 89–106). New York: Guilford Press.

Wilson, T. D., & Gilbert, D. T. (2003). Affective forecasting. In M. P. Zanna (Ed.), *Advances in experimental social psychology* (Vol. 35, pp. 345–411). San Diego, CA: Academic Press.

Wilson, T. D., & Gilbert, D. T. (2005). Affective forecasting: Knowing what to want. *Current Directions in Psychological Science, 14*(3), 131–134.

Wilson, T. D., Gilbert, D. T., & Centerbar, D. B. (2003). Making sense: The causes of emotional evanescence. In I. Brocas & J. D. Carrillo (Eds.), *The psychology of economic decisions: Vol. 1. Rationality and well being* (pp. 209–233). New York: Oxford University Press.

Wilson, T. D., Wheatley, T., Meyers, J. M., Gilbert, D. T., & Axsom, D. (2000). Focalism: A source of durability bias in affective forecasting. *Journal of Personality and Social Psychology, 78*(5), 821–836.

Wittgenstein, L. (2001). *Tractatus logico-philosophicus.* New York: Routledge. (Original work published 1922)

Wood, J. V. (1989). Theory and research concerning social comparisons of personal attributes. *Psychological Bulletin, 106*(2), 231–248.

Young, J. E., Klosko, J., & Weishaar, M. (2003). *Schema therapy: A practitioner's guide.* New York: Guilford Press.

Zajonc, R. B. (1980). Feeling and thinking: Preferences need no inferences. *American Psychologist, 35*(2), 151–175.

Zauberman, G. (2003). The intertemporal dynamics of consumer lock-in. *Journal of Consumer Research, 30*(3), 405–419.

# Index